T0248690

Global Views on Emergency Medicine

Global Views on Emergency Medicine

Edited by **Abby Cusack**

New Jersey

Published by Foster Academics,
61 Van Reypen Street,
Jersey City, NJ 07306, USA
www.fosteracademics.com

Global Views on Emergency Medicine
Edited by Abby Cusack

International Standard Book Number: 978-1-63242-197-5 (Hardback)

Contents

Preface

It is often said that books are a boon to mankind. They document every progress and pass on the knowledge from one generation to the other. They play a crucial role in our lives. Thus I was both excited and nervous while editing this book. I was pleased by the thought of being able to make a mark but I was also nervous to do it right because the future of students depends upon it. Hence, I took a few months to research further into the discipline, revise my knowledge and also explore some more aspects. Post this process, I begun with the editing of this book.

Global views on emergency medicine are provided in this descriptive book. Emergency medicine is an emerging area that has spread beyond the shores of North America and has acquired different characteristics around the world. While, many emergency practitioners face similar constraints, the field and its principles have adapted to local needs and resources. This book intends to educate readers not only on emergency medicine theory, science and practice, but also reflects on the multinational nature of emergency medicine, allowing readers to learn from experiences of others. This book exhibits a true international prospect of emergency medicine practice and science that will be educational for any reader.

I thank my publisher with all my heart for considering me worthy of this unparalleled opportunity and for showing unwavering faith in my skills. I would also like to thank the editorial team who worked closely with me at every step and contributed immensely towards the successful completion of this book. Last but not the least, I wish to thank my friends and colleagues for their support.

Editor

Emergency Medicine in China

Xiang-Yu Hou

School of Public Health, Queensland University of Technology, Brisbane,
Department of Emergency Medicine, Royal Brisbane and Women's Hospital, Brisbane,
School of Medicine, The University of Queensland, Brisbane,
Australia

1. Introduction

With the world's largest population of 1.3 billion, China is a rapidly developing country. In line with this development, China's enormous health system is experiencing an unprecedented series of reforms. According to a recent official government report, China has 300, 000 health organizations, which include 60, 000 hospitals and a total number of 3.07 million beds (China NBoSoP 2006). To provide health services for the national population, as well as the substantial number of visitors, China has 1.93 million doctors and 1.34 million registered nurses (China NBoSoP 2006). From 1984 to 2004, the number of inpatients grew from about 25 to 50 million, with outpatient figures increasing from 1.1 to 1.3 billion (China MoH 2006). The scale of the health system is likely bigger than in any other countries in the world, but the quality of medical services is still among the levels of developing countries. In 2005, approximately 3.8% of inpatients (about 1.5 million)(China NBoSoP 2006) were admitted because of injury and poisoning, which created significant load for the acute health system. These increased figures are at least partly because of the development of the health system and technological health-care advances but, even with such advances, this rapid change in emergency health-care demand has created a very significant burden on existing systems.

The Chinese Emergency Medical Service system is primarily composed of three sectors: pre-hospital care, hospital Emergency Departments (EDs) and hospital intensive care units (ICU). While pre-hospital care systems development in China, especially the workforce status, has been reported and discussed before (Hou and Lu 2005), the purpose of this book chapter is to introduce the development of emergency medicine (EM) in China, including the role of traditional Chinese medicine, which is based mainly on hospital ED. EDs in hospitals are like the window of the world where the health problems in the community would show among the ED patients (Hou and Chu 2010), therefore an in-depth understanding of the hospital EDs in different countries would enhance the appreciation of the general health system in other countries.

2. Brief history of emergency medicine development in China

Development of Chinese hospital ED over the past two decades has been characterized by two main factors: establishment of a professional body of Emergency Medicine (EM) practitioners and the institution of ED in all county-level hospitals nationally. The professional association of EM was officially founded in 1986, as a recognized specialty branch of the China Medical Association. This EM branch has eight specialty groups, including prehospital, resuscitation, trauma, intensive care, acute poisoning, paediatric EM, disaster medicine and ED quality control (Jiang 2004). Professor Jiang has described EM as consisting of three integral and interrelated sections – prehospital care, hospital ED and critical care in ICU wards (Jiang 2004). From the late 1990s onward, all county-level hospitals in China established ED, with urban hospitals having already done so through the 1980s. For example, Tongji Hospital in Wuhan city (a relatively well-known large tertiary hospital) established its ED in 1986 (Bai, Li et al. 2004). According to its Health Bureau, even Guangxi Province, a relatively low socioeconomic area, had established a Department of Emergency Medicine in all county-level hospitals by 2003 (Lu and Qin 2005).

At pace with the rapid economic development of the country, Chinese hospital EDs have been equipped with 'hardware' equipment that is often state-of-the-art. However, because of underdeveloped 'software', such as clinical and technical expertise and fully functional management systems, equipment might not be used or maintained appropriately. This disparity has occurred largely because of an outdated economic health-care system that has not kept pace with the political and socioeconomic change in China.

A unique characteristic of the health care system in China is that Traditional Chinese Medicine (TCM) and western medicine are practised at almost all levels of the health care delivery system including hospital EDs. Almost every city in China has a TCM hospital, and almost every TCM hospital has an ED. Among the hospitals practising western medicine approximately 95% have a TCM outpatient clinic as well as an inpatient ward (Hesketh and Zhu 1997). There were over 300,000 TCM practitioners in China in 1995 and the number could be grown significantly since the Chinese central government continued its policy to expand TCM in China (Hesketh and Zhu 1997). The rapid expand of hospital EDs inevitably caused some concern in risk management at some county level TCM hospitals (Liu 2010) which could be due to the problems such as young nurses working at the front line who did not have enough working experiences in dealing with acute illness (Liu 2010), under-resourced in the number of clinicians and equipment, no standardised clinical procedure and not sufficient herbal remedies for their hospitals (Wu 2009).

It is not only the political will, but also the grass root demand among the general population of Chinese, that made the further grow of TCM possible. It was reported that in 1992 in Jiangsu province (a relatively richer and more sophisticated province in China) about 10 million patients chose to be treated by TCM (not western medicine) at hospitals (Hesketh and Zhu 1997). It was reported that TCM treatments including herbal remedies, acupuncture, massage, and moxibustion, accounted for approximately 40% of health care delivered in China (Hesketh and Zhu 1997). For example, the First Affiliated Hospital ED at Guangzhou TCM University, established in 1965 (Zhou 1996), has a historical record showing the process how TCM saved a patient's life from snake bite. This is an example of evidence regarding the perception of TCM among the general population in China.

It needs to be noted that TCM has always been part of the Chinese history and culture. Here is an example to illustrate this. The author of this chapter's first name is Xiang-Yu (Pinyin from the Shandong dialect, and Xiang-Ru in mandarin) which is a Chinese herb 香薷 (picture below) that all its leaves, flowers, and roots can be used for herbal medicine treating patients with a range of health problems. The author's father, who was a school teaching in Chinese literature, hoped that his daughter would make the society a better place, just like this herb to the patients.

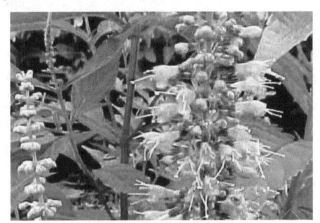

The Chinese herb Xiang-Ru

Therefore, TCM has been a well accepted practice among the Chinese population for over thousands of years. Under this macro environment combined with political will, there is no doubt that a profession will develop speedily when political will and population demand are available. Dept of TCM at China Ministry of Health held a forum in Chongqing city in November 1983 to discuss the development of Traditional Chinese Emergency Medicine (TCEM) in all TCM hospitals in China (Luo 2010). There were seven groups established during that Forum to focus on different acute health problem. This was later formally announced in 1985 at a Shanghai TCEM Meeting (Luo 2010). The focus groups included high fever, stroke, stomach-aches, and blood group. Among each group, there were 8 -10 provincial TCM hospitals to lead research related activities (Luo 2010). Two years later, the first China national scientific TCEM conference was held in Changchun in 1987; followed by the second conference in 1992 in Guangzhou (Luo 2010). Through a lot of hard work and discussion among the TCEM professionals, the TCEM practice guideline was then finalised and published in 1996 (Luo 2010).

A couple of years later, the Emergency Medicine Branch of China Traditional Chinese Medicine Association was established in 1997 (Chao, Jiang et al. 2010) with eleven TCEM Centres assembled in all over the country. This was officially announced on the 5th January 1998 (Luo 2010).

Here is an example to demonstrate the rapid development of TCEM in China. The Jiangsu Province TCM Hospital ED was established on the 5th June 1963, with a couple of TCM practitioners (Xi 2008). By 2006, the number of ED patients was over 100,000. It was reported that the successful rescue rate was approximately 92% (assuming general mortality at this ED in 2006 was about 8%), and the TCM treatment was applied to 90% of the patients (Xi 2008). By 2008 this TCM hospital ED had 60 clinic beds, 12 beds in observation ward, and four ICU beds. Considering the relatively small market for TCM in the health system in modern China, this Jiangsu Province TCM Hospital ED is an example of the rapid development of TCEM in China.

3. Current emergency medicine practice among Chinese hospitals

The current ED practice among hospitals in China will be discussed in three parts: financial, clinical and education and training of health professionals. This is mainly due to the availability of published literature and its importance in affecting the ED practice in hospitals in China.

Part I: the financial situation of China hospital ED

As a result of comprehensive macro-level trade and economic reform since the 1980s, China has essentially developed a market economy. The effect of this economic reform on the health-care system was that the Chinese government dramatically reduced hospital funding, from almost 100% of the premium to about 10–20%. The 80–90% balance of hospital premiums are now borne by the patients themselves, who are obliged to pay for most of their own health-care costs through a fee-for-service system (Yang, Huo et al. 1999). Figure 1 was a picture taken at a teaching hospital ED in Beijing which is a notice to all ED patients saying they need to purchase a card to process payment while at ED and the deposit for the card could be refunded when leaving ED. Thus, the number of patients attending any hospital and the value of services rendered directly determine the hospital's income and viability. With about 40% of a typical hospital's income resulting from emergency presentations, responsibility for ensuring viability of hospital services rests largely with ED (Yang, Huo et al. 1999).

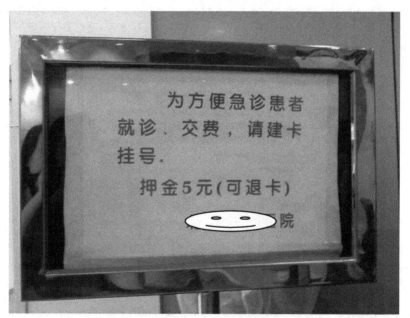

Fig. 1. Notice to ED patients about establishing a card for payment.

Further, financial 'success' of hospitals has become fundamentally linked to effective marketing strategies, particularly those highlighting emergency services. The need for hospitals to survive in a competitive health-care market has significantly contributed to the establishment and effective marketing of ED in Chinese hospitals. For example, Shanghai Changhai Hospital, Shanghai, China, has been enormously successful in the fee-for-service health-care market, and has attributed this success to factors such as quality of ED clinical services, patient-focused service, reasonable costs, media and marketing (Yang, Huo et al. 1999). In addition, its success is thought to be essentially related to provision of aesthetic features in the ED, including large-screen televisions in the intravenous therapy day-room, a facility that services around 500 patients per day (Yang, Huo et al. 1999). Such factors are believed to have accounted for around a 10% annual increase in this hospital's ED patient number (Yang, Huo et al. 1999). Figure 2 provides a general idea what an intravenous therapy day-room is like in China hospitals. At the other end of the spectrum, negative publicity resulting from emergency clinical mistakes can be devastating for hospital business, and is actively avoided.

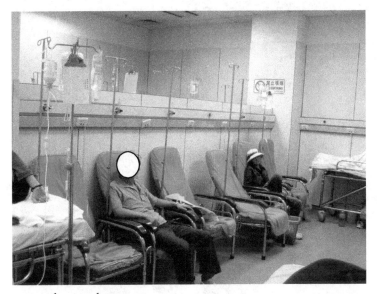

Fig. 2. Intravenous therapy day-room.

Therefore, to make patients happy becomes the first priority for the medical service providers. This is simply because those happy patients will come back to the same hospital to pay for the medical services again, then reputation spreads and more financial return is feasible.

When we visited a few EDs in Shenyang city in China in 2006, we did question the ethical issues of providing intravenous antibiotics to common cold or influenza patients. We were told by the doctors that they are well aware of the potential problems in overusing antibiotics, but the demand from the patients makes it impossible to refuse as 'Clients are God' in a market system plus that the direct financial return for their hospitals is also a consideration. The bigger size & better service from the hospital ED, the more crowded the hospital ED partly due to the market mechanism. Figure 3 and 4 were taken from a tertiary teaching hospital ED in Beijing where patients were treated in the corridor or intravenous treatment room where usually no beds are available.

In summary, the market system and financial responsibility of ED to their hospitals make it difficult for emergency health-care providers to develop and deliver a high-quality clinical service to their patients.

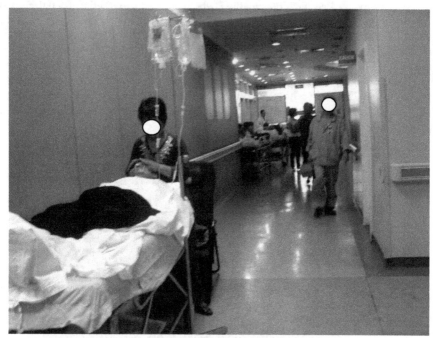

Fig. 3. ED patient being treated at the corridor.

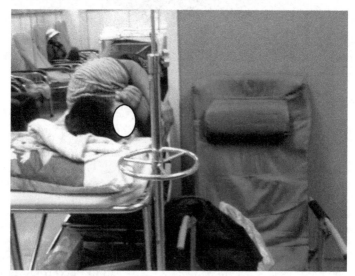

Fig. 4. ED patient on a temporary bed at an IV room.

Part II: the clinical practice situation of China hospital ED

The current configuration of hospital ED in China reflects the conceptualization of these units as places from which patients can be allocated to appropriate departments as soon as possible, with little treatment actually provided in the ED themselves. The concept of ED as a kind of 'transit lounge' has resulted in the coining of the term 'Green Channel' by Chinese health professionals (Luo 2003). The Green Channel implies rapid transit to the inpatient services for patients, with little intervention in the ED, like green lights in the traffic. Dr Luo, from Zhejiang University, one of China's leading education institutions, has described emergency clinicians' dissatisfaction with the 'Green Channel' ED conceptualization (Luo 2003). Other surveys (e.g. two studies (Wang 2000; Liu, Xie et al. 2002) have also highlighted clinicians' concerns that patients awaiting allocation to other departments often suffer complications, arising from delays and disagreements between departments about which will receive them. This was believed to be the case even for trauma patients and patients with life-threatening conditions, resulting in considerable preventable mortality (Wang 2000). Figure 5 is an example of a hospital ED where different health problems are allocated to different departments. For example, Department One was for neurological medical problems, Department Seven was for neurological surgical problems, and Department eight was for orthopaedics problems.

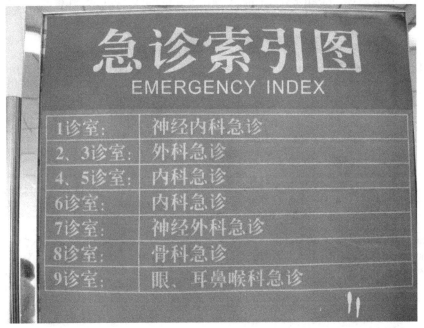

Fig. 5. An ED index directory informing patients which room to go for what type of emergency problem.

Another issue is the limited facilities available in many EDs, largely because of the 'Green Channel' concept described above. For example, only 38% of EDs in county-level hospitals in Guangxi Province had surgical facilities in 2005 (Lu and Qin 2005). This is largely because patients requiring such treatment would be expected to be transferred to surgical departments immediately following their arrival in the ED, rather than being assessed in the ED and prepared for the operating theatre there. For example, a survey of a convenience sample of 2183 patients presenting to the Shanghai Ruijin Hospital ED (a leading hospital ED in Shanghai) in June 2008 showed that following triage, patients were predominantly referred to an internist (41%), neurologist (14%), pulmonologist (11%), or general surgeon (9%) (Lammers, Folmer et al. 2011). One of the founders of Chinese EM, Professor Yitang Wang, has argued that future ED should include full surgical facilities, including operating theatres (Wang 2001). This sentiment has been supported by other scholars since (Sun, Tang et al. 2006).

The body of knowledge in EM in China is somehow behind the world as well. For example, a research paper written by a leading expert in EM in China and published by the national leading EM peer-reviewed journal, discussed the concept of triage. The article showed a lack of understanding of the importance and role of triage in emergency and disaster management (Wang 2002).The author believed that just to rush all the victims to a hospital would be the right strategy if there were many severely damaged patients and a hospital close to the site. This level of triage awareness demonstrated the underdeveloped body of knowledge in EM, as the statement from a developed country in 2002 described that the most significant advance in EM has been formalization and application of triage (Jelinek, Cameron et al. 2002).

Another example of the low standard in clinical practice in China is in the area of chemical poisoning treatment. Chemical poisoning is a leading cause of poisoning patients attending the ED in hospitals in China. Averagely about 500 patients attend each hospital in China (Zhou, Chen et al. 2004). Most alcohol poisoning happened in the east, west and south parts of China whereas most carbon oxide poisoning happened in middle and north part of China (Zhou, Chen et al. 2004). There are an estimated 170, 000 deaths annually from pesticide poisoning, mainly from Organic Phosphates (OP)(Little and Murray 2004).The mortality of OP pesticide poisoning in China was about 10% whereas overseas report of 2% (Wang, Wang et al. 2006). The author reported that among the 10% of patients who died, 60% of them died of atropine poisoning when atropine was overdosed during treatment. The consensus guidelines on reasonable precautions that should be taken when managing these patients, developed by Dr Little, could be of significant help to Chinese doctors (Little and Murray 2004).

The current clinical practice standards in China hospital ED are alarming when considering a pandemic situation. To apply World Health Organization's international standards, such as the International Health Regulations 2005 (Bradt and Drummond 2006), China needs to develop its EM practice to the world's standard as fast as possible. Developed countries with mature EM practice, such as Australia, New Zealand, USA and UK, could contribute to this development significantly to benefit the global community of emergency medicine professionals.

Part III: the education and training situation of China hospital ED

Although there have been dramatic improvements and advancements in recent years, the Chinese education and training system for Emergency Medicine is not yet fully developed. Thus, insufficient numbers of high-quality EM specialists have thus far been produced.

Another factor that limits the development of the specialty is the fact that doctors working in the ED often do not do so as their primary area of specialization. They are commonly specialists in other departments, such as medicine and surgery, who work in the ED on a rotating roster. The proportion of doctors and nurses who are employed to work in the ED on ongoing appointments varies across hospitals, and has been estimated to be from 50% (Xu 2000) to 60% (Luo 2003). This situation causes problems for the career development of clinicians and the absence of a clear career path for those aspiring to specialize in Emergency Medicine is likely to act as a deterrent. A recent survey found that Chinese clinicians clearly felt that this was the case (Bai, Li et al. 2004).

Three different types of Chinese hospital EDs have been described: dependent, semi-dependent and independent, with the type determined by allocation of human resources (Fan, Li et al. 2000). In the 'dependent' type of ED, only the ED director holds an ongoing appointment, with all other staff rostered on a rotational basis from other hospital departments. In the 'semi-dependent' type of ED, the director and some other staff members hold ongoing ED appointments. On the other hand, 'independent' types ED are staffed completely by doctors and nurses with ongoing ED appointments. Fan *et al.* surveyed 53 tertiary-level hospitals in China (termed San-Ji-Jia-Deng in Chinese), with an average inpatient bed number of 895, average day patient number of 2,168 and mean staffing of 1,556 health professionals. Among all of these hospitals, only three were identified as having 'independent' type ED, highlighting the slow development in terms of the Chinese EM workforce (Fan, Li et al. 2000).

Evidence-based training and practice are a concept that has been welcomed and widely accepted by Chinese clinicians (Song and Fan 2003). Consequently, educational institutions have been involved in a complete overhaul of their curricula over the past 20 years, and many courses at Chinese universities can now be described as among the best in the world. However, specialty training in some postgraduate areas is still often sought abroad, in part as a result of underdeveloped courses and academic expertise.

Tertiary educational programs in Emergency Medicine in China began in 2002 with the establishment of an EM major within the clinical degree program in Nanjing Medical University (Wang 2002). However, it has been acknowledged that one of the main reasons for the continuation of such majors is to ensure a supply of qualified ED staff, as the perception remains that ED is one of the least attractive hospital areas for medical graduates, despite the fact that ED doctors could master the essential clinical skills including eight medical skills and eight surgical skills (Wen 2005).

It was proposed that it takes three years for a clinician with a doctoral degree, and 5 years if bachelor or masters degree, to specialize as a specialist in Emergency Medicine (Bai, Li et al. 2004). However, the duration of training is still an question of debate, as some experts believe that it takes five years to master the necessary knowledge and skills and it makes no difference whether you have a bachelor or master degree (Wan and He 2006). The content of the training program has not been standardized in China, which varies in time duration and content of training in a range of departments in hospitals (Wan and He 2006).

It was argued among the Chinese health professionals whether it was appropriate to develop a major of EM in clinical medicine (Song 1999). The argument result was summarized in Table 1.

	Specialists of emergency medicine	Specialists in other clinical areas and roster in ED
Cost/benefit ratio	Low	High
Clinical service quality	General high	General low
	Specific case low	Specific case high
ED management	Easy	Difficult
EM as a specialty to develop	Fast	Slow
Acceptance	Difficult	Easy
To develop	Initially difficult	Initially easy
	Later easy	Later difficult

Table 1. With or without emergency medicine specialists in hospital EDs.

The author is from Hainan Province People's Hospital, Hainan, China, and actually supported the idea of developing EM as a specialty area among clinical medicine in China (Song 1999).

China is not a leading country in Asia in developing EM in many ways, but is considerable ahead of some countries, such as India (David 2007) where the medical system is governed by a single, central, regulatory body known as the Medical Council of India (MCI) which oversees all specialities. Multiple representations have attempted to enlighten MCI regarding the need for postgraduate training in EM. However, no positive notes of response have been forthcoming, by November 2006 (David 2007). The author described that without the consent of the MCI, a recognized postgraduate training in EM cannot be started in the country (David 2007), while emergency physicians cannot play a significant role in persuading the government.

By all estimates, the pace of growth of EM in China will continue to accelerate as China's economy and demographics approach those of the west, but the final form they will take is still uncertain (Ali 2001). The certain point is that China is taking the parts of the western system it can use and implementing its own methods in the overall practice of EM (Clem, Thomas et al. 1998).

4. Traditional Chinese Emergency Medicine (TCEM) in hospital EDs

4.1 Brief theory and current situation

Traditional Chinese Medicine (TCM) is based upon descriptive metaphors for human energies that do not translate well into the English terms, and very often some meanings are lost in the process of translation. The basic concept in TCM is that a vital force of life surges through the body called Qi. Any imbalance in Qi can cause illness or diseases. TCM focus on the whole body, not just the foot or head where the illness is located (Zhang, Wang et al. 2007). For example, pain is the result of conflict between blood and Qi (Dillard and Knapp 2005). The treatment in pain using TCM would then include balancing the energy, nourishing the blood, and building up deficient blood using herbal remedies, acupuncture, massage, and moxibustion.

The importance of TCM application in Emergency Departments at TCM hospital in China has been demonstrated by some academics who believe that "no western medicine if TCM works; and TCM first, western medicine later" (in Chinese, it says "能中不西，先中后西")

(Wu 2011), seeing western medicine as the "opposition". However, some TCM clinicians are more positive towards western medicine and believe that western medicine could compliment TCEM in diagnosis and treating acute illness and trauma patients (Liu 2008) which may be due to the slow development in TCEM regarding its limited facility and equipment and staff's low capacity (Su, Ding et al. 2002). It is not surprising that some TCM practitioners, maybe the most of TCM practitioners, believe that clinicians should use whatever the best for the patients whether it was TCM or western medicine or both (Sun and Xi 2006) (Su, Ding et al. 2002).

To apply the essential concept of TCM as the holistic approach in treating a patient, the nurses in charge of PCI patients practised the "emotional nursing" which was to look after the patients prior, during, and post the operation regarding their emotional status and concerns. It was demonstrated that the patients' general outcome was improved after the intervention (Wang 2011). Similar outcome was also reported in PTCA older patients (Liu and Lin 2009), the hysteria patients (Cheng and Lu 2011) and suicidal attempt patients attending the emergency departments in a TCM hospital (Zhou 2007).

Similar to the development in emergency medicine among the emergency physicians, doctors specialising in Traditional Chinese Emergency Medicine (TCEM) should be able to deal with all acute illness and trauma whether it was medicine, surgery or obstetrics problems (Jiang, Chen et al. 2007) which was supported by the ED development at Guangdong Province Fe-Shan TCM hospital (He, Zhang et al. 2004).

Due to the large number of universities delivering western medicine courses, most ED doctors working in TCM hospitals have the degree in western medicine, which equals the Bachelor of Medicine and Bachelor of surgery (MBBS) program in medical schools in Australia. For example, in Kunming City TCM Hospital ED, there were 20 doctors. Fifteen of them were trained in western medicine, and 12 out of these 15 doctors graduated with the second degree in TCM (Liu, Xie et al. 2002).

Herbal medicine is a large part of TCM. China TCM Management Bureau, the highest level of TCM professional organisation in China, publishes the recommended herbal remedies list for Emergency Departments at TCM hospitals. There were 15 products in the list published on 9th January1993 (Wu 1997), and 50 in 1997 (China-TCM-Management-Bureau 1997). The list has been updated every two years. There were about 134 injection type of herbal remedies being used in western medicine practice in China (Luo 2010). These herbal remedies for injection use included anaesthetic, anti-bacteria, anti-shock, treating coronary heart problems, pain reliever, stop-bleeding, anti-cancers and improving immune system (Luo 2010). It was believed that a well performed TCM hospital ED should use all the products in the list regularly, and that Chongqing TCM Hospital ED used about 42% of the list products (Li, Cheng et al. 2006) was regarded as a low level performance and needed to increase the number of the used herbal remedies rapidly.

5. Diagnosis and treatment

The traditional diagnosis method in TCM is called Four Diagnosis Method, namely inspection (望), listening and smelling （闻）, inquiring （问） and palpation （切）(Wei and Su 2010). Applying this "Four Diagnosis " method in triage in emergency medicine in TCM hospitals (Chen 2010) , its accuracy rate was 90.3% as good as non-TCM hospitals

(Zhang 2007). This finding was supported by a report about Four Diagnosis method applied in Triage for abdominal pain patients (Tao 2003).

It was reported that there were three ways to make a diagnosis in TCEM: to borrow the western medicine diagnosis; to use the TCM diagnosis only; and to combine TCM with western medicine to generate a diagnosis (Liu, Wang et al. 2010). It would not make any sense for a western medicine practitioner to read a diagnosis in TCM. For example, diagnosis of unconscious patients in TCM has six types, all of them are in TCM terms and no translation to English was available to understand them (Zhang 2010). The author of this book chapter was educated in western medicine in China and has very little idea what the diagnosis really mean regarding the concept of diagnosis in western medicine. This "confusion" among the practitioners trained in western medicine was also supported in a general discussion paper about principles of diagnosis in TCEM (Zhong 1983). It would not surprise the western medicine colleagues that misdiagnosis would be more often in TCM, which could be a result of the many factors including the limitation in TCEM diagnosis; limitation in herbal remedies treatment; weak concept of "emergency"; and under-equipped with modern facilities (Liu and Cui 2004).

Despite the confusion in understanding the TCM diagnosis, its application in successfully treating a range of acute illness for patients attending TCM hospital EDs has been reported in the Chinese literature. These include dizziness patients (Lan and Lin 2009), headache, and head injury patients (Gao 2009) (YAN, HAN et al. 2008), nose bleeding (YAN, HAN et al. 2008), chest pain patients (Shen and Han 2009) (Gao 2009), acute myocardial infarction patients (Wang and Chen 2009), intoxicated carditis with shock (Tan and Mei 1995), haemorrhoid (Deng and Zheng 1997), acute pneumonia and acute pancreatitis, (YAN, HAN et al. 2008), pain from cancer (Xu and Liu 1994) and even fracture (Jin 1982). It was reported that acupuncture was effective and fast in treating acute stomach pain, high fever, hysteria, and hiccup (Ni 1998); and acupressure was impressively effective in treating angina, hiccup and cough (Jiang, Tang et al. 1992).

In many cases, the treatment for the patients attending a TCM hospital ED was a combination of TCM and western medicine. Researchers believe that the application of TCM in treating SARS (Severe Acute Respiratory Syndrome) in 2003, swine influenza in 2004 and H1N1 influenza in 2010, had demonstrated the feasibility of combining TCM with western medicine to improve the treatment outcome for patients with virus infections (Luo 2010) (Jiang, Tang et al. 1992).

6. Teaching

The general perception is that where there is a university teaching western medicine, there is a university teaching TCM. For example, in the capital city of Beijing, there is a Beijing Medical University (now called Health Science Centre of Peking University) and there is also a Beijing TCM University. Therefore, there are quite a few publications in Chinese language about teaching TCM and its vital role in keeping the TCM practice alive and continues to develop. It needs to be noted that universities in China now have a major in Chinese-Western combined medicine where students learn both the TCM and the western medicine (Sun and Xi 2006); and that the first group of doctorate students undertaking research in the area of Traditional Chinese Emergency Medicine at Guangzhou TCM

University graduated in 1996 (Zhou 1996). These are important milestones for the TCEM teaching and research in China.

Regarding the teaching content in knowledge, it was important to teach the intern students at Emergency Department in TCM hospitals the essential knowledge of the Four Diagnosis in TCM, especially now most county TCM hospitals have emergency departments (Zhou and Zhang 2011) and the recognition of these skills in ED triage (Lin and Liu 2003). It was recommended to combine the concept and theory of TCM with western medicine (Wu 2011). Some leading experts in TCM believe that an essential part to further develop TCEM was to ensure the TCEM practitioners are experts in western emergency medicine although that how to achieve this objective was still unclear (Jiang 2009). For example, to treat bacteria infectious patients with fever, both antibiotics to kill the bacteria and herbal remedies to build the body's immune system should be considered (Wu 2011). However, in reality of current teaching practice, the education and training of western medicine in TCM teaching was not sufficient enough to provide students enough acute clinical skills, partly because some TCM clinicians tend to only use TCM in treating acutely ill patients (Zhang, Zhang et al. 2010). Nurses are important part of this team and it is also important to train the nurses for the core capacity at ED in TCM hospitals (Chen, Wang et al. 2011) as well as their capacity in triage and legal practice (Chang, Pang et al. 2010).

Regarding the teaching content in skills, reports suggest that students graduated from TCM universities have a good understanding of the TCM theories but low clinical practice skills at EDs which explained why a standard set of teaching and training criteria was required for the intern students at ED in TCM hospitals (Li 2011). Some academics believe that students' critical thinking capacity is as important as their emergency medicine clinical skills (Wu 2011), which would be accepted by most western medicine practitioners.

Regarding the teaching method, it was reported that to employ Problem Based Learning method in teaching TCEM could activate students' interests in studying this area, improve their general understanding of the subjects, and enhance their critical and clinical thinking capacity (Li, Yang et al. 2010) (Li, Han et al. 2009).

Continuing professional education is important for any health profession. To send TCEM practitioners in low level TCM hospitals to western medicine hospitals to learn and update their knowledge, skills and practice in western emergency medicine was regarded as an important measure for the TCEM development strategy (Ding 2005).

7. Research

Published literatures in Chinese language in the area of Traditional Chinese Emergency Medicine (TCEM) are relatively few and without strong research designs in the concept of western medicine research. Some TCEM researchers in China even believed that it is not appropriate to apply western medicine methods to assess the effectiveness of the TCEM treatments (in Chinese, it says"道不同理能清吗?") and that the challenges from western medicine was a barrier for the TCEM development in China (Chao, Jiang et al. 2010).

Here is an example to illustrate the research status of TCEM in China. Almost ten out of ten clinicians agree to use western medicine to treat acute cardiac failure, but ten out of ten would not agree to try TCM herbal remedies (such as Gan-Cao-Gan-Jiang-Tang) to rescue patients (Zhao and Fu 2008). It was described that clinicians did not like to try the TCM because they were not sure if it would work and asked "what would you do if it failed and patient died?" Then the author argued that it was as if patients did not die under the treatment of western medicine; if that was the case, "why the bigger the hospital the bigger the dead house size?" (Zhao and Fu 2008). It would be such an obvious point that the bigger the hospital, the higher proportion of severe patients, the higher general mortality for the hospital. This article demonstrated the status of evidence based practice in TCEM in China.

There are leaders in TCEM research in china who advocate the fact that without strong scientific research, TCEM would not develop further in the future in China (Chen 2001). A leading member from the Chinese Association of Combined TCM with Western Medicine reported that evidence is what TCEM needed the most at the time, such as research about time-effectiveness and dose-response of the herbal remedies (Chen 2001).

To better coordinate the research outcome, the Emergency Medicine Branch of China Traditional Chinese Medicine Association published their research priorities which were stroke, infectious fever, shock, lung diseases, cardiac attack, and virus diseases (Chao, Jiang et al. 2010). The significant research outcome in TCEM including the establishment of the TCEM peer reviewed journals such as Chinese Journal of TCM and Shanghai Journal of TCM. The first TCEM book in history titled "Traditional Chinese Emergency Medicine", over one million Chinese words, initiated and monitored by China TCM Management Bureau, was published in 1995 after three years of hard work from the TCM practitioners and researchers (Wang and Wang 1995).

The relatively active research was conducted in acupuncture due to its wide accepted effect in treating acute and chronic pain, including osteoarthritis, back pain, dysmenorrhea, and migraints (Dillard and Knapp 2005). A lot of research activities have been undertaken trying to understand the mechanism of how acupuncture works in treating pain, and they have found the improvement in immune system, neurochemical and hormone functions, and pain pathways (Dillard and Knapp 2005). However, the exact mechanism of how acupuncture works specifically remains unclear.

The challenge in further developing TCEM research included no vision and long term strategies, weakness in research to provide strong evidence, and the capacity in teaching and training to produce quality TCEM practitioners (Chao, Jiang et al. 2010).

8. Overseas TCM

Alternative and complementary medicine has been used among populations in a range of countries and will always be there in the future. The National Centre for Complementary and Alternative Medicine (NCCAM) outlined six categories, which are mind-body interventions, diet lifestyle modification, herbal remedies, manual healing, bioelectromgnetics, and pharmacologic-biologic treatments (Dillard and Knapp 2005). There is no doubt that TCM is one of the options when people turn to alternative and complementary medicine. For example, acupuncture gained attention in USA in the 1970s when China and USA started the diplomatic relationship (Dillard and Knapp 2005). There were approximately 10,000 certified acupuncturists practice in USA in 2005 and increasing number of those acupuncturists are physicians who have incorporated acupuncture into their daily practice (Dillard and Knapp 2005).

TCM was commonly used among the Chinese immigrants living in other countries such as USA, Canada, UK and Australia. A survey using a convenience sample of first- and second-generation adult Chinese immigrants (Pearl, Leo et al. 1995) attending at an Emergency Department in a hospital in New York, found that 43% had used traditional Chinese therapy within one week of the ED visit. Therefore, emergency physicians treating Chinese-Americans should be aware of the medical and social implications of alternative medical therapies.

9. Opportunities and challenges for the future development of emergency medicine in China among this global medicine community

In this globalization environment, international organizations and health professionals have started to be involved in the development of EM in China. For example, a description of the US emergency physicians' experience as consultants at a new ED and in establishing an EM residency program in Hangzhou, China was reported about 13 years ago (Clem, Thomas et al. 1998). A total of seven months were spent in the observation, identification and development of a basic framework of emergency care at a new hospital in Hangzhou (Clem, Thomas et al. 1998). About six years ago, a collaborative partnership between the Johns Hopkins Hospital, Chaoyang Red Cross Hospital in Beijing and Chinese Ministry of Health was established to initiate EM administrative training in Beijing, China (Hsu, Dey et al. 2005). The Emergency Medical Education and Training Center (EMETC) at Chaoyang Red Cross Hospital was opened as a training facility to foster EM administrative curriculum development and training nationwide. A six-step approach with problem identification, needs assessment, goals and objectives, educational strategies, implementation and evaluation was used to form a locally adapted curriculum (Hsu, Dey et al. 2005). With a train-the-trainers model, the EMETC sponsored several EM administration courses, the first of their kind in China. Since its inception, the EMETC has trained 95 persons from throughout China in EM administration. An EM administration curriculum has been developed and refined. The author believes that an international partnership between academic hospitals, supported by the local Ministry of Health, to develop a national training facility using this six-step approach might be an attractive strategy for dissemination of EM administration principles (Hsu, Dey et al. 2005).

Emergency physicians from Hong Kong also believe that they could contribute to the fast development of EM as a specialty area in mainland China (Fu, Chan et al. 1998). Queensland University of Technology has signed a Memorandum of Understanding with China Medical University to work together to develop award courses and training programs in EM in China (Figure 6).

Considering the development of EM in Australia, health professionals working related to hospital EDs are well placed to contribute their knowledge and skills to assist in the development of ED in hospitals in China. As early as ten years ago, Dr Chris Curry (Curry 2001) described his vision that 'there is much new territory to be explored: in refugee and developing world medicine; in travel medicine and public health; in providing services to remote locations on the ground, water or ice; and at a distance by telemedicine. Emergency physicians have been making contributions in trouble spots like Bosnia, Timor, Myanmar, the Kenya/Sudan border, Afghanistan. We are joining with developing neighbours like New Guinea and the Pacific Islands. We are going to the outback, we are going to sea, we

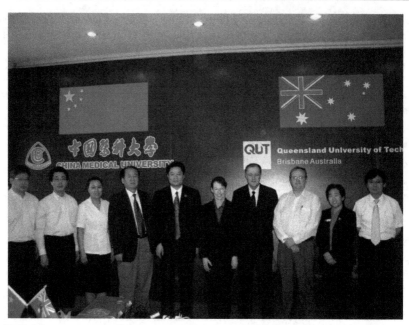

Fig. 6. QUT delegation visited China Medical University in 2006 (the second right is the author).

are developing EM links with China, South-East Asia, and the Middle East" (Curry 2001). The Australian emergency physicians are proud of their achievement, for example, Dr Cox's wonderful work in Tanzania, East Africa (Cox 2007), Australia's contribution to the EM work in post-tsunami Thailand (Liew and kennedy 2007) and Dr Frieda Law from Australia being the invited guest editor for the *Chinese Journal of Emergency Medicine (Jiang 2006)*. Australasian emergency physicians have connections with more than 30 developing countries in the Pacific, Asia and Africa by 2006 (Curry 2007). However, we would definitely achieve more if we could link more closely to our neighbour developing countries, such as China.

The 11th National Emergency Medicine Conference was held in Dalian in May 2006 and the President Professor Jiang Guanyu expressed his excitement of holding the 17th World Congress in Disaster and Emergency Medicine in China in 2011. He expected a rapid development in EM in the coming years to prepare for the world congress, especially now China has its EM professional association, EM is a major in medicine and doctors' career path is clearer than ever (He 2006).

It is believed that TCEM will continue to provide acute care to the population in China. An health official from China TCM Management Bureau suggested to build the TCEM in the 21st century, health professionals need to (Yang 2001) combine the tradition with innovation; the characteristics with its strength; align the ED development with the hospital development; clinical practice with clinical quality governess; research in herbal remedies; education and training in TCEM; and to combine TCEM with information technology and related regulations (Yang 2001). Modernisation was not regarded as the appropriate choice for TCEM's future and it actually could kill TCM as a whole (Su, Ding et al. 2002); TCM should stand on its own feet while learning the high technology from the western medicine (Su, Ding et al. 2002).

There is no doubt that China EM will develop dramatically in a short period of time, in this global environment with contributions from developed countries. Developed countries such as Australia, being China's neighbour and friend, would be well placed to play a significant role in this Emergency Medicine development.

10. Competing interests

I declare that there are no competing interests, such as financial support or relationships that might pose conflicts of interests during writing this book chapter.

11. Acknowledgment

I sincerely acknowledge the financial support from the School of Public Health at Queensland University of Technology and the generous support from Dr Jingzhou Zhao and Ms Shuang Zhong who helped me in building the Endnote library including the references in Chinese language.

12. References

Ali, R. (2001). "Emergency medicine in China: redefining a specialty." *J Emerg Med* 21(2): 197-207.

Bai, X., Z. Li, et al. (2004). "The theory and practice of multi-trauma treatment in emergency department in hospitals." *Chin. J. Emerg. Med* 13: 863-864.

Bradt, D. A. and C. M. Drummond (2006). "Avian influenza pandemic threat and health systems response." *Emerg Med Australas* 18(5-6): 430-443.

Chang, L. J., Y. B. Pang, et al. (2010). "The difficulties and countermeasures of the clinical teaching to emergency nurses from TCM hospitals." *China Prac Med* 5(35): 261-262.

Chao, E. X., L. D. Jiang, et al. (2010). "Research report on development of the subject of emergency medicine in TCM." *Chinese Medicine Modern Distance Education Of China* 8(17): 164-166.

Chen, L. F., Y. Y. Wang, et al. (2011). "Discuss the training methods for core capability of nurses from emergency departments of TCM hospitals." *Journal of Emergency in Traditional Chinese Medicine* 20(2): 338-339.

Chen, Q. Z. (2010). "The application of the "four diagnostic" method from TCM in the triage of emergency department at a TCM Hospita." *Modern Journal o f Integrated Traditional Chinese and Western Medicine* 19(25): 3223-3224.

Chen, S. K. (2001). "Promote the continuous development of traditional Chinese emergency medicine and related subjects." *Journal of Emergency in Traditional Chinese Medicine* 10(1): 2-4.

Cheng, H. and Y. H. Lu (2011). "The application of emotional nursing in 96 emergency hysteria patients." *Modern Journal o f Integrated Traditional Chinese and Western Medicine* 20(7): 889.

China-TCM-Management-Bureau (1997). Herbal Medicine list for Emergency Departments in TCM Hospitals in China in 1997. *Chin J Inf Tradit Chin Med* 4: 5-6.

China MoH. (2006). "2005 Report of China Health." from
http://www.moh.gov.cn/news/search_index.aspx.

China NBoSoP. (2006). "2005 Report." from http://www.stats.gov.cn/was40/gjtjj_detail.jsp?
searchword=%BB%A4%CA%BF&presearchword=%D2%BD
%C9%FA&channeled=6697&record=26.

Clem, K. J., T. L. Thomas, et al. (1998). "United States physician assistance in development of
emergency medicine in Hangzhou, China." *Ann Emerg Med* 32(1): 86-92.

Cox, M. (2007). "Emergency medicine development in Tanzania, East Africa." *Emerg. Med.
Australas* 19(s1): A19.

Curry, C. (2001). "Journey with emergency medicine." *Emerg. Med. Australas* 13(1): 1-4.

Curry, C. (2007). "Emergency medicine in the Developing World." *Emerg. Med. Australas*
19(s1): A18.

David, S. (2007). "The challenges of developing emergency medicine in India." *Emerg. Med.
Australas* 19(s1): A18.

Deng, F. Y. and A. F. Zheng (1997). "95 cases of emergency treatments of TCM for embedded
hemorrhoids." *Fujian Journal of Oct ober* 28(6): 21.

Dillard, J. N. and S. Knapp (2005). "Complementary and alternative pain therapy in the
emergency department." *Emerg Med Clin North Am* 23(2): 529-549.

Ding, S. X. (2005). "Suggestions for the work of emergency in TCM hospitals " *Management
of Chinese Medicine* 4(2): 35-36.

Fan, X., C. Li, et al. (2000). "The current situation and development strategy of emergency
medicine in China." *J. Emerg. Med* 9: 364-366.

Fu, t., K. Chan, et al. (1998). "Emergency medicine in Hong." *Ann. Emerg. Med* 32(1): 83-85.

Gao, Z. L. (2009). "Three ruls for the application of the angry machine method in TCM
emergency." *Chinese Journal of ethnomedicine and ethnopharmacy* 7: 53.

He, M. F., Y. J. Zhang, et al. (2004). "Chinese and western in hand, into the modern
emergency system- -the discussion of the emergency mode in TCM hospitals in
Foshan city, Guangdong province." *Journal of Emergency in Traditional Chinese
Medicine* 13(1): 43-44.

He, X. (2006). "Report of the national 11th conference on emergency medicine." *Chin. J.
Emerg. Med* 15: 666-668.

Hesketh, T. and W. X. Zhu (1997). "Health in China. Traditional Chinese medicine: one
country, two systems." *BMJ* 315(7100): 115-117.

Hou, X.-Y. and K. Chu (2010). "Emergency Department in Hospitals: Window of the world -
A preliminary comparison between Australia and China." *World Journal of
Emergency Medicine* 1(3): 180-184.

Hou, X. Y. and C. Z. Lu (2005). "The current workforce status of prehospital care in China."
Journal of Emergency Primary Health Care 3: Article 990127.

Hsu, E. B., C. C. Dey, et al. (2005). "Development of emergency medicine administration in
the People's Republic of China." *J Emerg Med* 28(2): 231-236.

Jelinek, G. A., P. A. Cameron, et al. (2002). "Emergency medicine." *Med J Aust* 176(1): 11.

Jiang, G. (2004). "The theory and practice of emergency medicine." *Chin. J. Emerg. Med* 13(1):
5-6.

Jiang, G. (2006). "20 years of emergency medicine in China: past and future." *Chin. J. Emerg.
Med* 15(1): 5.

Jiang, J. Z., H. Y. Chen, et al. (2007). "Discuss the construction of emergency departments in TCM hospitals." *Journal of Emergency in Traditional Chinese Medicine* 16(6): 718.

Jiang, L. C., S. Y. Tang, et al. (1992). "Application of accupressure in emergency departments at hospitals" 4(4): 239.

Jiang, S. M. (2009). "Discussion of TCM emergency " *Journal of Emergency in Traditional Chinese Medicine* 18(12): 1933-1934.

Jin, D. S. (1982). "The preliminary study of carrying out emergency in TCM." *Hubei Journal of Traditional Chinese Medicine*(5): 38-39.

Lammers, W., W. Folmer, et al. (2011). "Demographic analysis of emergency department patients at the ruijin hospital, shanghai." *Emergency Medicine International* 2011: 748274.

Lan, L. H. and W. Lin (2009). "Characteristics of TCM dialectical triage and protection for emergency patients with vertigo." *Journal of Liaoning University of Traditional Chinese Medicine* 11: 200-201.

Li, X. L., N. L. Han, et al. (2009). "Discuss the application of PBL teaching method in the teaching of clinical emergency in TCM." *Journal of Emergency in Traditional Chinese Medicine* 18(10): 1663-1665.

Li, Y. (2011). "Study and practice of standardized training and assessment of clinical skills for emergency medecine of TCM " *Guide of China Medicine* 9(22): 176-177.

Li, Y., Y. F. Cheng, et al. (2006). "The analysis of the application of emergency necessary proprietary from TCM." *Journal of Emergency in Traditional Chinese Medicine* 15(4): 385-386.

Li, Y., C. Z. Yang, et al. (2010). "Clinical teaching of TCM emergency medicine applying Problem Based Learning." *Education of Chinese Medicine* 29(5): 69-71.

Liew, D. and M. kennedy (2007). "Emergency medicine in post-tsunami Thailand: Australia's contribution." *Emerg. Med. Australas* 19(s1): A8.

Lin, Y. Z. and B. Liu (2003). "Discussion on triage in emergency departments of TCM hospitals " *Jilin Journal of Traditional Chinese Medicine* 23(2): 41.

Little, M. and L. Murray (2004). "Consensus statement: risk of nosocomial organophosphate poisoning in emergency departments." *Emerg Med Australas* 16(5-6): 456-458.

Liu, L. (2010). "Strengthening the thinking for the risk management of emergency in primary TCM hospitals " *Chinese Community Doctors* 12(6): 161-163.

Liu, M., D. Xie, et al. (2002). "Discussion and practice of models in emergency department in TCM hospitals " *Journal of Emergency in Traditional Chinese Medicine* 11(5): 401-402.

Liu, Q. Q. (2008). "Get to know the science of emergentology medicine of TCM." *GLOBAL TCM*(1): 11-13.

Liu, Q. Q., G. L. Wang, et al. (2010). "Talk about the core of clinical teaching of TCM from emergency medicine of TCM " *Chinese Medicine Modern Distance Education Of China* 8(18): 196.

Liu, X. R. and C. Y. Lin (2009). "The application of "sentiment nursing" from TCM in nursing of elderly patients who are in the use of PTCA emergency care." *Journal of Clinical Medicine in Practice* 5(5): 32-33.

Liu, Z. H. and Y. L. Cui (2004). "Misdiagnosis and prevention of emergency medicine of TCM." *Chinese Journal of Misdiagnostics* 4(8): 1161-1162.

Lu, Y. and L. Qin (2005). "A Situation analysis of medical resources in emergency department in Guangxi province in China." *Chin. J. Emerg. Med* 14: 1054.

Luo, K. (2010). "The application of emergency medicine and new dosage forms of TCM." *Chinese Medicine Modern Distance Education Of China* 8(18): 202-204.

Luo, X. (2003). "Discussions on the external environment of 'emergency department channel." *Chin. J. Emerg. Med* 12: 802.

Ni, L. Y. (1998). "Discuss the application of acupuncture in TCM emergency " *JOURNAL OF CLINICAL ACUPUNCTURE AND MOXIBUSTION* 14(1): 40-41.

Pearl, W. S., P. Leo, et al. (1995). "Use of Chinese therapies among Chinese patients seeking emergency department care." *Ann Emerg Med* 26(6): 735-738.

Shen, S. G. and X. J. Han (2009). "TCM emergency dialectical treatments for chest pain." *Journal of Emergency in Traditional Chinese Medicine* 18(10): 1628-1629.

Song, G. and X. Fan (2003). "The current situation and a few issues in emergency department in paediatrics." *Chin. J. Emerg. Med* 12: 293-294.

Song, W. (1999). "The theory and practice of emergency medicine development." *J. Emerg. Med* 8(6): 1.

Su, W. G., B. H. Ding, et al. (2002). "Applying modern emergency medicine system to promote traditional Chinese medicine." *Journal of Emergency in Traditional Chinese Medicine* 11(2): 77-79.

Sun, J. G. and Z. Q. Xi (2006). "In which direction is the way of emergency in TCM in the 21 st century?" *Chinese Journal of Integrated Traditional and Western Medicine in Intensive and Critical Care* 13(1): 63-64.

Sun, Z., L. Tang, et al. (2006). "The development of modern trauma rescue and treatment." *Chin. J. Emerg. Med* 15: 659-661.

Tan, R. Y. and G. Y. Mei (1995). "Construction and management of emergency department in TCM hospitals." *Chinese Journal of Hospital Administration* 11(4): 215-216.

Tao, X. Y. (2003). "The application of the "four diagnostic" from TCM in the triage of emergency abdominal pain." *Journal of Emergency in Traditional Chinese Medicine* 12(2): 188.

Wan, Z. and Q. He (2006). "The training of the residence doctors in emergency department in Huaxi hospital at Sichuan University " *Chin. J. Emerg. Med* 15: 183-185.

Wang, L. J. (2011). "The experience of "emotional nursing" for PCI patients at Emergency Department in a TCM Hospital " *The Qiqihar Medical School Journal*(14).

Wang, P. (2000). "Discussions on development of emergency department – to face 21st century and the newchallenges." *Chin. J. Emerg. Med* 9: 353-354.

Wang, R. P. and X. M. Chen (2009). "Building and the study of standardized evaluation of the green channel using emergency medicine of TCM for acute myocardial infarction." *Jiangsu Journal of Traditional Chinese Medicine* 41(10): 35-36.

Wang, Y. (2001). "Emergency department in city hospitals should develop a 5-year plan." *Chin. J. Emerg. Med* 10(1): 9-10.

Wang, Y. (2002). "To strengthen the basic construction in emergency medicine teaching: congratulations on the first bachelor course in emergency medicine in China." *Chin. J. Emerg. Med* 11: 272.

Wang, Z., Y. Wang, et al. (2006). "Mistakes in rescube and treatment of pesticide of organic phosphorus." *Chin. J. Crit. Care Med* 26: 442-443.

Wang, Z. P. and Y. Y. Wang (1995). "The first book of "Traditional Chinese Medicine (TCM) in emergency medicine "." *Chinese Journal of emergency medicine* 4(3): 140-141.

Wei, H. Q. and Y. H. Su (2010). "The application of the "four diagnostic" from TCM in the evaluation of patients of emergency departments " *JOURNAL OF LIAONING UNIVERSITY OF TCM* 12(10): 85-86.

Wen, L. (2005). "The establishment and development in emergency department and EICU." *Chin. J. Emerg. Med* 14: 699-700.

Wu, J. (2009). "Problems and countermeasures of emergency in primary TCM hospitals " *Journal of Emergency in Traditional Chinese Medicine* 18(1): 104-105.

Wu, k. (1997). "Development in applying herbal medicine in emergency departments at TCM hospitals." *Journal of Chinese tranditional emergency medical* 6(6): 243.

Wu, Y. (2011). "The thinking about teaching in emergency disciplines in TCM." *MEDICAL INFORMATION*(9): 4519-4520.

Xi, Z. Q. (2008). "The development and prospects of emergency medicine in TCM." *Journal of Emergency in Traditional Chinese Medicine* 17(4): 425-427.

Xu, F. (2000). "To develop rural emergency medicine and improve quality and team management." *Chin. J. Emerg. Med* 9: 281-282.

Xu, Z. Y. and J. X. Liu (1994). "TCM treatments for cancer pain." *Shanghai J Tradit Chin Med* (12): 6-8.

YAN, X. i., T. i. X. HAN, et al. (2008). "Discussi on of treatment determination in TCM emergency , from effects of medications will be detected after the first decoction and the disease can be cured after the second decoction." *JOURNAL OF TONG JI UN I VERSITY* 29(4): 136-140.

Yang, R., Z. Huo, et al. (1999). "To maintain the development of emergency medicine in the medical market competition through enhancing the awareness of the practice." *J. Emerg. Med* 8(3): 1.

Yang, R. C. (2001). "Construction of the 21st century traditional Chinese emergency medicine." *Zhejiang Traditional Chinese Medicine*(4): 175-176.

Zhang, C. H., W. X. Zhang, et al. (2010). "Exploration and practice of the training and thinking for undergraduate students in clinical emergency of TCM." *Li Shi Zhen Medicine And Materia Medicare Sesearch* 21(8): 2037-2038.

Zhang, M. (2007). "The experience by applicating TCM diagnostic methods in the triage work of emergency department " *Chinese Journal of Guang Ming Tranditional Chinese Medicine* 22(6): 79-80.

Zhang, Q. (2010). "The thought of TCM dialectical thought and the idea of diagnosis and treatment for emergency unconcious patients " *Chinese Journal of Guang Ming Tranditional Chinese Medicine* 25(9): 1582-1583.

Zhang, X. J., X. L. Wang, et al. (2007). "Brief introduction of the holistic approach in Traditional Chinese Emergency Medicine." *Journal of Xinjiang Tranditional Chinese Medicine* 25(4): 112-113.

Zhao, B. and Z. P. Fu (2008). "The status quo and thought of the work of emergency in TCM in Gansu." *Gansu Journal of TCM* 21: 54-55.

Zhong, M. L. (1983). "Preliminary discussion of dialectical emergency medicine treatment of TCM " *Qinghai Medicine* 61(3): 58-64.

Zhou, H. P. (1996). "Emergency medicine of TCM for 30 years." *The new journal of traditional Chinese medicine* 1(1): 37.

Zhou, J., S. Chen, et al. (2004). "The Investigation of chemical poisoning in emergency department in 25 comprehensive hospitals." *Chin. J. Emerg. Med* 13: 729-732.

Zhou, S. B. and W. Q. Zhang (2011). "The discussion of clinical teaching in emergency department of TCM hospitals " *Chinese Journal of Traditional Chinese Medicine* 9(16): 46-47.

Zhou, X. P. (2007). "Discuss the application of "seven emotions" to cure and cause diseases into TCM emergency nursing." *Journal of Guiyang College of Traditional Chinese Medicine* 29(6): 69.

Intensive Care Management of the Traumatic Brain Injury

Akarsu Ayazoglu Tülin[1] and Özden Nihan[2]
*[1]Chief Asistant Kartal Kosuyolu Highly
Specialized Education and Training Hospital İstanbul
[2]Göztepe Education and Training Hospital Istanbul
Turkey*

1. Introduction

Traumatic brain injury has been major cause of mortality and morbidity worldwide, especially in children and young adults and it has been continuing a difficult problem in intensive care units.

Brain trauma can be caused by a direct impact or by acceleration alone. In addition to the damage caused at the moment of injury, brain trauma causes secondary injury, a variety of events that take place in that minutes and/or days following the injury

Secondary brain injury is attributable to a decrease in cerebral oxygen delivery as a result of hypertension, hypoxia, cerebral oedema, intracranial hypertension or abnormalities in cerebral blood flow. Although the severity of primary brain injury cannot be reduced, secondary brain injury can be minimised if appropriate therapies are implemented in time.

The main aim in the traumatic brain injured patients must be to maintain a good result from primary injury caused by trauma and/or as a result of direct effect of trauma.

The second aim must be to prevent secondary brain injury caused by as results of the complications. The basic principle in the care and treatment of traumatic brain injury is to describe and begin the treatment these complications that worsen the primary injury and lead to secondary brain injury.

The main targets in these aims are:

1. Maintain the cerebral energy metabolism by maintaining needed systemic support,
2. Maintain cerebral perfusion pressure (CPP) in normal limits,
3. Maintain ICP in normal limits as possible.

The intensive care for traumatic brain injury should consist beside the control of ICP, respiratory system, central nervous system, and cirulatory system, it should also consist monitoring of metabolism especially glucose metabolism, temperature and electrolite balance in short intervals. With these invasive and noninvasive monitoring, all the precausions for the problems should be ready.

Beside heavy brain injury may result in a permanant neurologic sequale, it may also give a good results especially in young patients that aggresivelly lowered inreased ICP levels and optimized CPP and cerebral oxygenation by multidisiplinary approach with neurointensivist, neuroanesthesist and neurosurgeon.

In this chapter we will discuss the intensive care management of severe TBI with emphasis on the specific measures directed for prevention and/or treatment of secondary brain injury

2. Indication for admission to ICU

The role of an intensive care unit is to maintain a patient's normal physiological homeostasis while actively treating the underlying cause of any physiological derangement. Discussion will be targeted towards a number of areas; respiratory system, cardiovascular system, alimentary system, nasocomial infection and infection surveillance, anticoagulation, patient comfort.

Indication for admission to ICU include

- Impaired level of consciousness,
- Impaired airway protection
- Progressive respiratory impairment or the need for mechanical ventilation
- Seizures
- Clinical or computed tomographic (CT) evidence of raised ICP caused by a space occupying lesion , cerebral edema or haemorrhagic conversion of a cerebral infarct.
- General medical complications (for example, hyper/hypotension, fluid and electrolyte disturbances, aspiration pneumonia,sepsis, cardiac arrhytmias, pulmonary embolism)
- Monitoring (for example level of conciousness, respiratory function, ICP continuous electroencephalography(EEG)
- Specific treatments(for example , neurosurgical intervention, intravenous or arterial trombolysis)

Mechanical ventilation

Most patients admitted to neuro-intensive care require respiratory support because of hypoxaemia, ventilatory failure or due to treatment modalities requiring respiratory support.

The support may range from oxygen therapy by face mask, through non-invasive techniques such as continuous positive airways pressure, to full ventilatory support with endotracheal intubation.

Oxygen is usually given by face mask, although nasal prongs or cannulas may be well tolerated.

If the patient remains hypoxaemic on high flow oxygen (15 l/min) continuous positive airways pressure (CPAP) may be used. The continuous positive airways pressure mask often becomes uncomfortable and gastric distension may occur. Patients must therefore be cooperative, able to protect their airway, and have the strength to breathe spontaneously and cough effectively.

In patients with acute brain lesions at risk for cerebral ischemia, maintenance of adequate cerebral perfusion pressure (CPP), artificial ventilation for prevention of hypercapnia and deep sedation are all major determinants for actual strategies of a cerebroprotective therapy [1].

The patient who has an altered level of consciousness (GCS <8) and loss of gag/cough reflex often has deficits in a number of airway protection mechanisms or exhaustion need ventilatory support.

The goals of mechanical ventilation of acute severely brain injured patients are to improve gas exchange, to minimize intrathoracic pressure, to reduce the work of breathing and to avoid complications. These patients are also in the risk of developing neurogenic pulmonary edema, aspiration of oropharyngeal contents, pneumonia, and atelectasis.

Criteria for starting mechanical ventilation are difficult to define and the decision is made clinically. It is decided according to respiratory status.

Neurologic indications

- Altered level of consciousness (GCS <8) /airway protection.
- Brainstem dysfunction.
- Intracranial hypertension.
- Anticipated neurologic deterioration.

Respiratory indications

- Respiratory rate >35 or <5 breaths/ minute
- Exhaustion, with laboured pattern of breathing
- Hypoxia - central cyanosis, SaO_2 <90% on oxygen or PaO_2 < 8kPa
- Hypercarbia - $PaCO_2$ > 8kPa
- Tidal volume < 5ml/kg or Vital capacity <15ml/kg

Activity	Score
Eye Opening	
None	1= Even to supra-orbital pressure
To pain pressure	2=Pain from sternum/limb/supra-orbital
To speech	3=Non-specific response, not necessarily to command
Spontaneous	4=Eyes open, not necessarily aware
Motor Response	
None	1=To any pain; limbs remain flaccid
Extension	2=Shoulder adducted and shoulder and forearm internally rotated
Flexor response	3=Withdrawal response or assumption of hemiplegic posture
Withdrawal	4=Arm withdraws to pain, shoulder abducts
Localizes pain	5=Arm attempts to remove supra-orbital/chest pressure
Obeys commands	6=Follows simple commands
Verbal Response	
None	1=No verbalization of any type
Incomprehensible	2=Moans/groans, no speech
Inappropriate	3=Intelligible, no sustained sentences
Confused	4=Converses but confused, disoriented
Oriented	5=Converses and oriented

Table 1. Glasgow Coma Scale.

Intracranial physiology and mechanical ventilation

The goals of positive-pressure ventilation (PPV) in patients with multitrauma with head trauma are improving oxygenation and controlling arterial CO2 tension to minimise intracranial hypertension. PPV increases functional residual capacity (FRC) by improving alveolar recruitment, thus optimising oxygenation.

On the other hand, increased intrathoracic pressure (ITP) increases intracranial pressure (ICP) by these mechanisms:

- Direct transmission of ITP to the intracranial cavity via the neck.
- Increased ITP decreases venous return to the right atrium, and increases jugular venous pressure, thereby increasing cerebral blood volume (CBV) and ICP.
- Decreased venous return decreases cardiac output and mean arterial pressure (MAP). This results in decreased cerebral perfusion pressure (CPP) leading to compensatory cerebral vasodilation, increased CBF and potentially increased ICP, if cerebral autoregulation is impaired.

Mechanical ventilatory strategies[2]: conventional ventilation

Current practice guidelines for ventilatory management advocate protective lung strategies to prevent volutrauma, barotrauma, atelectrauma and biotrauma [3-5]. The principles are to use low tidal volumes (Vt) (5-6 ml/kg ideal body weight), maintenance of low mean airway pressures ≤ 30 cmH2O, judicious use of positive end-expiratory pressure (PEEP) with Δ pressure ≤ 18 cmH2O, higher respiratory rates and permissive hypercapnia. This is in direct conflict with the previous "brain-directed" ventilatory strategies that used Vt of 10 ml/kg, high FiO$_2$ and low PEEP or zero end-expiratory pressure. There is proven mortality benefit with the use of low Vt, but permissive hypercapnia may precipitate intracranial hypertension[3,6,7]. Animal studies indicate a higher incidence of severe pulmonary oedema and haemorrhage after exposure to injurious ventilation in the presence of brain trauma. High Vt independently predicts ALI/ARDS and poor outcome in brain trauma patients[8]. Haemodynamic fluctuations induced by mechanical ventilation may be detrimental in the brain with impaired autoregulation. That's why with starting mechanical ventilation, intravascular expansion and vasopressor may be necessary.

The role of PEEP

Lung protection strategy permising hypercapnia induces the development of cranial hyperemia and hypertension. On the other hand, "aggressive" ventilation with high tidal volume may aggravate lung injury and provoke ventilator-associated lung damage[9].

In mechanical ventilation treatment, PEEP improves oxygenation by recruitment of atelectatic alveolar units, improving FRC and preventing atelectrauma. Also it may have detrimental neurologic effects in certain clinical circumstances[10]. In a recent study in patients with traumatic brain injury shows that increasing PEEP up to 15 cm H2O to optimize oxygenation has not been associated with reduced cerebral perfusion pressure or acute intracranial hypertension [11]

In normal pulmonary compliance, PEEP is associated with increased ITP, decreased right atrial volume, decreased MAP and thus compromised CPP. This situation is not similar to non-compliant lungs, where there is a comparatively low ITP transmission to the cranium, therefore lesser effects on cerebral blood flow (CBF) and ICP. CPP may be indirectly affected by systemic effects of PEEP, but these effects still remain quantitatively modest. PEEP is therefore safe to apply as part of a ventilatory strategy to improve oxygenation.

Alveolar overdistension should be avoided and stable haemodynamic parameters should be maintained. Head position also needs attention. At least 30° head elevation promotes intracranial venous drainage via anterior neck veins, as well as the vertebral venous system - which is not majorly affected by ITP. Jugular veins collapse and act as resistors to some of the ITP transmitted. Tight endotracheal tube ties around the neck and extremes of neck rotation should be avoided

The Role of PaCO$_2$ control

Arterial CO$_2$ tension is a powerful modulator of cerebral vascular calibre, CBF and ICP [12-15.] While the mechanisms are incompletely understood, CO2 relaxes pial arterioles by interactions between the endothelium, vascular smooth muscle, pericytes, adjacent neurons and glial cells. Studies supported that cerebral vessels are sensitive to changes in extracellular pH, rather than a direct response to CO2 or bicarbonate. In the limits of physiological PaCO2, 20-60 mmHg, the relationship between PaCO2 and CBF is linear. Therefore, increased PaCO2 results in vasodilation of cerebral vessels and this leads to increase CBF, increase CBV, decrease intracranial compliance and increase ICP. The reverse mechanism is also true for low CO2 tension. This has been the reason for inducing hyperventilation in the patients with intracranial hypertension, but there is a risk for cerebral vasoconstriction precipitating cerebral ischaemia because pericontusional areas are sensitive to hyperventilation-induced ischaemia. The Brain Trauma Foundation management guidelines do not recommend hyperventilation for initial management of raised ICP, unless ICP is unresponsive to first-line therapy or hyperventilation is for very brief periods of time. Maintaining normocarbia is recomended.

Role of brain monitoring during ventilatory support in brain injury

It is essential to monitor intracranial pressure, CPP, and brain oxygenation during ventilatory support in the patients with traumatic brain injury. Brain oxygenation monitoring technics are jugular venous saturation monitoring, near-infrared spectroscopy and microdialysis catheters. Availability and cost of these devices are limiting factors to their use. The studies on brain trauma patients shows that there is no proven mortality benefit in continuous ICP monitoring.

Non-conventional ventilatory strategies

There are some ventilatory strategies that may be used for proper patients. These are prone position, recruitment manouvres, high frequency oscillatory ventilation (HFOV) and newer technics like extracorporeal CO2 removal (ECCO2R), pumpless extracorporeal lung assist (pECLA) and nitric oxide.

Prone ventilation[15- 18]

Benefits are:

• Recruitment of atelectatic lung units.
• Improved ventilation-perfusion matching.

- Improved drainage of secretions.
- Even distribution of mechanical ventilatory forces.

ICP and brain tissue oxygenation (PbtO2) monitoring are recomended. There are conflicting results on the effects of prone ventilation on ICP and CPP, but there are clear data on benefits for respiratory mechanics and oxygenation. Present studies shows that there is no mortality benefit to prone positioning.

Recruitment manoeuvres

In neurointensive patients with acute lung injury, achieving the goal of lung protection without threatening cerebral perfusion is very difficult. In patients with more refractory raised intracranial pressure, the optimal balance between brain and lung may not be well established. Multiple strategies are used to recruit atelectatic alveoli and improve oxygenation. Among them incremental levels of PEEP and high intermittent tidal volumes should require extend brain physiological monitoring.

High frequency oscillatory ventilation (HFOV) [18,19]

High frequency oscillatory ventilation (HFOV) forms high mean airway pressure with very small Vt of 1-5 ml/kg at a rapid rate. It's aim is to recruit alveoli, while preventing overdistension. Some studies have supported that HFOV is safe and effective in preventing ventilator-induced lung injury (VILI) and improving oxygenation in severe ARDS. There no sufficient studies supporting HFOV for the improvement of intracranial compliance.

Extracorporeal CO_2 removal (ECCO2R) [20]

Extracorporeal membrane oxygenators have been attempted in brain-injured patients to improve oxygenation. By using ECMO increased intracranial pressure may decrease in a normal limits and CPP is maintained. But anticoagulation requirement in that technic increases the risk of intracranial bleeding.

Pumpless extracorporeal lung assist (pECLA) [21]

pECLA has recently been utilised in small case series with promising results. Protective respiratory care can be maintained while CO2 removal is optimised. Patients treated by pECLA must be hemodynamically stable. So cardiovascular instability and shock are contraindications for pECLA. Anticoagulation is as for thrombo prophylaxis in immobilised patients. The risk of the device clotting is not entirely eliminated by impregnation with anticoagulant in the filter. Vascular injury, exsanguination and limb ischaemia are some of the recognised complications.

Nitric oxide

Nitric oxide improves oxygenation in ALI/ARDS with no survival benefit. There is potential to cause harm. There is no data for its use in ARDS with the patients with brain taruma.

Weaning [22-30]

Without resolving underlying pathological condition, weaning must not be thought. With prolongation ventilatory support, the respiratory muscles become weaken and atrophy of this muscles is inevitable. As a consequence, the duration of weaning period is often related to the duration and mode of ventilation. As possible as using assisted modes of ventilation and good nutritional support are essential to prevent atrophy of the respiratory muscles.

Critical illness polyneuropathy is seen in patients recovering from prolonged critical illness. In this condition, there is both respiratory and peripheral muscle weakness, with reduced tendon reflexes and sensory abnormalities. There is evidence that long-term administration of some aminosteroid muscle relaxants (such as vecuronium) may cause persisting paralysis. No absolute treatment is used for it except supportive therapy.

The plan for disengagement of the patient from mechanical ventilation should be made at initiation of ventilation therapy. The recognition of when mechanical ventilatory support should be reduced and ultimately discontinued is so important. Appropriate time for disengagement from ventilation has the following advantages:

- Decreased airway injury
- Decreased risk of VILI.
- Decreased risk of VAP.
- Decreased sedation requirements.
- Decreased delirium.
- Shortened ICU length of stay.
- Assessment for extubation criteria:
- Respiratory criteria.
- Haemodynamic criteria.
- Neurologic criteria. This includes stable neurological status, ICP ≤ 20 mmHg, CPP ≥ 60 mmHg.

Premature weaning and extubation may cause respiratory muscle fatigue, gas exchange failure and loss of airway protection.

There is clear benefit to weaning according to protocol. There should be frequent assessment of ventilatory support requirement and re-evaluation of factors contributing to ventilator dependence before ventilation is discontinued.

Indications for weaning

- Improving of underlying illness
- Respiratory function:
  Respiratory rate < 35 breaths/minute
  FiO_2 < 0.5, SaO_2 > 90%, PEEP <10 cmH$_2$O
  Tidal volume > 5ml/kg
  Vital capacity > 10 ml/kg
  Minute volume < 10 l/min
- Absence of infection or fever
- Cardiovascular stability, optimal fluid balance and electrolyte replacement

Prior to trial of weaning, there should be no residual neuromuscular blockade and sedation should be stoped or decreased in appropirate level so that the patient must be awake, cooperative and in a semirecumbent position. Weaning is likely to fail if the patient is confused, agitated or unable to cough.

Modes of weaning

There are several different approaches for the weaning that are not superior to others.

- Unsupported spontaneous breathing trials. The machine support is withdrawn and a T-Piece (or CPAP) circuit can be attached intermittently for increasing periods of time, thereby allowing the patient to gradually take over the work of breathing with shortening rest periods back on the ventilator.
- Intermittent mandatory ventilation (IMV) weaning. The ventilator delivers a preset minimum minute volume which is gradually decreased as the patient takes over more of the respiratory workload. The decreasing ventilator breaths are synchronised to the patient's own inspiratory efforts (SIMV).
- Pressure support weaning. In this mode, the patient initiates all breaths and these are 'boosted' by the ventilator. This weaning method involves gradually reducing the level of pressure support, thus making the patient responsible for an increasing amount of ventilation. Once the level of pressure support is low (5-10 cmH$_2$O above PEEP), a trial of T-Piece or CPAP weaning should be commenced.

Failure to wean

During the weaning process, the patient should be observed for early indications of fatigue or failure to wean. These signs include distress, increasing respiratory rate, falling tidal volume and haemodynamic compromise, particularly tachycardia and hypertension. At this point it may be necessary to increase the level of respiratory support as, once exhausted, respiratory muscles may take many hours to recover.

It is sensible to start the weaning process in the morning to allow close monitoring of the patient throughout the day. In prolonged weaning, it is common practice to increase ventilatory support overnight to allow adequate rest for the patient.

Tracheostomy in the intensive care unit [31-33]

The commonest indication of tracheostomy in an ICU setting is to facilitate prolonged artificial ventilation and the subsequent weaning process. Tracheostomy allows a reduction in sedation and thus increased cooperation to the weaning process. It also allows effective tracheobronchial suction in patients who are unable to clear pulmonary secretions either due to excessive secretion production or due to weakness following critical illness. Tracheostomy can be performed as a formal surgical procedure in theatre or at the bedside in the intensive care unit using a percutaneous method. Tracheostomy placement leads to earlier liberation from mechanical ventilation, but without any mortality benefit or effect on pulmonary infection rates.

Other indications for tracheostomy are to bypass an upper airway obstruction, protect the lungs from soiling if the laryngopharygeal reflexes are depressed or as part of a surgical or anaesthetic technique eg larygectomy.

Advantages of tracheostomy is summerized as decreased risk of self-extubation; decreased sinusitis; decreased airway resistance, dead space and breathing work ;better tolerance; less sedative requirements; potentially-reduced duration of mechanical ventilation.

Risks of tracheostomy is summerized as surgical site infection, airway haemorrhage, pneumothorax, oesophageal perforation.

Sedation in the Neuro-ICU[34-67]

Sedation is the important factor in comfort of brain trauma patients. Insuffient sedation causes hypertension, tachycardia, hypoxia, hypercapnia and uncomfortable with ventilator. On the other hand excess sedation causes hypotansion, bradycardia, coma, respiratory depresion, ileus, renal insufficiency, veinous stasis and immunosupression.

For the patients in the critical care unit firstly nonpharmacological method should be experinced for sedation. The patients should be frequently oriented. Sleep-awake cycling, proper enveriomental temperature, control of the noise aroused from alarms must be arranged.

Calling the family members, the relexing exercises, musical therapy, masaj and sitting exercises are important in control of anxiety and ajitation of patients.

Safe and effective management of the pain and anxiety needs a delicate balance for analgesia and sedation protocols while managing delirium status.

The weaning of patients from mechanical ventilation is often hampered by the sedation that they receive. Additionally, coordinated daily interruption of sedative infusions with objective re-titration in critically ill patients has been shown to decrease the durations of mechanical ventilation and length of ICU stay.

Consequences of agitation include self-extubation, removal of IV catheters, dyssynchrony with mechanical ventilation, and, perhaps, a long-term risk of psychiatric problems, such as delirium and posttraumatic stress disorder can be prevented by a proper sedation. Prolonged and excessive sedation are problematic too, interfering with weaning from mechanical ventilation and leading to increased rates of nosocomial pneumonia, prolonged ICU stays, and difficulty identifying new problems, such as myocardial infarction or stroke.

Sedation Indications in the Neuro-ICU

- Patient comfort
- Decreases anxiety and agitation
- Relieve fear
- Risk of self-injury or injury of others
- Withdrawal from alcohol or drugs
- Risk of self-extubation or removal of invasive monitors
- Suppreses stres response
- Increases the tolerance of ventilatory support
- Facilitates the cares like aspiration, invasive prosedures and dressing the wound
- Control of pain
- Facilitate mechanical ventilation
- Reduce oxygen extraction/ utilization in ARDS and Sepsis
- Brain protection (seizure control, decrease cerebral metabolism , control ICP)
- Blunting adverse outcome
- Provide hemodynamic stability; protection against myocardial ischemia

- Amnesia during paralysis with muscle relaxants
- During interventions (line insertion, tracheostomy)
- To prevent movement (during imaging and transfering of the patient)
- Facilitate sleep
- Facilitate nursing management

Properties of an ideal agent for neurointensive care sedation:

- Rapid onset and rapid recovery so that a neurologic evaluation can be conducted
- Predictable clearance independent of end-organ function, avoiding the problem of drug accumulation
- Easily titrated to achieve adequate levels of sedation
- Reduces intracranial pressure by cerebral blood volume reduction or cerebral vasoconstriction
- Reduces cerebral blood flow and cerebral metabolic rate of oxygen consumption, maintaining their coupling
- Maintains cerebral autoregulation
- Permits normal cerebral vascular reactivity to changes in arterial carbon dioxide tension
- Minimal cardiovascular depressant effects
- Easy control respiratory side-effects
- Inexpensive
- Adapted with permission.
- Both sedative and analgesic
- Lack of respiratory depression
- No tolerance over time
- Inactive or non harmful metabolites
- No interactions with other ICU drug
- Rapid onset and rapid recovery so that a neurologic evaluation can be conducted

General expectational situations:

- Equipment and personnel to intubate and mechanically ventilate must be readily available
- Decreased level-of-consciousness or obtundation
- Poor airway protection
- Respiratory depression, hypercarbia, and increased intracranial pressure (ICP)
- Impairment of neurological exam
- Hemodynamic instability

Sedation should be performed according to protocols standarized with scales. For this reason Ramsay Sedation Scale (RSS), Riker Sedation-Agitation Scale (SAS) and Richmond Agitation-Sedation Score (RASS) are used for planing treatment. For many years, the Ramsay Sedation Scale was the most commonly used tool to monitor sedation in the ICU. However, it cannot distinguish different levels of agitation, making it less useful than other available scales. Currently, two of the most commonly used techniques are the Riker Sedation-Agitation Scale (SAS) and the Richmond Agitation-Sedation Score (RASS).

Score Term Descriptor
1. Unarousable – Minimal or no response to noxious stimuli, does not communicate or follow commands
2. Very Sedated – Arouses to physical stimuli but does not communicate or follow commands, may move spontaneously
3. Sedated – Difficult to arouse, awakens to verbal stimuli or gently shaking, but drifts off again, follow simple commands
4. Calm and Cooperative – Calm, awakens easily, follows commands
5. Agitated – Anxious or mildly agitated, attempting to sit up, calms down to verbal stimuli
6. Very Agitated – Does not calm despite frequent verbal reminding of limits, biting ET
7. Dangerous Agitation – Pulling ET, trying to remove catheters, climbing over bedrails, striking at staff, thrashing side to side
Guidelines for SAS Assessment
1. Agitated patients are scored by their most severe degree of agitation, as described.
2. If patient is awake or awakens easily to voice ("awaken" means responds with voice or head shaking to a question or follows commands), that is a SAS 4 (same as calm and appropriate might even be napping).
3. If more stimuli such as shaking is required but patient eventually does awaken, that is a SAS 3.
4. If patient arouses to stronger physical stimuli (may be noxious) but never awakens to the point of responding yes/no or following commands, that is a SAS 2.
5. Little or no response to noxious physical stimuli is a SAS
6. This helps separate sedated patients into those you can eventually awaken (SAS 3), those you can not awaken, but can arouse (SAS 2), and those you can not arouse (SAS 1).

Table 2. Riker Sedation-Agitation Scale (SAS) (SAS Target Sedation = 3 to 4).

Score Description
+4Combative Overtly combative, violent, immediate danger to staff
+3 Very Agitated Pulls or removes tube(s) or catheter(s),aggressive
+2 Agitated Frequent non-purposeful movement, fights ventilator
+1 Restless Anxious but movements not aggressive vigorous
0 Alert and Calm
-1 Drowsy Not fully alert, but has sustained awakening (>10 seconds) (eye-opening/eye contact) to voice
-2 Light Sedation Briefly awakens with eye contact to voice (<10 seconds)
-3 Moderate Sedation Movement or eye opening to voice (but no eye contact)
-4 Deep Sedation No response to voice, but movement or eye opening to physical stimulation
-5 Unarousable No response to voice or physical stimulation

Procedure for RASS Assessment: The basis of the RASS assessment is to see what amount of stimulation is necessary to evoke a respons and evaluate sedation.
•   Observe patient.
a.   Patient is alert, restless, or agitated. (Score 0 to +4)
•   If not alert, state patient's name and say "open eyes and look (speaker)."
b.   Patient awakens with sustained eye opening and eye contact (Score –1)
c.   Patient awakens with eye opening and eye contact, but not sustained (Score –2)
d.   Patient has any movement in response to voice but no eye contact (Score –3)
•   When no response to verbal stimulation, physically stimulatepatient by shaking shoulder and/or rubbing sternum.
e.   Patient has any movement to physical stimulation (Score –4)
f.   Patient has no response to any stimulation (Score –5).

Table 3. Richmond Agitation Sedation Scale (RASS) (RASS Target Sedation = 0 to -3).

Even if the sedative strategy in the NICU shares the same general aims as general intensive care, the characteristics of the patients in the NICU present other unique challenges and specific indications, including intracranial pressure control, cerebral oxygen consumption and seizure reduction . Analgesic and sedative agents are used both to prevent undesirable increases in intracranial pressure and to reduce cerebral metabolic requirements. Intracranial pressure control cerebral autoregulation may be impaired in the traumatic brain injury. Therefore, agitation and associated blood pressure elevations directly determine intracranial pressure surges. Moreover, severe agitation increases intrathoracic pressure, reducing jugular venous outflow and increases cerebral metabolism with concomitantly increased cerebral blood flow (CBF). These potentially deleterious phenomena can lead to increase in intracranial pressure. This can trigger an additional cerebral vasodilator cascade, as cerebral perfusion pressure (CPP) is reduced.

Sedatives decrease the cerebral metabolic rate of oxygen consumption (CMRO2), and because the coupling of CBF and CMRO2 is usually maintained with these agents, CBF is reduced by increasing cerebral vascular resistance. The reduction in CBF results in a reduction of cerebral blood volume and, consequently, a decrease in intracranial pressure. In order to maintain adequate oxygen availability and energy production at the cellular level, treatment is directed to increase oxygen delivery by optimizing systemic hemodynamics and reduce cerebral metabolic demand. Sedative drugs confer a protective effect by reducing oxygen demand and increasing oxygen delivery (through improvement of central perfusion pressure and by inhibiting deleterious pathologic intracellular processes). The pharmacologic reduction in CMRO2 depresses either the basal or the activation components of cerebral metabolism. The metabolic suppression is dose dependent until the electroencephalogram becomes isoelectric. Beyond this level, no further suppression of cerebral oxygen consumption or blood flow occurs because energy expenditure, associated with electrophysiologic activity, has been reduced to close to zero, and the minimal consumption for cellular homeostasis persists unchanged.

There is no appropriate ratio for seizure activity in patients with brain trauma, seizures are a frequent complication in the NICU. Sedation appears to be an attractive option in reducing seizures in the NICU. Benzodiazepines increase the seizure threshold and are useful anticonvulsants. There are conflicting data on propofol, and, consequently, its ability to protect against seizures is less certain. Pharmacologic properties rapid onset and rapid recovery of hypnosis are the most important pharmacokinetic properties to consider when comparing different hypnotic alternatives.

The drug used for sedation in intensive care summarized in table below.

	Lorezepam	Midazolam	Fentanyl	Remifentanil	Propofol	Dexmedetomidine
IV bolus dose	0.02–0.06 mg/kg	0.02–0.08 mg/kg	25–125 µg	NR	NR	0.5–1mcg/kg
Continuous IV infusion	0.01–0.10 mg/kg/h	0.04–0.30 mg/kg/h	10–100 µg/h	0.05–.25µg/kg/min	5-200 mg/kg/min	0.2–0.7 µg/kg/h
Elimination half-time, h	10–20 0.	2.0–2.5	7	0.3	7.2	2
Clearance,ml/min/kg	75–1.00	4–8	13	44	24	8.2
Metabolic pathway	Glucuronidation	CYP3A4	CYP3A4	Plasma esterases	Hepatic	Glucuronidation and CYP2D6
Active metabolites	None	Yes	None	None	None	None
Cost	Inexpensive	Moderate	Inexpensive	Expensive	Expensive	Expensive

NR: Not recommended

Table 4. Pharmacokinetic parameters, dosing, and cost of sedative and analgesic agents.

For patients that are mechanically ventilated for three days or less, short acting agents should be used such as Propofol or Midazolam. For longer periods of mechanical ventilation, longer acting agents such as Lorazepam should be used. Patients that have been ventilated for long periods using the long acting agent Lorazepam may need to be switched to a shorter acting agent such as Propofol for optimal weaning purposes.

	Propofol	Midazolam	Lorazepam	Fentanyl	Remifentanyl
Rapid onset	+++	+++	+	+++	+++
Fast recovery	+++	++	+	++	+++
Easily titrated	+++	++	+	++	+++
ICP reduction	↓↓	↓	↓	↔/↓	↔/↓
CBF reduction	↓↓	↓↓	↓	↔	↔
CMRO2 reduction	↓↓	↓	↓	↓	↓
MAP	↓↓	↓	↓	↓	↓↓

↑, modest increase; ↑↑, pronounced increase; ↔, no clear effect; ↓, modest decrease; ↓↓, pronounced decrease; +++, very favorable; ++, favorable; +, not favorable; CBF, cerebral blood flow; CMRO2, cerebral metabolic rate of oxygen consumption; ICP, intracranial pressure; MAP, mean arterial pressure.

Table 5. Cerebral and systemic characteristics of the available molecules.

Barbiturate, benzodiazepins, propofol and narcotics are all used as a sedative agent.

Propofol is very lipid soluble, has a large volume of distribution, and can be given for prolonged periods of time without significant changes in its pharmacokinetic profile. Because propofol has no active metabolites, the termination of its clinical effect is dependent solely on redistribution to peripheral fat tissue stores. When the infusion is discontinued, the fat tissue stores redistribute. Because of its pharmacokinetics and specific effects on cerebral hemodynamic variables, preserving autoregulation and vasoreactivity to carbon dioxide, propofol approximates the ideal sedative. Intravenous bolus administration produces a dose-dependent, coupled decrease in CBF and CMRO2 similar to that described after barbiturate administration. The effects on CBF are probably secondary to a reduction in CMRO2. A strong linear correlation between CBF and CMRO2 has been demonstrated. The major cardiovascular effect of propofol is a profound decrease in mean arterial pressure, resulting from a decrease in systemic vascular resistance, cardiac contractility, and preload. A bolus dose of 2 to 2.5 mg/kg propofol results in a 25 to 40% reduction in systolic blood pressure. This potent effect on mean arterial pressure may affect CPP by one of two mechanisms. If autoregulation is intact, a reduction in mean arterial pressure will produce reflex cerebral vasodilatation and a possible increase in intracranial pressure. Alternatively, if autoregulation is impaied hypotension may produce a critical decrease in CPP and CBF. The risk of hypotension is greatest in the presence of hypovolemia.

Evaluations of the effects of benzodiazepines on cerebral physiology have involved primarily diazepam and midazolam. Both cause dose-dependent decreases in CMRO2 and CBF, and by increasing cerebral vascular resistance, decreases in intracranial pressure have been observed. Usually CPP is not compromised. Moreover, a "ceiling effect" in CBF and CMRO2 reduction has been described, suggesting a saturation of the benzodiazepine receptors. It appears that benzodiazepines are safe to administer to patients with intracranial hypertension without respiratory depression and associated increases in arterial carbon dioxide tension.

The cerebral physiologic effects of opioids are controversial. Morphine-related increases in CBF, as described in early reports, were probably secondary to an increaseing arterial carbon dioxide tension resulting from respiratory depression. In general, opioids slightly reduce CMRO2, CBF, and intracranial pressure, as long as normocapnia is maintained by mechanical ventilation. Opioids can produce short-lasting, mild decreases in mean arterial pressure and then, subsequently, can produce decreases in CPP. Furthermore, remifentanyl may cause decreases in both cerebral metabolic rate and intracranial pressure, with minimal changes in CPP and cerebral blood flow. Opioids lead to dose-dependent, centrally mediated respiratory depression. The carbon dioxide response curve is shifted to the right, and the ventilatory response to hypoxia is obliterated. For this reason, in spontaneously ventilating NICU patients, if opioids are administered, strict end-tidal carbon dioxide monitoring or frequent blood gas analysis must be implemented to identify rapid onset of respiratory depression. When opioids and benzodiazepines are administered concomitantly, they may exhibit a synergistic effect on hemodynamics. The reasons for this synergy are not entirely clear.

Hypnotics can decrease mean arterial blood pressure by both cardiac depression and peripheral vasodilatation. The decrease in blood pressure can cause an increase in intracranial pressure as a result of autoregulatory compensation (vasodilatory cascade) and consequently, can cause a reduction in CPP. The hemodynamic effects are usually dose dependent. Therefore, to avoid, or at least to limit, decreases in blood pressure, the patient should be euvolemic before the infusion is started, and slow boluses or continuous infusions are preferred.

Because no single drug can achieve all of the requirements for sedation and analgesia in the ICU, use of a combination of drugs, each titrated to specific end points, is a more effective strategy. This allows lower doses of individual drugs and reduces the problems of drug accumulation. In the acute phase (ie, first 48–72 hours or when intracranial hypertension is not controlled), a continuous infusion of a combination of propofol (1.5–6 mg/kg/h) and fentanyl (0.5–1.5 μg/kg/h) should be initiated.

In the subacute phase (ie, after 72 hours or when intracranial pressure is normalized), intermittent infusion of lorazepam (0.05 mg/kg every 2–6 h) should be initiated.

It is essential to contiue sedation until ventilatory support is required, and then sedation is stoped step by step to prevent withdrawal symptoms in 24 to 48 hours. No neuromuscular blocking drugs are routinely added, except in cases of severe, uncontrollable intracranial hypertension.

Neuromuscular blockers in the Neuro-ICU [68-71]

The routine use of neuromuscular blockers varies between centres. The routine use of muscle relaxants should be avoided, they can be useful to prevent peaks in ICP induced by the patient coughing or "straining" or in the face of patient-ventilator dysynchrony. However, muscle paralysis makes it clinically impossible to recognise and treat seizures. Prolonged administration of neuromuscular blockers by continuous infusion can also lead to significant long-term problems, such as critical illness polyneuropathy and myopathy.

Neuromuscular blockers indications

- Facilitation of intubation
- Facilitate mechanical ventilation
- To eliminate spontaneous breathing and promote mechanical ventilation
- During interventions (line insertion, tracheostomy)
- To prevent movement (during imaging and to permit transfer of the patient)
- Severe refractory intracranial hypertension
- Severe pulmonary disease with inability to mechanically ventilated
- Cause a pharmacologic restraint so patients do not harm themselves

General Precautions

- Patient must be intubated for mechanically ventilated
- Transient increase in ICP with depolarizing blockade (succinylcholine)
- Unexpected prolongation of neuromuscular blockade (e.g.,enzyme deficiencies, hepatic or renal dysfunction)
- Complete loss of neurological examination

Agent Onset of action Duration of action ED$_{90-95}$* (mg/kg)

Agent	Onset of action	Duration of action	ED$_{90-95}$* (mg/kg)
Short Acting			
Mivacurium (Mivacron)	2.5 min	15 - 20 min	0.07
Rapacuronium (Raplon)	Mean: 90 seconds (35 - 219 sec)	Mean: 15 min (6 - 30 min)	1.03
Rocuronium (Zemeron)	1 - 3 min	31 min (15 - 85 min)	0.3
Succinylcholine	30 - 60 seconds	5 - 8 min	0.3
Intermediate acting			
Atracurium (Tracrium)	2.5 - 5 min	20 - 45 min	0.2
Cisatracurium (Nimbex)	2 - 3 min	30 - 40 min	0.05
Pancuronium (Pavulon)	2 - 3 min	60 - 90 min	0.06
Vecuronium (Norcuron)	2 - 3 min	25 - 40 min	0.05
Long Acting			
Doxacurium (Nuromax)	6 min (2.5 - 13)	100 min (39 - 232)	0.025
Pipecuronium (Arduan)	2.5 - 5 min	75 min (35 - 175)	0.07
Tubocurarine	3 - 5 min	70 - 90 min	0.05

ED90-95 = Dose required to produce 90-95% suppression of muscle response

Table 6. Neuromuscular Blocking Agents.

Atracurium: initially 0.4 -0.5 mg/kg IV bolus, Maintenance infusion rates of 5 to 9 mcg/kg/min are usually adequate (Range:2 to 15mcg/kg/min). Toxic metabolite (laudanosine) may accumulate in renal failure

Doxacurium: initially, 0.05 mg/kg -0.08 mg/kg IV bolus, Maintenance, 0.005 mg/kg and 0.01 mg/kg IV to provide neuromuscular blockage for an average of 30 min and 45 min, respectively.

Rocuronium: initially, 0.6-1.2 mg/kg IV bolus. Maintenance, 0.1-0.2 mg/kg IV repeated as needed. Maintenance (continuous IV infusion): 0.01-0.012 mg/kg/minute.

Pancuronium: initially 0.1 to 0.2 mg/kg (usually 0.1) bolus, followed by 1 to 1.7 mcg/kg/min or 0.06 to 0.1 mg/kg/hr

Vecuronium: Initially 0.08 to 0.1 mg/kg IV bolus. (Higher initial doses-up to 0.3 mg/kg-may be used for rapid onset. Continuous infusion: 1 mcg/kg/min infusion, usual range: 0.8 to 1.2 mcg/kg/min).

Succinylcholine: Initially 0.3-1.1 mg/kg, bolus Infusion is 2.5-4.3 mg/min (cause refractory intracranial hypertension Succinylcholine should be avoided due to increased ICP)

Nutrition

Nutrition could also have an impact on the posttraumatic stress response, which is associated with adverse outcomes from TBI. The posttraumatic stress response is charaterized by increased blood levels of glucose, lactate, catecholamines, and cortisol. Nutrition support should be initiated as soon as possible following the head injury. Adequate nutrition is to provide the body healing. Early enteral nutrition (EN) support has been shown to attenuate the catabolic response and improve immune function and is associated with improved neurologic outcome[73,74] .If the digestive tract is functional, enteral nutrition, or nutrition given via a tube placed into the stomach, is the preferred route. Parenteral nutrition (PN) should be reserved for those patients with impaired gastrointestinal function or those who cannot meet their nutritional needs via EN alone.

The goal of nutritional support in patients who are critically ill is to provide protein and caloric replacement while attenuating a negative nitrogen balance. Incidence of malnutrition in hospitalized patients ranges between 30% to 55%. Delaying in the initiation of nutritional support may result in muscle and gastrointestinal atrophy, inability of weaning from ventilatory support, heart failure, impaired immunity, increase in the incidence of sepsis, length of hospital stay, morbidity and mortality and all of these resulte increase in costs [72].

At the begining, all patients admitted to the critical care unit should be screened for risk or presence of malnutrition. Critically ill patients with neurologic impairment often require specialized nutrition support because of needing intubation, dysphagia, or altered mental status.

The provision of adequate nutritional support is an essential component of caring the critically ill patient. During starvation, homeostatic mechanisms are designed to burn fat rather than protein as an energy source until the fat stores are significantly depleted. Especially in the begining of the infection, a catabolic state causing significant protein loss progresses. Plasma and urine levels of catecholamines and cortisol are elevated. Hyperglycaemia is frequently seen and causes ketone production and lactic acid production leading acidosis in brain cells. The studies show that the severity and duration of hyperglycaemia following head injury correlate with longer term outcome.

Enteral nutrition should be preferred in the critically ill patients[75,76]. This can be achieved by either nasal tube feeding or via a percutaneous gastrostomy (PEG) if prolonged feeding is envisaged. Standard enteral feeding regiments aim to provide 1500-2500 kcal in 24 hours with 70 g protein in a volume of 1.5-2 L.

A patient may require more calories for healing for the TBI. Patients with a GCS of 8 to 12 will require approximately 30 to 35 calories per kilogram of body weight per day. Patients with a GCS of 6 to 7 require 40 to 50 calories per kilogram of body weight per day.

The main goal of nutrition should be preserve muscle mass, and provide adequate fluids and strict electrolyte and glucose monitoring should be recommended.

It is prudent to consider postpyloric feeding in patient with neurological catastrophies, because gastric atony increases the risk of aspiration. Enteral feeding should be preferably done by continuous infusion with a volumetric pump.

In the average patient in the intensive care unit who has no contraindications to EN or PN, the choice of route for nutritional support may be influenced by several factors. Because EN and PN are associated with risks and benefits[77,78]

Advantages associated with enteral rather than parenteral nutrition include:

- Maintenance of mucosal integrity and prevention of villous atrophy
- Reduced infection rate
- Absence of requirement for central venous line
- Better maintenance of fluid balance
- Reduced cost

Contraindications to enteral feeding are few, particularly in the patient with isolated intracranial pathology, but include abdominal sepsis, obstruction, acut malabsorption and inflammatory syndromes and enteric fistulae. Only a short segment of small intestine (30 cm) is required for adequate absorption since hypertrophy will occur in response to lumenal nutrients. Neither bowel sounds nor flatus are required for successful enteral feeding. Enteral feeding should be started if gastric aspirates are less than 400 ml/day and there are no obvious contraindications. Commence with standard enteral feed at 25 ml/h, increasing the rate every 12 hours until 100 ml/h is achieved. Aspirate residual volume and rest for 1 hour in every 6 hours of feeding, and rest continuously for 8 hours overnight.

Complications of enteral feeding [79].:

- Large residual gastric volumes.
- Regurgitation and aspiration.
- Diarrhoea.
- Ulceration of nares.
- Contamination of feed (rare).

Gastric atony and delayed emptying may be seen during enteral feeding. For treating this unwanted result pro-kinetic agents can be used. Also nasojejunal tube bypassing pylorus should be inserted. The passage of nasal feeding tubes should be avoided in patients with facial injuries and basal skull fracture. Instate oragastric replacement should be used. Diarrhoea also may be seen during enteral feeding and may resolve with using a different formula of feed. But persistent diarrhoea should be thought infection with Clostridium difficile , particularly in patients receiving multiple antibiotics. A specimen should always be sent for microbiological culture.

Total parenteral nutrision (TPN) is prefered especialy enteral nutrision is imposible[80]. Protein calorie requirements are more easily met by parenteral nutrition comparing enteral nutrition. Excessive calorie intake, particularly consisting excessive carbohydrate increases oxygen consumption, carbon dioxide production, the respiratory quotient (RQ) and lipogenesis.

The calorie:nitrogen ratio for TPN should be 150:1 and it must be contain lipid, carbonhyrates, amino acids, electrolytes, trace elements and vitamins as much as needed.

Lipids are essential for cell wall integrity, prostaglandin synthesis and the action of fat-soluble vitamins, but should provide no more than 33% of the energy requirements. Intralipid, mixture of refined olive oil (approximately 80%) and refined soya oil (approximately 20%) (which may rarely cause severe hypersensitivity reactions), is an isotonic emulsion of soyabean oil with egg phosphatides and lecithin. The particle size of the emulsion is similar to a chylomicron, and the lipidis handled in a similar manner. The energy yield from fat is 9 cal/g, but the presence of the egg phosphatides increase the caloric value of intralipid to 11 cal/g. The lipid load should be decreased in the presence of sedation with propofol, severe jaundice ,severe hypoxamia, thrombocytopaenia and hypothermia .

Carbohydrate should be consist of two-thirds of the energy requirement and is in the form of glucose having 4cal/g energy. An insulin sliding scale will frequently be required to tightly control plasma glucose levels.

Protein is usually omitted from caloric calculations. A wide range of amino acids are supplied as the L-isomer in commercial preparations. Protein requirements increase in sepsis and burns and are 12–17 g nitrogen/day (1 g nitrogen=6.25 g protein).

Daily electrolyte requirements of sodium, potassium, calcium, phosphate, magnesium and chloride should be met by TPN. Trace elements essential for homeostasis include zinc, copper, manganese, iron, cobalt, chromium, selenium, molybdenum and iodine. Commercially prepared vitamin supplements contain most water-soluble and fat-soluble vitamins (A, D and E) with the exception of folic acid, vitamin B12 and vitamin K (fat-soluble).

Schedule	Enteral	Parenteral
Baseline	Electrolytes, BUN, Cr, Ca, Mg, PO4, glucose, albumin	Electrolytes, BUN, Cr, Ca, Mg, PO4, glucose, liver function tests, triglycerides, cholesterol, albumin
Daily	Intake and output, weight	Intake and output, weight
Daily until stable; then 2 to 3 times/week	Electrolytes, BUN, Cr, glucose	Electrolytes, BUN, Cr, glucose
Every other day until stable; then 1 to 2 times/week	Ca, Mg, PO4	Ca, Mg, PO4
Every 10-14 days	Albumin	Liver function tests, albumin, triglycerides
Weekly	PT, prealbumin	PT, prealbumin
BUN, blood urea nitrogen; PT, prothrombin time; Cr, creatinine; PO4, phosphate		

Table 7. Recommended monitoring guidelines for enteral and parental nutrition.

Increasingly, hospital pharmacies are supplying pre-mixed 'big bag' TPN containing the complete 24-hour nutritional requirements.

While receiving enteral or parenteral nutrition, the patient must be monitored for changes in body composition, blood chemistry, blood glucose, triglycerides, and protein synthesis. Electrolytes (Na, K, Cl, Mg, Phosphate, and Ca) and markers of renal function (blood urea nitrogen and creatinine) should be monitored routinely. Daily weight and the total volume of the patient's intake and output need to be monitored in addition to assessing other markers of hydration and volume status.

Management and treatment of intracranial hypertension

The principle focus of critical care management for traumatic brain is to limit secondary brain injury (SBI). On admission to the NICU, all patients after trauma are at risk of increasing ICP, and standard systemic monitoring; pulse oximetry, invasive arterial blood pressure with regular analyses of arterial blood gases and blood glucose and central venous access with central venous pressure monitoring must be established. End-tidal carbon dioxide monitoring is invaluable in this group of patients because it enables early correction of hypercapnia-induced rises.

For the treatment and prevention of SBI, using a neuroprotective strategy to maintain cerebral perfusion and maintaining intracranial pressure within normal limits are important. Beside this optimizing oxygenation and blood pressure are needed and temperature, glucose, seizures, and other potential secondary brain insults management are essential.

If GCS of the patients equal and below the 8, there are clinical symptoms like unilateral or bilaterally fixed and dilated pupils suggesting possible impending herniation from elevated ICP and/or decorticate or decerebrate posturing, bradycardia, hypertension, and respiratory depression progress, the treatment of head elevation, hyperventilation, and osmotic therapy (mannitol 1 g/kg iv) is planed urgently. With the treatment neuroimaging and other assessments are organized. The evaluation and management of increased ICP are discussed in detail below.

In traumatic brain injury, ICP and low CPP cause mass effect in the brain and is associated with more severe symptoms and more abrupt onset and poor outcome. The increased ICP is caused by increases in tissue volume, cerebral blood volume, or cerebrospinal fluid (CSF) volume. The pathophysiology and management of increased ICP is based on the Monro-Kellie doctrine.

Cerebral blood flow is maintained through adequate CPP, which is determined by the mean systemic arterial pressure minus intracranial pressure (CPP = MAP – ICP). Normal CPP values 80 mm Hg for adults, CPP > 50–60 mm Hg for children and CPP > 40–50 mm Hg for infants/toddlers.

If the CPP reduces below the value of 70 mmHg, it assosiated with high mortality and poor outcome[81-83] Especially the value reduces to less than 50 mmHg, metabolic evidence of ischaemia, reduced electrical activity and, ultimately, brain death are expected.

Normal values of ICP are within the range of 10 to 15 mm Hg for adults and older children, 3 to 7 mm Hg for young children, and 1.5 to 6 mm Hg for term infants[84]. Intracranial hypertension (ICH) is defined when the ICP values ebow 20 mm Hg. The values greater than 20 to 25 mm Hg require treatment in most circumstances. Sustained values of greater than 40 mm Hg indicate severe, life-threatening intracranial hypertension[76]. During intracranial hypertension, systemic hypotension or relative hypotension (insufficient to maintain adequate CPP due to increased ICP) lead to poor cerebral perfusion and ischemic insults and worse outcomes[81,85] and treatment is recommended [81,85,86] .

Sustained intracranial hypertension has a negative effect on cerebral blood flow and cerebral perfusion pressure and can cause direct compression of vital cerebral structures and lead to herniation. Appropriate management of intracranial hypertension begins with stabilization of the patient and simultaneous assessment of the level of sensorium and the cause of it.

Stabilization is initiated with securing the airway, ventilation and circulation[87]. The management of the patient involves the maintenance of an adequate CPP, prevention of intracranial hypertension and optimization of oxygen delivery. In patients with severe coma, signs of herniation or acutely elevated intracranial pressure, treatment should be started prior to plan imaging technics or invasive monitoring.

Indications for ICP monitoring, varing from unit to unit, may include traumatic brain injury, anoxic-ischaemic brain injury, intracerebral and subarachnoid haemorrhage, hydrocephalus, brain oedema after large strokes, hypoxic brain injury, central nervous system infections or fulminant hepatic failure[83,85].

The primary goals of ICP monitoring are identification of intracranial pressure trends and evaluation of therapeutic interventions. Intracranial hypertension compromises the relationship between systemic blood pressure and the resistance that must be overcome to accomplish cerebral perfusion. When cerebral perfusion pressure (CPP) falls below 50 mm Hg, secondary brain ischemia, herniation, and, ultimately, brain death occur. ICP monitoring allows for early detection of intracranial hypertension and subsequent aggressive management.

ICP monitoring helps the earlier detection of intracranial mass lesions and can limit the indiscriminate use of therapies to control ICP which themselves can be potentially harmful. It can also reduce ICP by CSF drainage and thus improve cerebral perfusion and helps in determining prognosis.

Currently, accurate monitoring requires invasive devices. Parenchymal pressure monitors (eg, Camino or Codman) measure ICP via a fiber-optic monitor placed in the subarachnoid space. Intraventricular catheters placed via ventriculostomy allow for both measurements of ICP and drainage of CSF. This device offers a therapeutic advantage over subarachnoid monitors but carries a higher incidence of infection[83,85].

Maintenance of adequate CPP[84,86, 89,90] is accomplished by reducing the ICP and ensuring adequate MAP. Adequate CPP and reducing ICP Interventions are used step by step.

The first step typically includes the use of analgesia and sedation, elevation of head, airway and ventilatory management and preferably with concomitant monitoring of jugular venous saturation[86,88-90] Obtunded patients, especially those with a GCS ≤ 8 require intubation for airway protection. Mechanical ventilation will also facilitate deep sedation and hyperventilation. During mechanical ventilation hypercarbia should be avoided because it causes vasodilation and may further increase ICP. Therapeutic hyperventilation decreases ICP via vasoconstriction cerebral vessels. Also it must be thought that hyperventilation is rapidly effective but may lead to reduce CBF and may not be a reasonable long-term strategy. Therefore, it is recommended that maintaining the PaCO$_2$ at the low end of normal level is more definitive strategies for reducing ICP.

The second step includes using mannitol or hypertonic saline infusions for refractory intracranial hypertension. In the third step rescue therapies such as high-dose barbiturate infusions and possibly decompressive craniectomy or hypothermia may be needed. Thus, interventions are traditionally chosen in the order of an increasing risk of complications. The goal for patients presenting with raised ICP is reduce ICP immediately (Table 8).

1.	Assessment and management of ABC's (airway, breathing, circulation)
2.	Early intubation if; GCS <8, evidence of herniation, apnea, inability to maintain airway
3.	Mild head elevation of 15–30° (Ensure that the patient is euvolemic)
4.	Hyperventilation: Target PaCO2:30–35 mm Hg (suited for acute, sharp increases in ICP or signs of impending herniation)
5.	Mannitol: Initial bolus: 0.25–1 g/kg, then 0.25–0.5g/kg,q 2–6 has per requirement, up to 48 h
6.	Hypertonic Saline: Preferable in presence of hypotension, hypovolemia, serum osmolality >320 mOsm/kg, renal failure, dose: 0.1–1 ml/kg/hr infusion, target Na+ 145–155 meq/L.
7.	Steroids: Intracranial tumors with perilesional edema, neurocysticerocosis with high lesion load, pyomeningitis, abscess
8.	Adequate sedation and analgesia
9.	Prevention and treatment of seizures: use lorazepam or midazolam followed by phenytoin as initial choice.
10.	Avoid noxious stimuli: use lignocaine prior to ET suctioning [nebulized (4% lidocaine mixed in 0.9% saline) or intravenous (1–2 mg/kg as 1% solution) given 90 sec prior to suctioning]
11.	Control fever: antipyretics, cooling measures
12.	Maintenance IV Fluids: Only isotonic or hypertonic fluids (Ringer lactate, 0.9% Saline, 5% D in 0.9% NS), No Hypotonic fluids
13.	Maintain blood sugar: 80–120 mg/dL
14.	Refractory raised ICP:
	• Heavy sedation and paralysis
	• Barbiturate coma
	• Hypothermia
	• Decompressive craniectomy

Table 8. Treatment to reduce intracranial pressure.

Osmotic Diuresis

Mannitol

The optimal dosing of mannitol is not known. Mannitol is used as a rapid and effective method for reducing ICP. It is given as a 0.5- to 1g/kg bolus and repeat every 6-8 hours to maintain serum osmolarity ebow the value of 310 mOsm/L. Mannitol results osmotic diuresis. The altered osmolar gradient facilitates fluid shifts and reduces cerebral edema. Similarly, furosamide increases intravascular oncotic pressure via hypoosmolar diuresis, which reduces cerebral edema and CSF production and is synergistic with mannitol. These agents should be used with caution because hypovolemia and hypotension may result, further impairing CPP[84,91,92]. Urine output should be matched with crystalloid replacement to maintain intravascular volume.

Attention has to be paid to the fluid balance so as to avoid hypovolemia and shock. There is also a concern of possible leakage of mannitol into the damaged brain tissue potentially leading to "rebound" rises in ICP [93]. For this reason, when it is time to stop mannitol, it should be tapered and its use should be limited to 48 to 72 h. Mannitol can also lead to hypokalemia, hemolysis and renal failure.

Hypertonic Saline

Hypertonic saline has an obvious advantage over mannitol in children who are hypovolemic or hypotensive. These may be preferred are renal failure or serum osmolality >320 mosmol/Kg too. It has been found effective in patients with serum osmolality of up to 360 mosmol/Kg[94]. The expected complications with the use of hypertonic saline are bleeding, rebound rise in ICP, hyperchloremic acidosis and hypokalemia, central pontine myelinolysis, acute volume overload, renal failure, cardiac failure or pulmonary edema [95-97]. In different studies the concentration of hypertonic saline used has varied from 1.7% to 30% [98]. There are also a variety of application method and evidence-based recommendations are difficult. It would be reasonable to administer hypertonic saline as a continuous infusion at 0.1 to 1.0 mL/kg/hr, to target a serum sodium level of 145–155 meq/L [99,100] Serum sodium level and neurological status should be closely monitored during treatment. While finishing hypertonic saline treatment, serum sodium should be slowly returned to normal values (hourly decline in serum sodium of not more than 0.5 meq/L) to avoid complications related to fluid shifts[101]. Monitoring of serum sodium and serum osmolality should be done every 2–4h till target level is reached and then followed up with 12 hourly estimations. Under careful monitoring, hypertonic saline has been used for up to 7 days [102].

Sedatives, analgesics, and neuromuscular blocking agents

Agitation and the painful stimuli may significantly increase ICP in traumatic brain injury patients, and therefore, the use of sedative agents is important in ICP management. A variety of pharmacological agents have been suggested to treat agitation. But no optimal sedative regimen has been exactly identified.

Sedatives, analgesics, and neuromuscular blocking agents are commonly used in the management of traumativ brain injury. This agents are used for two purposes, emergency intubation and management including control of ICP in the intensive care unit (ICU).

Pain and agitation produce sympathetic hyperactivity, resulting in an increase in heart rate, stroke volume, myocardial oxygen consumption and ICP and should be avoided. Analgesia and sedation reduce the neuro-endocrine response to stress by resulting an increase in adrenocorticotrophic hormone (ACTH), cortisol, antidiuretic hormone (ADH), growth hormone (GH) and glucagon. The stress response reduces insulin uptake, causing hyperglycaemia, relative glucose intolerance and insulin resistance, and promotes catabolism of proteins and lipids and a decrease in gastrointestinal motility and urine output.

Benzodiazepines

The benzodiazepines are the favoured group of drugs for sedation and are divided into short-acting, intermediate-acting and long-acting drugs. Among them midazolam, lorazepam and diazepam are mostly used.

Midazolam (Dormicum) is short-acting benzodiazepine and 2-3 times more potent than diazepam, and is available in three strengths. Midazolam is well known for its idiosyncratic effects. It has active metabolites, and can accumulate. Its duration of action is approximately 45 minutes. The adult loading dose is 2 mg intravenously over 30 seconds. The maximum effect is in 3 minutes. After 3 minutes, increments of 1 mg can be given every 3 minutes until the desired effect is achieved. Midazolam may cause respiratory depression. Elderly patients should be given half of the above recommended dosage. Midazolam can be used orally, rectally, intranasally, or intravenously in children. The recommended paediatric doses are as follows: intranasal 0.4 mg/kg, oral/rectal 0.5 mg/kg, intravenous 0.1 mg/kg.

Lorazepam (Ativan) is an intermediate-acting benzodiazepine which has no metabolites. It is useful in acute anxiety, acute phsychosis and status epilepticus. The maximum safe adult dosage is 4 mg and the minimum effective dose should be titrated to the individual patient's needs. The intravenous dose for children is 0.1 mg/kg.

Diazepam (Valium) is a long-acting benzodiazepine which is less potent than the previous two. It has active metabolites, and a sclerosing effect on veins. The intravenous dosage of 0.1 mg/kg applies to both adults and children, and the rectal dosage is 0.5 mg/kg.

α-2 receptors agonists

Sedative and hypnotic effects of these drugs are due to the action on α2-receptors in the locus ceruleus. Analgesic effect is maintened by an action on α2-receptors within the locus ceruleus and the spinal cord. These are dextmedetomidine and clonidine.

Dexmedetomidine (Precedex) is a new selective α-2 adrenoreceptor agonist drug. It has both anxiolytic and analgesic properties. It does not cause respiratory depression, and patients maintain cognitive function and are easily rousable. The bradycardia and hypotension may be seen as side effects. There is no effect on ICP, but CPP may decrease by virtue of decreasing MAP.

Anaesthetics

Propofol and thiopentone are used for sedation and lowering ICP in traumatic brain injuried patients.

Propofol

-   Mechanisms of actions:
-   Acts on GABAα receptors in the hippocampus.
-   Inhibition of NMDA receptors.
-   ↓ IOP, ICP & CMRO2

Propofol is widely used in the ICU to sedate intubated neurolojic patients with increased ICP[94]. Propofol has been shown to maintain or reduce ICP while maintaining an adequate

CPP[95]. Propofol has also neurovascular, neuroprotective, and electroencephalographical effects that are salutory in the patient in neurocritical care. The short half-life of propofol facilitates serial neurologic exams and is the prefered agent. However, excessive sedation and analgesia may mask examination findings and prolong the course of mechanical ventilation[82,88,104].

Propofol will be initiated at 25 mcg/kg/min and titrated to achieve an ICP < 20 mm Hg (up to a maximum of 75 mcg/kg/min). Propofol will be continued for up to 48 h or until removal of the ICP or when mechanical ventilation is discontinued.

Propofol is employed as a first-line sedative agent in neurosurgecal patients due to its favorable pharmacokinetic profile [105] . However, some patients require prolonged infusions and high rates of propofol. This has been shown increase their risk for development of a severe propofol-related infusion syndrome, which can be fatal. Propofol infusion syndrome is expected in ebow 5 mg/kg/hr infusion more than 48 hours. Its clinical features consist of cardiomyopathy with acute cardiac failure, myopathy, metabolic acidosis, hiperkalemia and hepatomegaly. Mechanism of this syndrome is by though inhibition of free faty acids entry into mitochondria and failure of its metabolism. Both barbiturates and propofol have favorable effects on cerebral oxygen balance, but propofol is more potent in this regard. Benzodiazepines and propofol have the added benefit of increasing the seizure threshold.

Barbiturates act on the GABA receptors and its mechenism of action in zero order kinetics. It provides a cerebral protection effect and uses in neurointensive care units in patients with high ICP and status epilepticus.

Barbiturates are less effective than mannitol for lowering ICP. Thiopentone can be used for this purpose and the dosing of the drug is adjusted to a target ICP as monitored on an ICP monitor. The drug is titrated to a 90% burst suppression (2–6 bursts per minute) using an EEG monitor. Monitoring in barbiturate coma should include EEG, ICP monitoring, invasive hemodynamic monitoring (arterial blood pressure, central venous pressure, SjvO2) and frequent assessment of oxygenation status. The complication rate of barbiturate therapy is high and includes hypotension, hypokalemia, respiratory complications, infections, hepatic dysfunction and renal dysfunction [106].

Opiods:

Morphine, fentanyl and remifentanil can be used not only pain management but also sedation effect. Morphine and fentanyl are the two most commonly used opioids for the analgesia of critically ill patients[107,108]. They are routinely used in patients with severe head injury as part of the management of increased intracranial pressure (ICP). However, the cerebrovascular effects of such drugs remain controversial. Studies in laboratory animals and humans have shown increases, decreases or no change in ICP after opioid administration[109-120]. Most of these studies find a concomitant decrease in systemic arterial pressure and, recently, it has been suggested that reduced MAP could in fact be responsible for the increases in ICP observed after the administration of potent opioids such as sufentanil[107]. In patients with low intracranial compliance and intact autoregulation, reduced MAP would be expected to result in vasodilation, increased blood volume, and thus increased ICP.

Remifentanil is a selective mu-opioid agonist with a context-sensitive half-time of 3 to 5 minutes, independent of dose or administration duration of. Its metabolism by nonspecific esterases results in rapid and uniform clearance leading to highly predictable onset and offset of action. Other desirable effects include decreased cerebral metabolism and decrease intracranial pressure (ICP) with minimal cerebral perfusion pressure changes .

Neuromuscular blockade

Neuromuscular blocking agents can facilitate mechanical ventilation and management of raised ICP, but their use should be reserved for specific indications. The depth and duration of neuromuscular blockade should be monitored and optimized, respectively. Although therapeutic paralysis may in a fall in ICP and prevents shivering if induced hypothermia is attempted. However, it may mask seizure activity, negates the physical exam potentially delaying early signs for deterioration, prolongs ventilation, and increases the risk for pressure ulcers and venothromboemboli [121]. Deep sedation may be safer while providing similar benefits[122].

Hypothermia

Hyperthermia increases ICP and should be prevented. Moderate hypothermia can help to control critically elevated ICP values in severe space-occupying edema.

The basic mechanisms through which hypothermia protects the brain are clearly multifactorial and include at least the following: reduction in brain metabolic rate, effects on cerebral blood flow, reduction of the critical threshold for oxygen delivery, blockade of excitotoxic mechanisms, calcium antagonism, preservation of protein synthesis, reduction of brain thermopooling, a decrease in edema formation, modulation of the inflammatory response, neuroprotection of the white matter and modulation of apoptotic cell death [123].

Hypotermia have some risks include coagulopathy and electrolyte abnormalities. Shivering may occur, which will increase ICP[88,124].

Glycemic control; Hyperglycemia has an adverse effect on outcomes in neurointensive patients and should be aggressively treated[125].

CSF drainage: The role of CSF drainage is to reduce intracranial fluid volume and thereby lower ICP. Removal of CSF through an intraventricular catheter reduces ICP. Drainage should be continued to maintained the ICP between 5 mm Hg and 15 mm Hg[126,127].

Craniectomy: Although drastic, bone and potentially brain removal are extremely effective in reducing ICP. Craniectomy greatly facilitates ICP management and may improve outcomes and is recommended if other therapies are not effective [128].

Intensive Care Unit Complications

Intensive care unit complications are very various because the illnesses affecting the various organ systems and the interventions put in the practise on the patients as a means of getting health. The patients being in neurointensive care unit would be expected more diferent diversty complications.

Pulmonary Complications

Pulmonary complications like nasocomial pneumonia, ARDS progressed in mechanicaly ventilated patients, neurogenic pulmonary oedema, pulmonary embolism are discussed below.

Nosocomial pneumonia

According to American Thoracic Society (ATS) guidelines, nosocomial pneumonia (also known as hospital-acquired pneumonia or health care–associated pneumonia) is defined as pneumonia that occurs more than 48 hours after hospital admission but that was not incubating at the time of admission.

Ventilator-associated pneumonia

Ventilator-associated pneumonia (VAP) is becoming common nosocomial infection in hospitals with devolopment of intensive care units[129]. VAP is defined as pneumonia that develops in 48 hours mechanicaly ventilated patients. The mechanism of VAP progresion is retrograde colonisation of the oropharynx caused by gastro-oesophageal reflux and possibly also cross colonisation from contaminated hospital personnel or equipment. In addition many mechanically ventilated patients are immobile and cannot expand the distal airways with sighs, deep breaths, and coughs. The main pathogens of VAP are Pseudomonas aeruginosa, Enterobacteriaceae, and other Gram-negative bacilli, Streptococcus faecalis, Staphylococcus aureus, Candida sp, Aspergillus sp, and episodes of polymicrobial pneumonia etc. Mortality rates, morbidity, and costs are all increased in the patient with VAP because the treatment of it is difficult and expensive. Early-onset VAP has almost no risk for having multidrug-resistant (MDR) pathogens. Currently recommended initial empiric antibiotics include ceftriaxone, fluoroquinolones, ampicillin-sulbactam or ertapenem. Late-onset VAP has a risk of having MDR pathogens. Their initial antibiotherapy may consist antipseudomonal cephalosporins (eg, cefepime, ceftazidime), antipseudomonal carbapenems (imipenem or meropenem), beta-lactam/beta-lactamase inhibitors (piperacillin-tazobactam) with an antipseudomonal fluoroquinolone (ciprofloxacin) or aminoglycoside plus linezolid or vancomycin (if risk factors for methicillin-resistant Staphylococcus aureus are present). If infection with Legionella pneumophila is suspected, the regimen should include a macrolide or fluoroquinolone rather than an aminoglycoside. Early administration of appropriate antibiotic regimens and with adequate dosing of antibiotics improve outcomes after VAP. Antibiotics should be further adjusted on the basis of culture results. The first antibiotic regimen must be optimized, because inappropriate initial therapy is associated with worsened outcomes, even if the regimen is subsequently changed on the basis of the microbiologic results.

Aspiration pneumonia

Aspiration pneumonia is usually caused by colonisation of aerobic bacteria from gastric and oesophageal flora because of repeated small volume aspiration during sleep, especially with impaired pharyngeal reflex [130]. It usually develops subclinically and fulminant aspiration syndrome is rare. There may be no symptoms before the development of transient hypoxaemia or infiltrates on x-ray. Increasing pulmonary artery pressure because of hypoxaemic vasoconstriction and pulmonary oedema developing secondary to acid induced lung damage. Chest X-Ray usually shows right lower lobe infiltration, atelectasis, and sometimes shows air bronchogram with bilateral, diffuse infiltrates. Treatment must be planed on the base of antibiograme results of tracheal and blood culture.

Adult respiratory distress syndrome

ARDS is a severe lung disease caused by a variety of directly and indirectly pertaining the lungs. It is characterized by inflammation of the lung paranchyme leading to impaired gas exchange with concomitant systemic release of inflammatory mediators causing inflammation, hypoxemia and frequently resulting in multiple organ failure. This condition is often fatal, usually requiring mechanical ventilation and admission to an intensive care unit. A less severe form of this fulminanat lung disease is called acut lung injury (ALI). Before thinking ARDS any cardiogenic cause of pulmonary edema should be excluded[131]. ARDS is a form of non-cardiogenic pulmonary oedema characterised by reduced respiratory compliance and increased work of breathing and V/Qmismatch, leading to an increased shunt and hypoxaemia. The definition of ARDS is based on the table below.

- Acute onset
- Pulmonary artery wedge pressure ≤18 mmHg or absence of clinical evidence of left atrial hypertension
- Bilateral infiltrates on chest radiography
- Acute lung injury (ALI) is present if Pao_2/Fio_2 ratio is≤ 300
- Acute respiratory distress syndrome is present if Pao_2/Fio_2 ratio ≤ 200

Table 9. ARDS criteria.

ARDS may follow any major illness, sepsis or surgery but is common following aspiration or septicaemia. Multiorgan failure may occur and is a common cause of death. The treatment of ARDS consist of apropirate managment of ventilatory support. Ventilatory support is arraenged for adequate oxygenation with different strategies. As saying baby lung ventilation with low tidal volumes between 5 and 6 mL/kg or predicted body weight are used. The aim this is to save the healty lung reagions from excessively high inflation pressures. The management depends on the recruitment of collapsed alveoli with PEEP to correct the pronounced ventilation–perfusion mismatch and to prevent compression atalectasis. The peak inspiratory (plateau) pressure should be kept below 30-35 cm water, and as possible as eucapnia should be maintained to avoid further increases in intracranial pressure. High levels of PEEP may be required to treat severe hypoxemia. Caution is advised, however, because PEEP can inhibit cerebral venous return and increase intracranial hypertension.

Neurogenic pulmonary oedema

Neurogenic pulmonary edema (NPE) is defined as an increase in pulmonary interstitial and alveolar fluid [132-135]developing after an acute injury to the brain or brainstem in patients with intracranial pathology, including subarachnoid haemorrhage, cerebral emboli, cerebral tumours, status epilepticus, and raised intracranial pressure (ICP). The increased intracranial pressure is thought to precipitate an increased central sympathetic nerve activity transmitted via peripheral alpha and beta-adrenergic receptors. Neurogenic pulmonary edema results from a predominant alpha-receptor stimulation with a significant increase in the preload and afterload. The patient may present with excessive sweating, hypertension, tachypnoea, and frothy sputum. Chest X-Ray shows diffuse pulmonary infiltrates, but the diagnosis depends on showing hypoxaemic respiratory failure with a normal pulmonary artery wedge pressure in the absence of a cardiac cause. Supplemental oxygen is required in most patients to correct hypoxemia. Mechanical Ventilation may be necessary, either noninvasive with a face mask or via an endotracheal tube. Neurogenic pulmonary oedema should be distinguished from aspiration pnomonia, ARDS, and other pulmonary diseases. Because treatment of NPE is different. Pharmacological agents are not used routinely in the treatment of neurogenic pulmonary edema. Several agents, such as alpha-adrenergic antagonists, beta-adrenergic blockers, dobutamine, and chlorpromazine, are advocated by some authors, but assessment of their effectiveness is difficult because neurogenic pulmonary edema is usually a self-limited condition that resolves spontaneously.

Pulmonary embolism

Patients with neurological disease are susceptible to deep vein thrombosis (DVT) and pulmonary embolism (PE) particularly if they are immobilised or paralysied. PE and DVT are two clinical presentations of venous thromboembolism (VTE) and share the same predisposing factors. In most cases PE is a consequence of DVT. PE is a relatively common cardiovascular emergency and a difficult diagnosis that may be missed because of non-specific clinical presentation[136]. Smaller emboli may cause few haemodynamic effects or may result in infarction of a section of lung tissue if collateral blood flow is inadequate. Large and/or multiple emboli might abruptly increase pulmonary vascular resistance to a level of afterload which cannot be matched by the right ventricle (RV) and right heart failure identified acute cor pulmonale may develope. Sudden death may occur, usually in the form of electromechanical dissociation[137].

The treatment of pulmonary embolism depends upon its size. Cardiopulmonary resuscitation may be necessary following a massive embolus with the patient in shock from acute cor pulmonale, justifying aggressive treatment with thrombolysis. Supportive treatment includes correcting hypoxaemia, intravenous fluid replacement, inotropic drugs, and analgesia. Mechanical ventilation may be necessary if the patient cannot maintain adequate oxygenation. Anticoagulation is usually begun with unfractionated heparin, the dose being titrated against the activated partial thromboplastin time. In ischaemic stroke, dosage should not be adjusted to lower levels for fear of haemorrhagic conversion as an inadequate dose increases mortality from pulmonary emboli. Warfarin administration should begin 48 hours after the start of heparin and continue for six months thereafter.

Hypovolaemia

Hypovolaemia often accompanies traumatic brain injury due to decreased intake and increased loss (vomiting, sweating). Fluid should be restricted to those who are in various grade of coma and central venous pressure can be measured to guide fluid therapy. Full maintenance of sodium should be given as hyponatraemia impairs cerebrovascular reactivity and serum sodium level should be maintained above 140mmol/l.

The choice of fluid replacement depends on a number of factors. If the patient is anaemic (haemoglobin < 8 g/dl), transfusion of red cells should be considered, especially if the patient has a history of ischaemic heart disease. If the patient's haemoglobin is above this value, blood volume may be increased by the use of colloids or crystalloid solutions. Colloids are expensive, carry the risk of anaphylaxis, and the absence of clotting factors may precipitate a coagulopathy. Generally, in neurointensive care practice, 0.9% sodium chloride solution is favoured over glucose or lactate containing solutions which have the potential to increase intracellular glucose concentrations and thus increase the risk of ischaemic damage.

Hypo/Hypertension[138-149]

For ensuring adequate organ perfusion, monitoring and maintenance of arterial blood pressure and blood volume in normal limits are essential. Arterial catheterization is indicated in ICU setting when abnormal blood pressure threatens to compromise blood flow to the brain, exacerbate high intracranial pressure. During hypotension, arterial and jugular venous oxygen contents significant decrease. Also hypotension causes inadequate blood flow to the brain, especially if intracranial pressure is already elevated. CVP monitoring, pulmonary pulmonary artery catheterisation and devices using Doppler principles are used to help untangle the explanation of hypotension and allow appropriate treatment.

Hypertension cause elevation of intracranial pressure and/or increase bleeding into the brain and surrounding compartments. Hypertension is a common sequelae of acute neurological events. When cerebral autoregulation is disturbed or its limits are exceeded, blood flow passively increases with increasing blood pressure. This in turn can increase intracranial pressure or cause breakdown of the blood–brain barrier with resultant transudation of intravascular fluid. Acute hypertension may also increase morbidity and mortality by exacerbating cerebral edema, raising intracranial pressure and bleeding. Treatment of hypertension requires carefull consideration. Causes of hypertension pertaning with acute neurological events are summerised at the below.

Causes of hypertension

Neurological disorders
- Increased intracranial pressure
  - Brain tumours
  - Encephalitis/encephalomyelitis
  - Respiratory acidosis
- Acute stress,
  - Psychogenic hyperventilation
  - After resuscitation
  - Hypoglycaemia
  - Hypoksemia
- Vasoconstrictors/Medications
  - Ephedrine
  - Phenylephrine
  - Pseudoephedrine
  - β-agonist bronchodilators
  - Glucocorticoids

On the other hand patients with raised ICP require an elevated MAP to maintain an adequate cerebral perfusion pressure, and any fall in cerebral blood flow may lead to global ischaemia. So treatment of hypertension must be planed according the situation of brain. Pharmacotherapy used to treat acute situation may have undesirable effects on cerebral perfusion pressure (CPP). Intravenous labetalol, hydralazine, and sodium nitroprusside are commonly used drugs. Longer term treatment includes oral β adrenergic receptor antagonists, angiotensin converting enzyme inhibitors, and calcium channel antagonists. Treatments are indicated if the mean arterial blood pressure is higher than 130 mm Hg or cerebral perfusion pressure is higher than 85 mm Hg.

Seizures

Seizures are a common complication of traumatic brain injury, and can occur immediately following the injury, or may develop later.The risk of post-traumatic seizure is generally related to the severity of the injury.

Hypo/hypernatremia, hypo/hyperglycemia, hypocalcemia, hypomagnesemia, hyperosmolarity, hypoxia and uremia can also lead to seizures. Many antibiotics often used in co-existant infections such as quinolones, third or fourth generation cephalosporins and meropenem may presipitate or aggrevate seizures.

Subclinical seizures or status epilepticus were associated with episodic clinically relevant increases in ICP. Often, subclinical status epilepticus is neither diagnosed nor treated in the ICU, and may be a target in neurointensive care for improving patient outcomes. Use of continuous EEG monitoring represents an important research priority.

As a complication of infection[150-154]seizure may seen only one single attact or may become a chronic epilepsy. Seizures may arise as an acute, subacute, or long- term consequence of an infectious state.

The patients with fever and having alteration in sensory status may be associated with focal neurological signs and seizures. Febrile seizures occur with a prodromal fever. A simple febrile seizure occurs as a brief generalized tonic clonic seizure occurring after the onset of fever. A complicated febrile seizure is occure with prolonged seizure activity or focal seizure activity.

The use of antiepileptic drugs to arrest the seizures and other general measures including the use of antibiotic and antiviral drugs, electrolyte and fluid management, blood pressure monitoring, respiratory monitoring and other aspects of intensive care are equally important. .

Management and goals of seizures

Treatment of a patients with seizures requires:
- Maintenance of vital functions
- Abolition of seizures
- Elimination of any precipitating factors
- Reversing correctable causes

Following protocols for management is vital.

The initial treatment is directed towards:

- Maintaining an airway.
- Supporting breathing and administration of oxygen.
- Support and maintenance of vital functions

The clinician should first search for underlying etiologies producing the seizures and treat it (hypoglycemia, hypocalcemia, sepsis). There are many different types of seizure medication used to treat many different types of seizures[155]. Examples of first -line medications are carbamazepine (Tegregol, Carbatrol), valproate (Depakote), phenytoin (Dilantin) and ethosuximide (Zarontin). Additional medications known as add-on medications or second-line therapy may be required in addition to first -line medications. Examples of second-line seizure drugs include gababentin (Neurontin), lamotrigine (Lamictal) and topiramate (Topamax). Loss of cerebral autoregulation and neuronal damage begin after 30 minutes of continuous seizure activity. Lorazepam is better than diazepam or phenytoin alone for cessation of seizures and carries a lower risk of continuation of status epilepticus requiring a different drug or general anaesthesia.

Fever [156-162]

Fever is among the most frequently detected abnormal physical signs in critically ill patients and may arise due to infectious or noninfectious etiologies. Fever is a complex adaptive response involving elaborate interactions between the immune and nervous systems. High temperatures inhibit growth of microorganisms, may reduce the expression of virulence factors, increase susceptibility to anti-microbials and enhance host immune responses. At the same time fever can worsen primary brain damage. Because increase in cerebral oxygen consumption may leads to increase in blood flow and accordingly in blood volume. This increase potentiates neurologic injury and causes brain edema. Fever is deleterious in patient with low cerebral compliance and generate dangerous intracranial pressure rises accelerating the terminal stages of fulminant infections (through cytokine-induced tissue injury).

Non-infectious causes of fever are common in the ICU. Transfusion reactions and drug hypersensitivity, in particular to anti-microbial agents, are frequent causes. Deep vein thrombosis, pulmonary embolus/infarct, myocardial infarction and acute haemorrhage may also cause fever. Neurogenic fever usually is caused by damage to the hypothalamus from CNS trauma, intracerebral bleeding, or an increase in intracranial pressure. Neurogenic fevers are characterized by a high temperature that's resistant to antipyretic therapy and isn't associated with sweating.

Fever treatment methods may include direct cooling and anti-pyretic medications such as acetylsalicylic acid, non-steroidal anti-inflammatory agents and acetaminophen. An alternative method for temperature management may be an intravascular approach.

Direct cooling is done by many methods for example reducing the ambient room temperature, application of cool external substances such as mist, ice packs, wet sponges and cooling blankets, and administration of cooled intravenous fluids[161,162]. A number of newer techniques have evolved including cooling jackets and intravascular catheter-based heat exchange systems. Convective cooling (ie, blowing cold air) is thought to be more effective than cooling blanket for decreasing body temperature and is also thought to be more comfortable for patients. Administration of ice cold intravenous fluid also directly cools core tissues and has been used for his purpose in physiologic studies. The method is obviously restricted by the volume that can be administered without overloaing the cardiovascular system.

Aggressive fever treatment strategy ; Acetaminophen (Adults 0.5-1 gm, every 4-6 hours upto a maximum of 4 gms. Children 10 mg/kg, every 4-6 hours) for fever >38.5°C and a cooling blanket added if >39.5°C) .Routes of Administration Oral, Parenteral (I.M.). Never IV use with great caution in patients with hepatic dysfunction and in alcoholics.

Intensive Care Nursing

Traumatic Brain İnjury can be fatal if it is not diagnosed and treated promptly; even with treatment, some patients have CNS damage and serious permanent neurologic problems at the end of disease.

The critical-care nurse must be alert with the potential problems encountering the brain-injured patient, who has the risk of sudden deterioration at any time.

Managing a patient with TBI requires a well-defined plan, plenty of resources, and an organized team to prevent secondary injuries. Nursing interventions for TBI are performing frequent vital signs and neurologic assessments for signs of disease progression, such as decreased level of consciousness and assessing mental status, muscle strength, headache severity, and pupillary reactions. An important nursing care for TBI is raising the head of the bed 30 degrees, these intervention promote cerebral venous drainage and to prevent increased ICP. Routine caring like maintaining a patent airway, suctioning the patient as needed and positioning him to encourage drainage of oral and nasal secretions is also essential. Monitorizing oxygenation, administering supplemental oxygen if indicated and monitorizing arterial blood gas analysis results is needed for planing of treatment. Reducing stimuli around the patient, and avoiding Valsalva maneuver, i.e., coughing, sneezing and straining during bowel movements are important intervention in progression of TBI . Keeping the patient's room quiet and darkened can make more comfortable and reduce agitation. An indwelling urinary catheter for accurate intake and output monitoring should be performed.

Patients with TBI frequently have hyperthermia, or fever. Nursing interventions includes reducing fever, not only for a patient's discomfort, but because fever causes increase in intracranial pressure. Nursing care plans that for reducing hyperthermia in TBI patients should include monitoring body temperature every four hours, administering antipyretics and cooling baths as ordered by the physician, and monitoring the patient for signs of dehydration. TBI can cause severe headaches and nursing interventions must be planed as completly pain-free. Positioning (if it is not contraindicated by ICP) and administering mild analgesics to combat discomfort are that can be doing for pain management. It may be helpful to cover the patient's eyes with a cool cloth because this will reduce unnecessary stimuli and photophobia.

Many patients may need mechanical ventilation and endotracheal tube/suctioning can increase ICP so that the use of lidocaine IV %2 1.5 – 2 mg/kg iv prior to endotracheal suctioning to attenuate the ICP response.

3. Conclusions

Traumatic brain injury is a serious public health problem all over the world. Each year, traumatic brain injuries contribute to a substantial number of deaths and cases of permanent disability. Management of TBI in intensive care is very difficult. Management is becoming more difficult when the pulmonary complications and organ dysfunctions added. Disease spesific applications are needed in treatment of mechanical ventilation. The aim of mechanic ventilation is to maintain adaquate oxgenation and ventilation without increasing ICP. Nurition strategy in these patients must be planned to support immune system without loading CO_2.

In conclusion, with the proper support therapy and close management, the mortality and morbidity of TBI patients can be decreased.

4. Abbreviations

TBI: traumatic brain injury; PaO_2: arterial partial pressure of oxygen; PEEP: positive end-expiratory pressure; PbtO2; brain tissue oxygenation, VILI: ventilator-induced lung injury; ICP:intracranial pressure; CBP:cerebral blood flow; CPP: cerebral perfusion pressure; MAP: mean arterial pressure; GCS; Glascow coma scale; PECLA:Pumpless extracorporeal lung asist; VAP:Ventilatory Associated Pneumonia; ITP: intrathoracic pressure; IV:intravenous; ALI:Acute lung injury; ARDS: Acute respiratory distress syndrome; PaO_2 : partial pressure of arterial oxygen; FiO_2:percentage of inspired oxygen; SBI: secondary brain injury; CMRO2: cerebral metabolic rate of oxygen consumption; PbtO2:brain tissue oxygenation; TPN: Total parenteral nutrition; EN:Enteral nutrition, PN: Parenteral nutrition , MDR:multidrug-resistant , DVT: Deep vein thrombosis, PE: Pulmonary embolism

5. References

[1] Pelosi P, Severgnini P and Chiaranda M. An integrated approach to prevent and treat respiratory failure in brain injured patients. Current Opinion in Critical Care. 2005; 11:37-42.

[2] Refresher Course: Mechanical ventilation and the injured brain. South Afr J Anaesth Analg 2011;17(1): 76-80

[3] Stevens RD, Lazaridis C and Chalela JA. The role of mechanical ventilation in acute brain injury. Neurologic Clinics. 2008; 26:543-563.

[4] Mascia L. Acute Lung Injury in Patients with Severe Brain Injury: A Double Hit Model. Neurocrit Care. 2009; 11:3, 417-426

[5] Nyquist P, Stevens RD and Mirski MA. Neurologic injury and mechanical ventilation. Neurocritical Care. 2008; 9:400-408.

[6] Bratton SL, Chestnut RM, Ghajar J, et al. Hyperventilation. Journal of Neurotrauma. 2007; 24 (1):87-90.

[7] Lapinsky SE, Posadas-Colleja JG and McCullagh I. Clinical review: ventilatory strategies for obstetric, brain-injured and obese patients. Critical Care. 2009; 13(2):206-213.

[8] Bratton SL and Davis RL. Acute lung injury in isolated traumatic brain injury. Neurosurgery. 1997; 40:707-712.

[9] Ricard JD, Dreyfuss D, Saumon G. Ventilator-induced lung injury.Current Opinion in Critical Care. 2002;8:12-20.

[10] Huyn T, Messer M, Sing RF, Miles W, Jacobs DG, Thomason MH. Positive end-expiratory pressure alters intracranial and cerebral perfusion pressure in severe traumatic brain injury. The Journal of Trauma. 2002;53:488-493.

[11] Davis DP. Early ventilation in traumatic brain injury. Resuscitation. 2008; 76:333-340.

[12] Gelb AW and Chan MTV. Hyperventilation -an ill wind that sometimes blows good. Canadian Journal of Anaesthesia. 2008; 55(11):735-738.

[13] Warner KJ, Cuschieri J, Copass MK, Jurkovich GJ and Bulger EM. Emergency department ventilation effects outcome in severe traumatic brain injury. Journal of Trauma. 2008; 64(2):341-347.

[14] Lee SW, Hong YS, Han C, et al. Concordance of end-tidal carbon dioxide and arterial carbon dioxide in severe traumatic brain injury. Journal of Trauma. 2009; 67(3):526-530.

[15] Pelosi P, Brazzi L and Gattinoni L. Prone position in acute respiratory distress syndrome. European Respiratory Journal. 2002; 20(4):1017-1028.

[16] Gattinoni L, Tognoni G, Pesenti A, et al. Effect of prone positioning on the survival of patients with acute respiratory failure. New England Journal of Medicine. 2001; 345(8):568-573.

[17] Reinprecht A, Greher M, Wolfsberger S, et al. Prone position in subarachnoid haemorrhage patients with acute respiratory distress syndrome: effects on cerebral tissue oxygenation and intracranial pressure. Critical Care Medicine. 2003; 31(6):1831-1838.

[18] Lo TM, Jones PA, Freeman JA, McFazcan and Minns RA. The role of high frequency oscillatory ventilation in the management of children with severe traumatic brain injury and concomitant lung pathology. Paediatric Critical Care Medicine. 2008; 9(5): 38-42.

[19] Salim A, Miller K, Dangleben D, Cipolle M and Pasquale M. High-frequency percussive ventilation: an alternative mode of ventilation for head-injured patients with adult respiratory distress syndrome. Journal of Trauma. 2004; 57:542-546.

[20] Bein T, Scherer MN, Philipp A, Weber F and Woertgen C. Pumpless extracorporeal lung assist in patients with acute respiratory distress syndrome and severe brain injury.Journal of Trauma. 2005 ; 58(6):124-127.

[21] Reng M, Philipp A, Kaiser M, Pfeifer M, Gruene S, Schoelmerich J. Pumpless extracorporeal lung assist and adult respiratory distress syndrome. Lancet. 2000;356:219-220.

[22] Ngubane T. Mechanical ventilation and the injured brain. South Afr J Anaesth Analg. 2011;17(1) 76-80.

[23] Feeley TW, Saumarez R, Klick JM, McNabb TG, Skillman JJ. Positive end-expiratory pressure in weaning patients from controlled ventilation. A prospective randomised trial. Lancet 1975; 2: 725-729.

[24] Ely EW, Baker AM, Dunagan DP, et al. Effect on the duration of mechanical ventilation of identifying patients capable of breathing spontaneously. N Engl J Med 1996;335: 1864-1869.

[25] Kollef MH, Shapiro SD, Silver P, et al. A randomized,controlled trial of protocol-directed versus physician-directed weaning from mechanical ventilation. Crit Care Med 1997; 25: 567-574.

[26] Esteban A, Anzueto A, Frutos F, et al. Mechanical Ventilation International Study Group. Characteristics and outcomes in adult patients receiving mechanical ventilation: a 28-day international study. JAMA 2002; 287:345-355.

[27] Tobin MJ. Mechanical ventilation. N Engl J Med 1994; 330:1056-1061

[28] Esteban A, Frutos F, Tobin MJ, et al. A comparison of four methods of weaning patients from mechanical ventilation. Spanish Lung Failure Collaborative Group. N Engl J Med 1995; 332: 345-350.

[29] Vallverdu I, Calaf N, Subirana M, Net A, Benito S, Mancebo J. Clinical characteristics, respiratory functional parameters, and outcome of a two-hour T-piece trial inpatients weaning from mechanical ventilation. Am J Respir Crit Care Med 1998; 158: 1855-1862.

[30] Brochard L, Rauss A, Benito S, et al. Comparison of three methods of gradual withdrawal from ventilatory support during weaning from mechanical ventilation. Am J Respir Crit Care Med 1994; 150: 896–903.

[31] Scales DC, Thiruchelvam D, Kiss A and Redelmeier DA. The effect of tracheostomy timing during critical illness on long-term survival. Critical Care Medicine. 2008; 36(9):2547-2557.

[32] Combes A, Luyt CE, Nieszkowska A, Trouillet JL, Gibert C and Chastre J. Is tracheostomy associated with better outcomes for patients requiring long-term mechanical ventilation? Critical Care Medicine. 2007; 35(3): 802-807.

[33] Clec'h C, Alberti C, Vincent F, et al. Tracheostomy does not improve the outcome of patients requiring prolonged mechanical ventilation: A propensity analysis. Critical Care Medicine. 2007; 35(1):132-138.

[34] Ostermann ME, Keenan AP, Seiferling RA, Sibbald WJ. Sedation in the intensive care unit. JAMA 2000; 283:1451-1459.

[35] Rotondi AJ, Chelluri L, Sirio C, et al. Patients' recollections of stressful experiences while receiving prolonged mechanical ventilation in an intensive care unit. Crit Care Med 2002; 30:746-752.

[36] Soltész S, Biedler A, Silomon M, Schöpflin I, Molter GP. Recovery after remifentanil and sufentanil for analgesia and sedation of mechanically ventilated patients after trauma or major surgery. Brit J Anaesth 2001; 86:763-768.

[37] Park G. Improving sedation and analgesia in the critically ill. Minerva Anestesiol 2002; 68:505-512.

[38] Muellejans B, Lopez A, Cross MH, et al. Remifentanil versus fentanyl for analgesia based sedation to provide patient comfort in the intensive care unit: a randomized, double blind controlled trial. Crit Care 2004; 8(1) 1-11.

[39] Schelling G, Richter M, Roozendaal B, et al. Exposure to high stress in the intensive care unit may have negative effects on health related quality of life outcomes after cardiac surgery. Crit Care Med 2003; 31:1071-1079.

[40] Devlin JW, Fraser GL, Kanji S, Riker RR. Sedation assessment in critically ill adults. Ann Pharmacother 2001; 35:1624-1632.

[41] Akçabay M. Yoğun bakım ünitesinde sedasyon ağrı kontrolü ve paralitik ilaç kontrolü. Yoğun Bakım Dergisi 2002; 2:151-161.

[42] Baillaard C, Cohen Y, Toumelin PL, et al. Remifentanil-Midazolam compared to sufentanil-midazolam for ICU long term sedation. Annales Franc ̧aises d'Anesthe ́sie et de Re ́animation 2005; 24: 480–486.

[43] Cohen IL, Abraham E, Dasta JF, et al.: Management of the agitated intensive care unit patient. Crit Care Med 2002, 30:116-117.

[44] Blanchard AR: Sedation and analgesia in intensive care. Medications attenuate stress response in critical illness. PostgradMed 2002, 111:59–60, 63–4,67–70 passim.

[45] Gemma M, Tommasino C, Cerri M, et al.: Intracranial effects of endotracheal suctioning in the acute phase of head injury. J Neurosurg Anesthesiol 2002,14:50-54.

[46] Hurford WE: Sedation and paralysis during mechanical ventilation. RespirCare 2002, 47:334-346.

[47] Gehlbach BK, Kress JP: Sedation in the intensive care unit. Curr Opin Crit Care 2002, 8:290-298.

[48] Kress JP, Pohlman AS, Hall JB: Sedation and analgesia in the intensive care unit. Am J Respir Crit Care Med 2002, 166:1024-1028.

[49] Ostermann ME, Keenan SP, Seiferling RA, et al.: Sedation in the intensive care unit: a systematic review. JAMA 2000, 283:1451–1459.

[50] Mirski MA, Muffelman B, Ulatowski JA, et al.: Sedation for the critically ill neurologic patient. Crit Care Med 1995, 23:2038–2053.

[51] Sessler CN, Gosnell MS, Grap MJ, et al. The Richmond Agitation-Sedation Scale: validity and reliability in adult intensive care unit patients. Am J Respir Crit Care Med 2002; 166:1338-1344

[52] Riker RR, Picard JT, Fraser GL. Prospective evaluation of the Sedation-Agitation Scale for adult critically ill patients. Crit Care Med 1999; 27:1325-29

[53] Ely EW, Truman B, Shintani A, et al. Monitoring sedation status over time in ICU patients-reliability and validity of the Richmond Agitation-Sedation Scale (RASS). JAMA 2003; 289:2983-91.

[54] Simmons LE, Riker RR, Prato BS, et al. Assessing sedation during intensive care unit mechanical ventilation with Bispectral Index and the Sedation-Agitation Scale. Crit Care Med 1999; 27:1499-1504

[55] Devlin JW, Boleski G, Miynarek M, et al. Motor activity assessment scale: a valid and reliable sedation scale for use with mechanically ventilated patients in an adult surgical intensive care unit. Crit Care Med 1999; 27:1271-1275

[56] Lemos de.J , Tweeddale M, Chittock D. Measuring quality of sedation in adult mechanically ventilated critically ill patients: the Vancouver Interaction and Calmness Scale. J Clin Epidemiol 2000; 53:908-919

[57] Detriche O, Berre J, Massaut J, et al. The Brussels sedation scale: use of a simple clinical sedation scale can avoid excessive sedation in patients undergoing mechanical ventilation in the intensive care unit. Br J Anaesth 1999; 83:698-701

[58] Ramsay MA, Savege TM, Simpson BR, et al. Controlled sedation with alphaxalone-alphadolone. Br Med J 1974; 2:656-659

[59] Jacobi J, Fraser GL, Coursin DB, et al. Clinical practice guidelines for the sustained use of sedatives and analgesics in the critically ill adult. Crit Care Med 2002; 30:119-141

[60] Oertel M, Kelly DF, Lee JH, et al.: Metabolic suppressive therapy as a treatment for intracranial hypertension—why it works and when it fails. Acta Neurochir Suppl 2002, 81:69–70.

[61] Robertson CS, Cormio M: Cerebral metabolic management. New Horiz. 1995, 3:410–422.

[62] Clausen T, Bullock R: Medical treatment and neuroprotection in traumatic brain injury. Curr Pharm Des 2001, 7:1517–1532.

[63] Grasshoff C, Gillessen T: The effect of propofol on increased superoxide concentration in cultured rat cerebrocortical neurons after stimulationof N-methyl-D-aspartate receptors. Anesth Analg 2002, 95:920–922.

[64] Starbuck VN, Kay GG, Platenberg RC, et al.: Functional magnetic resonance imaging reflects changes in brain functioning with sedation. Hum Psychopharmacol 2000, 15:613–618.

[65] Hanley DF, Pozo M: Treatment of status epilepticus with midazolam in the critical care setting. Int J Clin Pract 2000, 54:30–35.

[66] Magarey JM: Propofol or midazolam–which is best for the sedation of adult ventilated patients in intensive care units? A systematic review. Aust.CritCare 2001, 14:147–154.

[67] Cremer OL, Moons KG, Bouman EA, et al.: Long-term propofol infusion and cardiac failure in adult head-injured patients. Lancet 2001, 357:117–118

[68] Prielipp RC, Coursin DB. Sedative and neuromuscular blocking drug use in critically ill patients with head injuries. New Horizons. 1995;3(3):456–468

[69] Lowson SM, Sawh S. Adjuncts to analgesia: sedation and neuromuscular blockade. Crit Care Clin. 1999;15:119–141

[70] Coursin DB, Prielipp RC. Use of neuromuscular blocking drugs in the critically ill patient. Crit Care Clin. 1995;11:957–981

[71] Hsiang JK, Chesnut RM, Crisp CB, Klauber MR, Blunt BA, Marshall LF. Early, routine paralysis for intracranial pressure control in severe head injry: is it necessary? Crit Care Med. 1994;22:1471–476

[72] Riley KO, May AK, Hadley MN: Neurological injury and nutritional support. In: Batjer HH and Loftus CM (eds) Textbook of Neurological Surgery, Lippincott Williams & Wilkins, Philadelphia, PA. In press, 2001.

[73] Roger Härtl, ,Linda M. Gerber, ,Quanhong Ni, Jamshid Ghajar, Effect of early nutrition on deaths due to severe traumatic brain injury J Neurosurg . 2008;109:50-56

[74] Marik PE, Zaloga GP: Early enteral nutrition in acutely ill patients: a systematic review. Crit Care Med 2001; 29:2264–70

[75] K.G. Kreymanna, M.M. Berger, N.E.P. Deutz, M. Hiesmayr, P. Jolliet G. Kazandjiev, G. Nitenbergg, G.et al. ESPEN Guidelines on Enteral Nutrition:Intensive care Clinical Nutrition :2006; 25: 210–223

[76] Moore FA, Feliciano DV, Andrassy RJ, et al. Early enteral feeding, compared with parenteral, reduces postoperative septic complications. The results of a meta-analysis. Ann Surg 1992;216:172–183.

[77] Adams S, Dellinger EP, Wertz MJ, Oreskovich MR, Simonowitz D, Johansen K. Enteral versus parenteral nutritional support following laparotomy for trauma: a randomized prospective trial. J Trauma 1986;26:882–891

[78] Braunschweig CL, Levy P, Sheean PM, Wang X. Enteral compared with parenteral nutrition: a meta-analysis. Am J Clin Nutr 2001;74:534–542

[79] MD Bastow. Complications of enteral feeding Gut. 1986 ; 27(1): 51–55.

[80] Andre ´ Van Gossuma, Eduard Cabre, Xavier He ´buterne , Palle Jeppesen , Zeljko Krznaric ,Bernard Messing , Jeremy Powell-Tuck , Michael Staun , Jeremy Nightingale ESPEN Guidelines on Parenteral Nutrition: Gastroenterology Clinical Nutrition 2009;28 415-27

[81] McGraw C P. "A cerebral perfusion pressure greater than 80 mmHg is more beneficial." Intracranial Pressure VII. Edits. Hoff J T & Betz A L. 1989; 839-41. Springer-Verlag, Berlin.

[82] Rosner M J, Rosner S D & Johnson A H. "Cerebral perfusion: management protocol and clinical results." J.Neurosurgery 1985; 83: 949-962.

[83] Welch K. The intracranial pressure in infants. J Neurosurg.1980;52:693-699.

[84] Castillo LR, Gopinath S, Robertson CS. Management of intracranial hypertension. Neurol Clin. 2008;26:521-541.

[85] Juul N, Morris GF, Marshall SB, Marshall LF. Intracranial hypertension and cerebral perfusion pressure: influence on neurological deterioration and outcome in severe head injury. The Executive Committee of the International Selfotel Trial. J Neurosurg. 2000;92:1-6.

[86] Lane PL, Skoretz TG, Doig G, et al. Intracranial pressure monitoring and outcomes after traumatic brain injury. Can J Surg. 2000;43:442-448.

[87] Vincent JL, Berre J. Primer on medical management of severe brain injury. Crit Care Med 2005; 33:1392-1399

[88] Guha A. Management of traumatic brain injury: some current evidence and applications. Postgrad Med J. 2004;80:650-653.

[89] Signorini DF, Andrews PJ, Jones PA, et al. Adding insult to injury: the prognostic value of early secondary insults for survival after traumatic brain injury. J Neurol Neurosurg Psychiatry. 1999;66:26-31.

[90] Skippen P, Seear M, Poskitt K, et al. Effect of hyperventilation on regional cerebral blood flow in head-injured children. Crit Care Med. 1997;25:1402-409.

[91] Mendelow AD, Teasdale GM, Russell T, et al. Effect of mannitol on cerebral blood flow and cerebral perfusion pressure in human head injury. J Neurosurg. 1985;63:43-48.

[92] Muizelaar JP, Lutz HA, Becker DP, et al. Effect of mannitol on ICP and CBF and correlation with pressure autoregulation in severely head injured patients. J Neurosurg. 1984;61:700-706.

[93] Kaufmann AM, Cardoso ER. Aggravation of vasogenic edema by multiple –dose mannitol. J Neurosurg. 1992;77:584-589.

[94] Ziai WC, Toung TJ, Bhardwaj A. Hypertonic saline: first-line therapy for cerebral edema? J Neurol Sci. 2007;261:157-166.

[95] Doyle JA, Davis DP, Hoyt DB. The use of hypertonic saline in the treatment of traumatic brain injury. J Trauma. 2001;50:367-383.

[96] Himmelseher S. Hypertonic saline solutions for treatment of intracranial hypertension. Curr Opin Anaesthesiol. 2007;20:414-26.

[97] Suarez JI. Hypertonic saline for cerebral edema and elevated intracranial pressure. Cleve Clin J Med. 2004;71:9-13.

[98] Strandvik GF. Hypertonic saline in critical care: a review of the literature and guidelines for use in hypotensive states and raised intracranial pressure. Anaesthesia. 2009;64:990-1003.

[99] Larive LL, Rhoney DH, Parker D, Coplin WM, Carhuapoma JR. Introducing hypertonic saline for cerebral edema. Neurocrit Care.2004;1:435-440.

[100] Qureshi A, Suarez J, Bhardwaj A, et al. Use of hypertonic saline/ acetate infusion in the treatment of cerebral edema: effect on intracranial pressure and lateral displacement of the brain. Crit Care Med. 1998;26:440-446.

[101] Peterson B, Khanna S, Fischer B, Marshall L. Prolonged hypernatremia controls elevated intracranial pressure in head injured pediatric patients. Crit Care Med. 2000;28:1136-1143.

[102] Marcoux KK. Management of increased intracranial pressure in critically ill child with acute neurological injury. AACN Clin Issues. 2005;16:212-231.

[103] Kelly DF, Goodale DB, Williams J, et al. Propofol in the treatment of moderate and severe head injury: a randomized, prospective double-blinded pilot trial. J Neurosurg 1999; 90: 1042-1052.

[104] McKeage K, Perry CM. Propofol: a review of its use in intensive care sedation of adults. CNS drugs 2003; 17: 235-272.

[105] Johnston AJ, Steiner LA, Chatfield DA, et al. Effects of propofol on cerebral oxygenation and metabolism after head injury. Br J Anaesth. 2003;91:781-786.

[106] Shapiro BA, Warren J, Egol AB, Greenbaum DM, Jacobi J, Nasraway SA, Schein RM, Spevetz A, Stone JR: Practice parameters for intravenous analgesia and sedation for adult patients in the intensive care unit: An executive summary. Crit Care Med 1995; 23:1596-1600

[107] Hans P, Martin C: La sédation du traumatisé crânien. Cahiers d'Anesthesiologie 1994; 42:521-24

[108] Sperry RJ, Bailey PL, Reichman MV, Peterson JC, Petersen PB, Pace NL: Fentanyl and sufentanil increase intracranial pressure in head trauma patients. Anesth.1992; 77:416-420

[109] Trindle MR, Dodson BA, Rampil IJ: Effects of fentanyl versus sufentanil in equianesthetic doses on middle cerebral artery blood flow velocity. Anesth. 1993; 78:454-460

[110] Albanèse J, Durbec O, Viviand X, Potie F, Alliez B, Martin C: Sufentanil increases intracranial pressure in patients with head trauma. Anesth. 1993; 79:493-497

[111] Werner C, Kochs E, Bause H, Hoffman WE, Schulte am Esch J: Effects of sufentanil on cerebral hemodynamics and intracranial pressure in patients with brain injury. Anesth. 1995; 83:721-726

[112] Mayberg TS, Lam AM, Eng CC, Laohaprasit V, Winn R: The effect of alfentanil on cerebral blood flow velocity and intracranial pressure during isofluorane-nitrous oxide anesthesia in humans. Anesth. 1993; 78:288-294

[113] Scholz J, Bause H, Schulz M, Klotz U, Krishna DR, Pohl S, Schulte am Esch J: Pharmacokinetics and effects on intracranial pressure of sufentanil in head trauma patients. Br J Clin Pharmac 1994; 38:369-372

[114] Jamali S, Ravussin P, Archer D, Goutallier D, Parker F, Ecoffey C: The effects of bolus administration of opioids on cerebrospinal fluid pressure in patients with supratentorial lesions. Anesth Analg 1996; 82:600-606

[115] Warner DS, Hindman BJ, Todd MM, Sawin PD, Kircner J, Roland CL, Jamerson BD: Intracranial pressure and hemodynamic effects of remifentanil versus alfentanil in patients undergoing supratentorial craniotomy. Anesth Analg 1996; 83:348-353

[116] Herrick IA, Gelb AW, Manninen PH, Reichman H, Lownie S: Effects of fentanyl, sufentanil and alfentanil on brain retractor pressure. Anesth Analg 1991; 72:359-363

[117] Moss E, Powell D, Gibson RM, McDowall DG: Effects of fentanyl on intracranial pressure and cerebral perfusion pressure during hypocapnia. Br J Anaesth 1978; 50:779-784

[118] Moss E: Alfentanil increases intracranial pressure when intracranial compliance is low. Anaesthesia 1992; 47:134-136

[119] Albanèse J, Viviand X, Potie F, Rey F, Alliez B, Martin C: Sufentanil, fentanyl, and alfentanil in head trauma patients: A study on cerebral hemodynamics. Crit Care Med 1999; 27:407-411

[120] Tipps LB, Coplin WM, Murry KR, Rhoney DH. Safety and feasibility of continuous infusion of remifentanil in the neurosurgical intensive care unit. Neurosurgery 2000 ;46(3):596-601; discussion 601-602.

[121] Prough DS, Joshi S. Does neuromuscular blockade contribute to adverse outcome in head-injured patients? J Neurosurg Anes. 1994;5:135

[122] Hsiang JK, Chesnut RM, Crisp CB, et al. Early, routine paralysis for intracranial pressure control in severe head injury: is it necessary? Crit Care Med. 1994;22:1471-1476.

[123] Ahuquillo J, Vilalta A. Cooling the injured brain: how does moderate hypothermia influence the pathophysiology of traumatic brain injury. Curr Pharm Des 2007;13(22):2310-2322

[124] Jiang JY, Xu W, Li WP, et al. Effect of long-term mild hypothermia or short-term mild hypothermia on outcome of patients with severe traumatic brain injury. J Cereb Blood Flow Metab. 2006;26:771-776.

[125] Vogelzang M, Nijboer JM, van der Horst IC, et al. Hyperglycemia has a stronger relation with outcome in trauma patients than in other critically ill patients. J Trauma. 2006;60:873-877.

[126] Mokri B. The Monro-Kellie hypothesis: applications in CSF volume depletion. Neurology. 2001;56:1746-1748

[127] Polin RS, Shaffrey ME, Bogaev CA, et al. Decompressive bifrontal craniectomy in the treatment of severe refractory posttraumatic cerebral edema. Neurosurgery. 1997;41:84-92.

[128] Vincent JL Ventilator-associated pneumonia . J Hosp Infect. 2004; 57(4):272-280.

[129] Fagon JY, Chastre J, Hance A, et al. Nosocomial pneumonia in ventilated patients: a cohort study evaluating attributable mortality and hospital stay.Am J Med 1993;94:281-288.

[130] Bernard GR, Artigas A, Brigham KL, et al. The American-European consensus conference on ARDS. Definitions, mechanisms, relevantoutcomes, and clinical trials co-ordination. Am J Respir Care Med1994;149:818-824.

[131] Chang CH, Smith CA. Postictal pulmonary edema.Radiology 1967; 89:1087-1089.

[132] Lagerkranser M, Pehrsson K, Sylven C. Neurogenic pulmonary oedema, a review of the pathophysiology with clinical and therapeutic implications. Acta Med Scand 1982; 212:267-270.

[133] Rogers FB, Shackfor SR, Trevisani GT, et al. Neurogenic pulmonary edema in fatal and non fatal head injuries. J Trauma 1995;39:860-866.

[134] Baumann A, Audibert G, McDonnell J, Mertes PM Neurogenic pulmonary edema. Acta Anaesthesiol Scand. 2007;51(4):447 -455

[135] Fletcher SJ, Atkinson JD. Use of prone ventilation in neurogenic pulmonary oedema. Br J Anaesth. Feb 2003;90(2):238-240

[136] Carson JL, Kelley MA, Duff A, et al. The clinical course of pulmonary embolism. N Engl J Med 1992;326:1240-1245

[137] Morpurgo M, Marzagalli M. Death in pulmonary embolism. In: Morpurgo M, editor. Pulmonary Embolism. New York: Marcel Dekker; 1994. p. 107-114.

[138] Hravnak M, Boujoukos A. Hypotension. Am Assoc Crit Care Nur 1997;8:303-318

[139] Jones AE, Aborn LS, Kline JA. Severity of emergency department hypotension predicts adverse hospital outcome. Shock 2004;22:410-414.

[140] Robertson CS, Clifton GL, Taylor AA, et al. Treatment of hypertension associated with head injury. J Neurosurg 1983;59:455-460.

[141] Heyka RJ. Evaluation and management of hypertension in the intensive care unit. In: Irwin RS, Rippe JM (eds). Irwin and Rippe's Intensive Care Medicine. 6th ed. Philadelphia: Lippincott Williams and Wilkins, 2008:391-98.

[142] Alexander SC, Lassen NA: Cerebral circulatory response to acute brain disease: Implications for anesthetic practice. A nesthesiology 1970; 32 (1):60-68

[143] Fieschi C, Agnoli A, Battistini N, Bozzao L, Prencipe M: Derangement of regional cerebral blood flow and of its regulatory mechanisms in acute cerebrovascular lesions. Neurology 1968; 18 (12):1166-1179

[144] Skinhoj E, Strandgaard S: Pathogenesis of hypertensive encephalopathy. Lancet 1973; 1(801):461-462

[145] Strandgaard S, MacKenzie ET, Sengupta D, Rowan JO, Lassen NA, Harper AM: Upper limit of autoregulation of cerebral blood flow in the baboon. Circ Res 1974; 34 (4):435-440

[146] Hatashita S, Koike J, Sonokawa T, Ishii S: Cerebral edema associated with craniectomy and arterial hypertension. Stroke 1985; 16 (4):661–668

[147] Schutta HS, Kassell NF, Langfitt TW: Brain swelling produced by injury and aggravated by arterial hypertension: A light and electron microscopic study. Brain 1968; 91 (2):281–294

[148] Ekstrom-Jodal B, Haggendal E, Johansson B, Linder LE, Nilsson NJ: Acute arterial hypertension and the blood-brain barrier: An experimental study in dogs, Cerebral Circulation and Metabolism. Edited by Langfitt TW, MacHenry LC Jr, Reivich M, Wollman H. New York, Springer-Verlag, 1977, pp 7–9

[149] Van Aken H, Cottrell JE, Anger C, Puchstein C: Treatment of intraoperative hypertensive emergencies in patients with intracranial disease. Am J Cardiol 1989; 63 (6):43–47

[150] McGrath N, Anderson NE, Croxson MC, Powell KF. Herpes simplex encephalitis treated with acyclovir: diagnosis and long term outcome. J Neurol Neurosurg Psychiatry 1997;63:321–326.

[151] Hsieh WB, Chiu NC, Hu KC, Ho CS, Huang FY. Outcome of herpes simplex encephalitis in children. J Microbiol Immunol Infect 2007;40:34–38.

[152] Gourie Devi M, Ravi V, Shankar SK. Japanese encephalitis an overview. In: Clifford Rose F, editor. Recent advances in tropical neurology. Elsevier; 1995. p.211–35.

[153] Misra UK, Kalita J. Seizures in Japanese encephalitis. J Neurol Sci 2001;190:57–60.

[154] Kalita J,Misra UK, Pandey S, Dhole TN. A comparison of clinical and radiological findings in adults and children with Japanese encephalitis. Arch Neurol 2003;60:1760–1764

[155] Prasad K, Al-Roomi K, Krishnan PR, Sequeira R. Anticonvulsant therapy for status epilepticus. Cochrane Database of Systematic Reviews 2005, Issue 4. Art. No: CD003723

[156] Larke DE, Kimelman J, Raffin TA: The evaluation of fever in the intensive care unit.Chest 1991; 100:213–220

[157] Cunha BA, Shea KW: Fever in the intensive care unit. Infect Dis Clin North Am 1996;10:185–209

[158] Toltzis P, Rosolowski B, Salvator A: Etiology of fever and opportunities for reduction of antibiotic use in a pediatric intensive care unit. Infect Control Hosp Epidemiol 2001; 22:499–504

[159] Kilpatrick MM, Lowry DW, Firlik AD, et al: Hyperthermia in the neurosurgical intensive care unit. Neurosurgery 2000; 47:850–855; discussion 855–856

[160] Cunha BA: Fever in the intensive care unit. Intensive Care Med. 1999; 25:648–651

[161] Cornelia W Hoedemaekers, Mustapha Ezzahti, Aico Gerritsen and Johannes G van der Hoeven. Comparison of cooling methods to induce and maintain normo-and hypothermia in intensive care unit patients: a prospective intervention study. Crit Care 2007;11(4):R91.

[162] E Baumgardner, D Baranov, D S Smith, E L Zager The effectiveness of rapidly infused intravenous fluids for inducing moderate hypothermia in neurosurgical patients Anesthesia & Analgesia 1999 : 89(1): 163-169

3

Lumbar Puncture: Techniques, Complications and CSF Analyses

Ali Moghtaderi[1], Roya Alavi-Naini[2] and Saleheh Sanatinia[2]
[1]Neurology Department, Zahedan University of Medical Sciences
[2]Research Center for Infectious Diseases and Tropical Medicine,
University of Medical Sciences, Zahedan,
Iran

1. Introduction

Lumbar puncture (LP) is one of the well-known ancillary procedures in clinical neurology performed for a variety of functions such as spinal anesthesia, intrathecal administration of drugs, myelography, obtaining cerebrospinal fluid (CSF) samples and measuring pressure since more than 100 years ago. The question that who was really the discoverer of LP is still under debate. Most authors assume that it was Heinrich Irenaeus Quincke (1842-1922) a German internist who was introduced the procedure to medicine in 1891, however, some authors mentioned the American neurologist James Leonard Corning (1855-1923) as the first one who performed LP using birds quills in 1885 (Frederiks et al., 1997; Dakka et al., 2011).

The technique was passed on through generations of physicians to the next but the rules are the same. Quincke's aim on performing LP was to treat patients with hydrocephalus. In 1898 August Bear's assistant attempted to administer a spinal anesthetic to Dr. Bear which was never completed because the syringe did not fit the already implanted spinal needle. However, continued CSF leakage through the dural puncture site was the cause of post lumbar puncture headache (PLPH), discussed later in this monograph (Raskin, 1990).

2. Before beginning the procedure

Before performing LP it is important to think cautiously about the indications and the required diagnostic studies. Patient should be examined especially for papilledema; and cranial CT scans or MRI should be reviewed carefully. Obtaining a cranial CT scan before performing LP in all patients if possible is mandatory especially in patients with papilledema, loss of consciousness, focal neurologic deficit, new seizure onset, and inability to visualize optic fundi (Kastenbauer et al., 2002; Roos, 2003).

In adults with suspected meningitis, clinical features can be used to differentiate between patients with abnormal findings in their CT scans of the head. Clinical features at baseline that are associated with an abnormal findings in CT scans of the brain were an age of at least 60 years, immunocompromised patients and a history of CNS disease (Hasbun et al., 2001). A cranial MRI is an important diagnostic procedure when patient had symptoms and signs of a lesion in posterior fossa. Both CT scan and MRI should be reviewed especially for finding mass or signs of raised intracranial pressure (RICP) in posterior fossa and quadrigeminal cistern. Physician should carefully consider on the indications of the procedure and do other studies which are essential to perform simultaneously like measuring serum glucose and CSF pressure.

Patients should be carefully informed; explaining the procedure to the patient/ care giver/ next of kin completely and signing an informed consent for back pain, leg pain, headache, bleeding, infection, and death are important legal issues. To prevent hemorrhage platelet count and International Normalized Ratio (INR) should be more than 50,000 and less than 1.5, respectively (Table 1).

Full neurological examination especially for papilledema, hemiparesis and focal neurologic deficits
Cranial CT and/or MRI in all patients with papilledema, focal neurologic deficit, recent epileptic episodes
Obtain cranial MRI in all patients with posterior fossa lesions
Check for visualization of quadrigeminal cistern and fourth ventricle especially in patients with bacterial meningitis
Correct bleeding diatheses such as thrombocytopenia and INR>1.5
Careful consideration for indications or contraindications of LP
Obtaining informed consent from the patient/care giver for the procedure

Table 1. Steps prior to lumbar puncture.

3. Technique of the procedure

Experience will teach us the importance of meticulous of each technique. With a thorough knowledge of the contraindications, regional anatomy and rationale of the technique, and adequate prior skill, lumbar puncture can be carried out safely and successfully. Lack of knowledge may lead to a higher mortality and morbidity rate. It was mentioned that the most important elements of procedural competency are the cognitive aspects and anatomy plays a major role in this domain (Boon et al., 2004). There are two different positions for performing LP. For diagnostic LP, the left lateral recumbent position (for right-handed physicians) is preferred. Patient's knee and neck are flexed to overcome the lumbar lordosis that narrows the interspace between adjacent spinous processes and lamina. Sometimes they are in seated position and only the neck is fully flexed. Ill patients are unable to sit up and for pressure measurement the patient should be in recumbent position. In preterm infants it was suggested that the sitting or modified lateral recumbent, without knees-to-chest position, which results in less hypoxemia with the neck maintained in the neutral position is better than the classic position (Weisman et al., 1983).

Proper positioning is critical to success the procedure and the coronal plane of the trunk should be on right angle to the floor, one hip should stay exactly above the other, and the back should be close to the edge of bed because of pouring CSF in to the tube is easier (Fig.1). Inward rotation of the patient makes it difficult to obtain the CSF therefore it is necessary to place a pillow under the ear of the patient in lat recumbent position (Fig.2). In one study it was shown that fluoroscopy guided lumbar puncture may decrease the frequency of traumatic LP from 10.1% to 3.5% (Eskey et al., 2001). However, the patient charges for standard lumbar puncture and fluoroscopy-guided lumbar puncture were $393 and $559, respectively. Ultrasound machines with linear array transducers can also localize spinal interspaces noninvasively, in 2-3 minutes, exclusive of the time for setting up the ultrasound machine (Peterson et al., 2005).

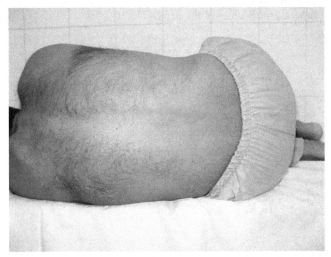

Fig. 1. Proper positioning of the patient for lumbar puncture. The pelvis is vertical and close to the edge of the table.

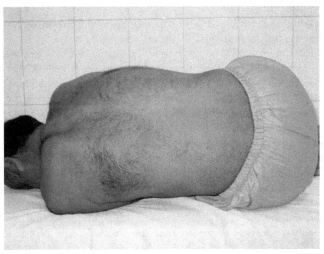

Fig. 2. Incorrect positioning of the patient due to inward rotation of the upper shoulder.

For the safety of both patient and physician the procedure should be done under sterile conditions. At least physician should wear sterile gloves, eye glasses and a mouth mask. Wearing a gown especially for patients with meningitis or meningoencephalitis is considered mandatory. The area should be cleaned and sterilized with 10% povidone iodine

(Betadine) and draped with a sterile towel with a whole in the middle which is large enough to visualize and find the correct place for insertion of the needle (Fig.3). It is better to anesthetize only the subcutaneous tissue of the intervertebral space by 1% to 2.5% lidocaine; however, experienced physicians especially in thin patients do not need it. Warming of the analgesic by rolling the lidocaine vial between the palms may diminish the burning sensation after cutaneous infiltration of the drug.

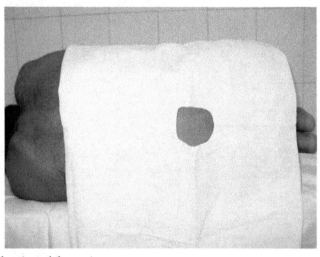

Fig. 3. Correct draping of the patient.

The best intervertebral space is L4-L5 but one space lower (L5-S1) or higher (L3-L4) may be used. In 94% of individuals conus medullaris will extend in to the L1-L2 interspace. In the remaining 6% it extends to the L2-L3 interspace (Fishman, 1992b). The possibility of injury in to the spinal cord will increase with performing the procedure at the L1-L2 or L2-L3 interspaces. In newborns and infants it is safer to use the lowest interspace. The needle is passed horizontally, parallel to the floor. Lumbar puncture is performed by inserting an 18 to 25 gauge needle. The smaller the gauge number, the bigger the diameter of the needle. The size of needle with gauge number 18 indicates that the diameter of the needle is 1/18 inch and for the gauge number 25 indicates 1/25 inch. For diagnostic collection of CSF, a larger gauge needle (18, 19 or 20 standard gauge needles; 22 G, 3.5-cm long needle for neonates; 20 G, 5-cm long needle for children) should be used. Finding the L4-L5 interspace in recumbent position is not very difficult by placing the index finger on the superior part of the upper iliac crest, then drawing an imaginary line between to upper and lower crests (Tuffier's line) and put the thumb of the same hand (for right handed individuals use the left hand and vice versa) in the interspace that the Tuffier's line is crossed with (Boon, Abrahams et al., 2004).

The standard needle for LP is Quincke needle with a bevel sharp tip at the end of the needle. The smaller the diameter the lowest risk for post lumbar headache but the procedure, obtaining CSF and measuring pressure will be more difficult. The bevel head of the needle must be parallel to the longitudinal fibers of the dura mater. It should be inserted at the superior aspect of the inferior spinous process, aimed to the umbilicus (15° cephaled).

There are two types of atraumatic needles, Whitacre pencil-point needle which is available since 1951 (Hart et al., 1951) and Sprotte needle since 1979 with a duller tip and a small oval opening proximal to the tip (Fig.4) (Sprotte et al., 1987). It should be pointed out that Sprotte needle is a modification of the Whitacre needle with larger laterally placed opening. Because of its dull head it needs an introducer which should not shear the dura, therefore it is technically more difficult to use, however, majority of physicians use Quincke needle nowadays. When using Quincke needle the flat portion of the bevel tip should be in line with and parallel to the longitudinal fibers and the hub's notch of the stylet should point to the lateral side of the patient (Evans, 1998).

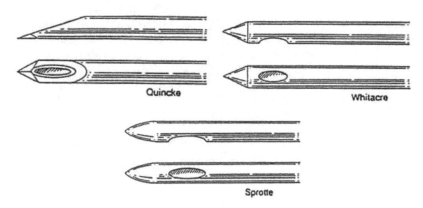

Fig. 4. Three types of spinal needles: Quincke, Whitacre and Sprotte.

When the needle pierces the supraspinous ligament and ligamentum flavum a sudden yielding sensation is often felt often referred by clinicians as a "pop". After entering the ligamentum flavum (1cm thick), the stylet should be removed each 2 mm, however, if the fluid is not appeared in the hub, stylet should be replaced again and the needle rotates 90 degrees, till the bevel head be in the way of CSF. Then, if the fluid does not appear again, the needle should pierce a few millimeters more and a second "pop" may be felt again. If the procedure fails again, the needle should be withdrawn almost under the skin where it can possible to redirect the needle without making another painful needle insertion. The stylet should always be removed slowly from the needle in order to avoid sucking a nerve root in to the lumen and/or causing radicular pain.

When the fluid appears in the hub, a three-way stopcock will be fixed at the hub and a manometer will be attached. A slow raise in the CSF pressure may indicate the obstruction of the tip of the needle with meningeal membranes or nerve roots. Normal CSF pressure in adults is 100-180 mmH$_2$O (8-14 mmHg) and 30-60 mmH$_2$O in children (Ropper et al., 2009). Sometimes a firm abdominal pressure, with the help of an assistant and rapid rise and fall in the pressure indicate the free flow of the CSF (Fishman, 1992b). Aspiration of the CSF by a syringe may increase the risk of subdural hemorrhage or root herniation through the opening of the needle and it is not recommended routinely. The rationale for using a stylet when inserting a non-cutting needle (Sprotte) into the subarachnoid space is the possibility of introducing a small piece of epidermoid tissue in to the subarachnoid space and increasing the risk of development of an epidermoid tumor. Reinserting the stylet before removing the needle may prevent a thread of arachnoid membrane to be withdrawn and CSF leakage will be shorter. Therefore the stylet should always be reinserted before the needle is withdrawn especially in non-cutting needles. Patient may remain flat for 4-24 hours and can take fluid liberally (Roos, 2003). The "dry tap" is almost always due to improper placement of the needle especially when the needle is placed far laterally than to the obliteration of the subarachnoid space by a compressive lesion in the cauda equina or lumbar arachnoiditis (Ropper and Samuels, 2009).

4. Bed rest after the procedure

There is not any firm recommendation for bed rest after LP and there is also no preference how to lie after the procedure on the side, supine or on the face. Spriggs *et al.* (Spriggs et al., 1992) performed a randomized study to assess the immediate effect of mobilization with 4 hours bed rest on the incidence of PLPH. They did not found any difference between the mobile (54 cases) and bed rest (56 patients) groups in the incidence of PLPH (32% versus 31%, respectively). The report of the Therapeutics and Technology Assessment Subcommittee of the American Academy of Neurology (Evans et al., 2000) recommendation noted that Class 1 evidence shows no benefit for the prevention of PLPH after 24 hours bed rest. In our department we ask patient to be at bed for one hour and after that they can walk at their will but we recommend them to be at rest during the remainder of the day. This is a successful practice till now in our department.

5. Transient complications

One of the most frequent transient complications is transient stabbing pain in the territory of sensory nerve root(s) due to contact of the spinal root with the needle. However, pain may be revealed with patient repositioning. In one study it was occurred in 13% of patients during LP (Dripps et al., 1951) but permanent motor or sensory loss is extremely rare (Dahlgren et al., 1995). It seems to be that analgesia is underused in infants and children, however, it should be mentioned that sometimes it takes less than an hour to be efficacious (Baxter et al., 2004). In case of severe nerve injury, pain may persist for a longer time. In the seated position, a drainage headache may be felt and the risk of faint is higher in this group of patients. Men are more sensitive to pain and may show a vasovagal syncope especially when they are seated. Infusion of intravascular normal saline before starting the procedure may decrease the risk of this problem (Table 2). Dysfunction of the 3rd to 8th cranial nerves has been reported in many case reports but they are transient and reversible complications probably secondary to the traction of the nerve over the cranium (Broome, 1993; Lybecker et al., 1995a).

Post-Lumbar Puncture Headache (PLPH)
Cerebral (brain) herniation
Infection
Backache
Subdural or epidural hematoma
Subarachnoid hemorrhage
Implantation of epidermoid tumor
Root irritation/Radicular pain

Table 2. Potential complications of lumbar puncture.

6. Post–Lumbar Puncture Headache (PLPH)

Post-lumbar puncture headache (PLPH) is the most frequent complication (40%) after performing diagnostic LP (Evans, 1998). Headache worsens 15 minutes after sitting or standing and improves within 15 minutes after lying down in the bed and it should be accompanied with one or more of symptoms such as neck stiffness, tinnitus, hypacusia, photophobia and nausea (Dakka, Warra et al., 2011). Tourtellotte *et al.*(Tourtellotte et al., 1972) reported that the average frequency of PLPH after diagnostic LP (excluding myelography and pneumoencephalography), obstetric spinal anesthesia and non-obstetric spinal anesthesia was 32%, 18%, 13%, respectively. In patients received special measures to prevent headache, the average frequency of PLPH in the above groups was decreased to 6.0%, 6.2% and 5.5%, respectively.

PLPH is more frequent in young individuals, thin women (Kuntz et al., 1992) and patients with previous headache (Evans, Armon et al., 2000). It occurs two times more in women than in men (Kuntz, Kokmen et al., 1992) and most of the increased frequency has been seen in child bearing age (18 to 30 years old) (Tourtellotte, Henderson et al., 1972). The frequency is lower in children less than 14 years (Bolder, 1986) and adults more than 60 years (Tourtellotte, Henderson et al., 1972). In a prospective study of 239 patients, pain was located within the region innervated by the trigeminal nerve in 49% of the patients, within the occipital and/or suboccipital region in 11%, and within the combined trigeminal/occipital region in 39% (Vilming et al., 1998). Temporal region is the most frequent place. The intensity of associated symptoms was positively correlated to PLPH severity. However, the classic feature of the headache is a bilateral generalized throbbing or pressure sensation which is increased with sneezing, sitting, coughing or straining especially 48-72 hours after the procedure. Associated symptoms were experienced by 85% of patients, nausea in 73% and dizziness in 60% being the most frequently reported. Those symptoms are more present during the upright position. It may be associated with neck stiffness, nausea and vomiting. Quite rarely there are unilateral or bilateral 6th palsy even at times without headache (Ropper and Samuels, 2009). The pain is revealed after lying down again in the bed (Vilming and Kloster, 1998; Roos, 2003). In particular, PLPH is a constant headache appearing or worsening significantly when standing and resolving or improving significantly upon lying down, however, the severity of the headache has not been defined completely (Lybecker et al., 1995b).

Muller *et al.*(Muller et al., 1994) in a double blind placebo controlled study showed that only 2 out of 42 patients, using Sprotte needle, had PLPH, backache or orthostatic hypotension comparing to the 15 patients out of 48 remaining patients whom experienced Quincke needle for LP. Convincing Class 1 evidence shows that the thicker Quincke needle is associated with more PLPH (Lybecker et al., 1990) from 70% when using 16-19 G to 12% when using 24-27 G needle (Evans, Armon et al., 2000). In another study it was shown that the frequency of PLPH will decrease from 18.9% after using Quincke needle 22 G comparing to 2.3% of PLPH with a 27 G needle. The frequency of PLPH after using atraumatic needles with the same gauges were 6.7% and 0.4% respectively (Carson et al., 1996). It is consistent with the theory of CSF leakage from the puncture site and intracranial hypotension due to presence of a whole in the dura. Thinner needles are harder and more difficult to use, unsatisfactory for measuring CSF pressure and sometimes it requires a syringe to drain CSF, however, it is more useful in performing spinal epidural anesthesia and lumbar myelography. Actually needles thinner than 20 G may not be practical until a small amount of fluid is needed.

There is Class 1 evidence that in the case of parallel insertion of the bevel head of Quincke needle with longitudinal dural fibers rather than perpendicular insertion may be associated with a lesser incidence of PLPH because the dural fibers run parallel to the long axis of the spine (Flaatten et al., 1998). When the bevel head is perpendicular to the dural fibers more of them will be severed and the risk of PLPH is 50% more in this group of patients comparing to the parallel group. Norris *et al.* in their study reported that fourteen of 20 women in the group in which the needle bevel was perpendicular to dural fibers developed a moderate to severe headache, whereas only five of 21 in the group in which the needle bevel was parallel to dural fibers did so (Norris et al., 1989).

The incidence of PLPH is lesser when the stylet reinserts before withdrawing the needle. Strupp *et al.* in a randomly assigned trial in 600 patients reported that the incidence and severity of PLPH was decreased from 16% to 5% after replacement the stylet (Strupp et al., 1998). They used Sprotte needle for performing LP in their 600 patients. Despite there is not any clear evidence for reinserting stylet before withdrawing a Quincke needle but it seems that it is safer to insert the stylet in all types of needles. The main disadvantage of Sprotte spinal needle is that it is technically more difficult to use than Quincke standard needle. Sprotte needle needs an introducer to insert up to the dura. It should not be pierce dura; therefore, the best results with atraumatic needles are depended in the experience of the physician. Sometimes it is not possible to perform LP with Sprotte needle and the physician has to change into the Quincke needle (Jager et al., 1993). It is possible that Sprotte needle will be damaged during the procedure because it needs more pressure and the sensation of cutting dura is different from the Quincke standard model (Benham, 1996).

The "pencil point" non-cutting needles of Whitacre or Sprotte had dull tips and an oval opening just proximal to the tip in contrast to the Quincke classic needles. Contrary to common use of those needles by anesthesiologists, many neurologists never heard anything about such needles and only 2% of neurologists use such needles (Evans, Armon et al., 2000). There are some reports confirming the use of small gauge non-cutting needle for spinal anesthesia especially in patients prone to PLPH (Halpern et al., 1994).

The amount of spinal fluid removed is not a risk factor for PLPH (Kuntz, Kokmen et al., 1992). There is not any Class 1 evidence confirming the effect of duration of recumbency in the bed after LP for preventing PLPH one century after Bier's recommendation (Bier, 1899) for staying in the bed at least for 24 hours (Corbett et al., 1983; Spriggs, Burn et al., 1992). However, many physicians still advise their patients staying in the bed for some hours. The role of psychological factors in the development of PLPH appears to be minimal. The frequency of PLPH without any awareness of the procedure was the same as in patients who were aware of the procedure (Raskin, 1990). The majority of headaches is self limited and will be resolved in 5 days. Bed rest is the simplest way of treatment. The patient stays on recumbent position and liberally takes fluids with a simple analgesic like acetaminophen, codeine, caffeine benzoate. Parenteral use of analgesics such as intravenous caffeine sodium benzoate by inactivating brain adenosine receptors may cause vasoconstriction (Raskin, 1990) and decreasing CSF pressure. Intramuscular NSAIDs such as piroxicam or diclofenac may be effective.

Injection of 20-30 ml of saline making an epidural saline patch may cause an increase in epidural pressure and stop headache abruptly (Bart et al., 1978; Baysinger et al., 1986). In refractory cases an epidural blood patch or epidural saline close to the site of puncture will be useful (Evans, Armon et al., 2000). The best place for administration of blood patch is the same interspace level of LP but in case of any problem it is better to use one space lower than the puncture site. In multiple punctures the lowest interspace is the best one (Evans, 1998). The recommended amount of the blood is 15-20 ml with a rate of 0.5 ml/sec. to achieve maximal benefit it would be better that the patient stays in decubitus position for 1-2 hours. The reported success rate is about 95% and it should not be earlier than 24 hours after LP (Tarkkila et al., 1989). Prophylactic epidural patch does not recommend and does not prevent PLPH (Berrettini et al., 1987). Epidural injection of blood may form a gelatinous tamponade over the dural hole that prevents CSF leakage and immediately stop headache (Raskin, 1990). Currently the cost of blood patch in the United States is about $1500 each time (Dakka, Warra et al., 2011). There is not any evidence for using oral or intravenous fluids to diminish headache after LP (Table 3).

Bed rest: Majority of patients are being improved in two days
Intravenous caffeine benzoate sodium (500 mg intravenous infusion)
Caffeinated beverages
Epidural blood patch
Epidural saline injection

Table 3. Treatment of post-lumbar puncture headache (PLPH).

7. Cerebral herniation

Another important and not commonly occurred complication of LP is cerebral (brain) herniation due to asymmetric increase in cranial vault or highly severe symmetrically increase in intracranial pressure. Theoretically, when the CSF is under increased pressure and there is an obstruction to the free flow between the supratentorial space and the thecal sac surrounding the spinal cord, removing spinal CSF under these circumstances would decrease the pressure below the tentorium cerebelli and allow the temporal lobes to be herniated downward, impinging on the brainstem. Increased intracranial pressure without the obstruction of CSF circulation usually does not have this catastrophic effect, for instance, in pseudotumor cerebri or acute bacterial meningitis (ABM) (Archer, 1993). In ABM brain herniation occurs in 5% of patients in which accounts for a significant proportion of deaths due to ABM (Joffe, 2007).

Rebaud et al. (Rebaud et al., 1988) in their study in a group of children with ABM reported that 86% had raised intracranial pressure (RICP). Intracranial hypertension defined as increased mean pressure more than 15 mmHg. Totally they analyzed intracranial pressure in 14 children with Glasgow Coma Scale (GCS) less than 7. The mean opening pressure in survivors and nonsurvivors were 14 ±6 and 55 ±25 mmHg, respectively. In another study Minns and his colleagues showed that 33 out of 35 patients with ABM had RICP (Minns et al., 1989). Those studies showed that RICP is common in ABM. This is attributed to hyperemia, impaired CSF outflow resistance and finally cerebral edema which is inflammatory in the earlier stages of the disease (Saez-Llorens et al., 2003). In most studies brain herniation defined as either pathologic confirmation at autopsy or at least two signs of herniation including loss of consciousness, asymmetric unresponsive pupillary dilatation, irregular respiration and/or respiratory arrest and finally decorticate/ decerebrate response or complete flaccidity (Rennick et al., 1993).

Korein *et al.* in a collection of 418 patients reported that only 1.2% of patients had brain herniation after LP (Korein et al., 1959; Joffe, 2007). It has been pointed out that regardless of ICP, LP may hasten herniation in patients with RICP only if brain shift is present. Sometimes it is a gradual process because of ongoing CSF leakage from the LP site or cerebral vascular engorgement and edema after LP (van Crevel et al., 2002). It should be reminded that herniation *after* LP does not necessarily means herniation *caused* by LP. It seems that LP cause herniation in patients with papilledema but it was not definitely approved (van Crevel, Hijdra et al., 2002).

There is strong evidence that when herniation occurs in ABM, it most often occurs shortly after an LP. Joffe in his review reported that 79% of cerebral herniation was occurred during the first 12 hours after LP, half of them in the first 3 hours (Joffe, 2007). The reported odds ratio for herniation occurring in the first 12 hours after the LP is 32.6 (95% CI, 8.5 to 117.3) (Rennick, Shann et al., 1993). Neuroimaging can provide the structural information from which pressure data must be inferred (Gower et al., 1987). Those findings include lateral shift of midline structures, loss of the suprachiasmatic and basilar cisterns, obliteration or shift of the fourth ventricle, obliteration of the superior cerebellar and quadrigeminal cisterns with sparing of the ambient cisterns. Fourth ventricle and quadrigeminal cistern should be visualized and open on CT; otherwise LP should not be done (Fig.5).

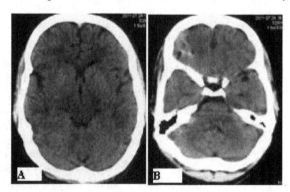

Fig. 5. Oblitration of quadrigeminal cistern (A) and fourth ventricle (B) in a patient with bacterial meningitis.

Only using very thin Quincke needles (26 G) or atraumatic Sprotte needles (22 G) reduce the incidence of herniation but it is unfeasible in practice but the incidence of brain herniation is not decreased by a head-down position (van Crevel, Hijdra et al., 2002). Therefore, a neuroimaging procedure is indicated prior to LP in all patients with papilledema, focal neurologic signs, significant altered level of consciousness or new onset seizure (during the last 24 hours) which are risk factors for abnormal CT scan (Kastenbauer, Winkler et al., 2002), however, very few patients in these studies had ABM. Patients with early signs of uncal or central cerebral herniation which is called "incipient herniation" are most vulnerable to complete the herniation process. Therefore, it seems that clinical signs and symptoms are the most reliable indicators of brain herniation after LP in the setting of ABM and normal brain CT scan (Joffe, 2007). The overall mortality of cerebral herniation after analysis of 8 articles was 60 out of 107 patients (56%). A good outcome for 51% of survivors (23 of 45) has been shown (Joffe, 2007). CT scan is more available in most emergency setting than MRI. However, CT cannot reliably estimate the risk of cerebral herniation after LP in ABM because of considerable variability in the size of lateral ventricles; decreased CSF absorption, decreased meningeal compliance due to meningeal inflammation and prevention of narrowing of the subarachnoid and ventricular spaces. Finally, a normal CTscan does not necessarily mean that an LP is safe. Avoiding LP also has two major risks. The first one is missing the exact cause of bacterial meningitis and appropriate treatment and the second one is misdiagnosis in some similar patients such as tuberculous meningitis (TBM), cerebral malaria, encephalitis and opportunistic infections in immunocompromised patients. Both consequences will postpone adequate therapy.

In conclusion, about 5% of patients with ABM have cerebral herniation, accounts for 30% of the ABM mortality. Although CT scan can reveal important data on the likelihood of herniation but a normal CT does not necessarily mean that LP is a safe procedure in ABM. Clinical correlation with impending signs of herniation is highly recommended for making decision. When herniation occurs it should be treated aggressively because there are many reports indicating good outcomes. In patients considered with signs of RICP, interventions to control ICP such as mannitol infusion (1gr/kg) and antibiotics should be started before a CT scan obtains and LP should *not* be performed. Hypertonic intravenous urea, mannitol, ventricular drainage, and in two studies, the "Lund protocol" of ICP management had been proposed for treatment of cerebral herniation after LP. The response to mannitol is often rapid. Some authors prescribe mannitol infusion 30-60 minutes before doing the procedure in patients with impending signs of herniation (Roos, 2003) but we do not recommend. Of course, the outcome is not dismal in many patients.

8. Bleeding (epidural or subdural hematoma/ subarachnoid hemorrhage)

Many patients complain back or low back pain after LP. Only simple reassurance and oral analgesics are enough except when there are neurological signs and symptoms concerning the involvement of spinal cord. Interventricular hemorrhage, subarachnoid hemorrhage (SAH) and spinal epidural hematoma have been reported after LP (Lee et al., 2009). Bleeding from small vessels of the ligamentum flavum or rupture of an epidural vein either by a sudden increase in the intra-abdominal pressure impacting on a previously damaged or weakened vein or by mild trauma can also cause spinal epidural hematomas (Gurkanlar et al., 2007). Sometime penetration of Adamkiewicz artery and/or vein is the responsible etiology (Scott et al., 1989). Progressive paraparesis, saddle anesthesia, low back pain and sphincter incontinence are the major neurological findings (Sweasey et al., 1992).

Those symptoms are completed in hours or days. Emergency MR scanning of the spinal cord is the first diagnostic procedure and early surgical decompression is mandatory. While patients with bleeding diathesis are more prone to local bleeding, SAH or intracranial subdural hematoma (uni- or bilateral) are usually seen in healthy individuals. The responsible mechanism is probably due to traction on bridging veins secondary to intracranial hypotension. Subdural hematoma may occur anywhere in the cranial vault but SAH may be presented in the territory of a fragile aneurysm (Vos et al., 1991).

9. Infection

Inadequate sterilization of the skin or a breach in the aseptic technique may induce rare but important complications of LP such as purulent meningitis or disc space infection. However, subcutaneous and/or epidural abscesses are sometimes reported. The most frequent causes are intravenous drug abuse, diabetes mellitus, trauma, alcohol abuse, wound infection, multiple medical illnesses and prior spinal surgery (Kamiyama, 2006). There are different ways to contaminate the skin: contamination of the skin site and subsequent spread along the needle track, by hematological spread, or by intraluminar contamination via a contaminated syringe or contaminated local anesthetic solution (Phillips et al., 2002).

Infectious complications ranging from vertebral osteomyelitis, discitis, epidural abscess, and bacterial meningitis have reported in the literature. In another study it was revealed that in consecutive neuroradiological procedures requiring LP, bacterial meningitis occurred with an incidence of 0.2% soon after the procedure (Domingo et al., 1994). The clinical signs and symptoms of vertebral discitis include pain, local tenderness, irritability, and spinal irritation usually two weeks after the procedure (Bhatoe et al., 1994). Lumbar puncture for analysis of CSF at different interspace other than the original puncture site is mandatory. The process of active degeneration to fusion takes about 6 to 24 months. One case report described retroperitoneal abscess that occurred after dural laceration and penetration of infected CSF to the abdominal cavity (Levine et al., 1982).

10. Contraindications

Lumbar puncture is an extremely safe procedure when performed by an experienced physician using standard methods and techniques (Table 4). LP is contraindicated in patients with asymmetric increase in cerebral pressure in one part of cranial cavity. It should not be performed when fourth ventricle or quadrigeminal cistern was not visualized. Other contraindications are spinal epidural abscess or subdural empyema because of telescopic herniation of the spinal cord or introducing infection into the spinal subarachnoid space when the abscess or empyema located in lumbar region. Lumbar puncture is also contraindicated in patients on coumadin therapy or platelet count less than 50,000/μL, shock with cardiorespiratory compromise and local superficial infection at the site where LP should be done. When there is thrombocytopenia and strong clinical indication for an LP, particularly in patients whose platelet count is below 20,000 per cubic milliliter, platelets should be transfused just prior to the procedure to reduce the risk of a procedure-related hemorrhage. Nevertheless, the risk of epidural or subdural hematoma should also be diminished before performing LP (Edelson et al., 1974).

Evidence of intracranial mass lesion
Evidence of midline shift on cranial CT/ MRI
Presence of posterior fossa tumor
Platelet count less than 50,000 per cubic milliliter
INR greater than 1.5
Poor visualization of quadrigeminal cistern or fourth ventricle
Known suppurative infection in the lumbar region
Presence of spinal subarachnoid block

Table 4. Contraindications to lumbar puncture.

11. Normal cerebrospinal fluid analyses

After performing LP the gross appearance of CSF should be noted. A complete CSF analysis can assist in the diagnosis and management of many central and peripheral nervous system disorders. Normally the CSF is clear and colorless. One of the strongest indications for urgent LP is suppurative infections of CNS. It should be examined for cells (white and red blood cells), microorganisms (bacteria, fungi, mycobacteria, cryptococcal antigen, herpes and cytomegalovirus DNA), protein and glucose content, gammaglobulines and cytological study for tumor cells. CSF will be changed in all patients with inflammatory, infectious, neoplastic and sometimes degenerative central or peripheral nervous system disorders.

11.1 Pressure and dynamics

An opening pressure should be measured in all patients with altered level of consciousness, papilledema, hydrocephalus and infections of the central nervous system. The upper limit of normal CSF pressure in lateral recumbent position is 110 mmH$_2$O in infants, 150 mmH$_2$O in children, 180 mmH$_2$O in adults and 200-250 mmH$_2$O in obese individuals (Corbett and Mehta, 1983). Pressure less than 50 mmH$_2$O indicates intracranial hypotension due to CSF leakage or severe dehydration. CSF must be measured in recumbent position. When it is measured in sitting position, the fluid may rise to the cisterna magna but not to the ventricle level because of presence of negative pressure in the closed cranial cavity. Pressure in this situation is about two times higher than recumbent position (Ropper and Samuels, 2009).

11.2 Cells

During the first month of life CSF contains a small number of leukocytes. Beyond this period, in uninfected CSF the number of leukocyte (WBC) count is zero to five mononuclear cells (monocytes or lymphocytes) per cubic milliliter. CSF should not contain polymorphonuclear (PMN) in the uninfected CSF. However, if the total number of cells is less than five, the presence of one PMN per cubic milliliter is not considered abnormal. Counting leukocytes needs an ordinary chamber but identification needs Wright stain of the centrifuged sediment. A "traumatic tap" will be occurred when a radicular artery or epidural venous plexus is penetrated with the spinal needle and blood is introduced into the spinal fluid. In this situation, to calculate the true number of WBC count in the CSF one WBC per cubic milliliter for every 700 RBC per cubic milliliter is subtracted from the total number of the WBC count in the CSF. In case of traumatic tap in the collection tube, a clot or a thread of blood will be seen in the CSF. When a small amount of blood entered into the CSF, it is possible to collect CSF after dripping for a few seconds but in case of more amounts of blood it is necessary to change the position of needle and enter into the another interspace. The presence of 200 RBC per cubic milliliter cause a ground-glass appearance, 1000-6000 RBC per cubic milliliter imparts a hazy pink to red color and several hundreds of WBC per cubic milliliter (pleocytosis) induces a slight opaque haziness of the CSF color, respectively (Ropper and Samuels, 2009).

To distinguish a traumatic (bloody) tap from SAH the number of RBCs and WBCs remains in the first and it will be diminished in third or fourth tube. In SAH the CSF color remains pink-tinged through all tubes and the supernatant is xanthochromic (yellow-brown) after CSF centrifuge. Xanthochromia will be occurred 2 to 12 hours after SAH and persists for a few weeks. The reason for rapid hemolysis of RBCs in the spinal fluid after SAH is not clear.

In case of multiple punctures of the radicular arteries of different interspaces it is possible that the CSF color became blood tinged due to entrance of RBCs in to the subarachnoid space. Special immunochemical staining and electron microscopy will be helpful for the diagnosis of malignant cells in the CSF (Bigner, 1992).

11.3 Glucose

The concentration of glucose in the CSF depends on the serum glucose. Normal CSF glucose concentration is between 45 and 80 mg/dL when the serum glucose is between 70 and 120 mg/dL or approximately two thirds of serum glucose (about 0.6 to 0.7 serum glucose). CSF glucose range is in parallel with higher level of blood glucose. With marked hyperglycemia the ratio is lower (0.5-0.6) and with marked hypoglycemia the ratio is greater (0.85). Hyperglycemia will mask hypoglycorrhachia, however, CSF glucose less than 45 mg/dL will be considered abnormal (Fishman, 1992a) and values less than 35 mg/dL are always abnormal (Ropper and Samuels, 2009). It takes 2-4 hours after intravenous glucose injection to have equilibrium with CSF glucose. Therefore it is mandatory to measure serum glucose level at the time of LP. In normal individuals CSF/serum glucose ratio is about 0.6 and CSF/glucose ratio less than 0.6 considered to be abnormal.

11.4 Protein

In contrast to the high concentration of protein in the blood (5500 to 8000 mg/dL) the protein concentration of CSF is low. Protein concentration is also diminished in a rostral-caudal direction in the neuroaxis. It reflects a ventriculo-lumbar gradient in the permeability of capillary endothelial cells to protein. The upper ranges of normal cisternal and lumbar CSF protein are 30 and 50 mg/dL in adults, respectively. The choroidal and meningeal perfusion is also increased in bacterial meningitis.

12. Cerebrospinal fluid analysis for bacterial meningitis

Independent of the causative agent of bacterial meningitis, CSF findings in acute bacterial meningitis are often similar. The major determinants of CSF profile are the time duration between performing LP and the onset of infection, severity of the disease, clinical setting in which the infection was acquired and the immune state of the patient (Venkatesan et al., 2009). The opening pressure is typically increased in almost all patients. In 90% of cases the opening pressure is over 200 mmH$_2$O, in 20% more than 400 mmH$_2$O and in 15% of patients it is more than 500 mmH$_2$O (Durand et al., 1993; Venkatesan and Griffin, 2009). Pressure will increase parallel with the progression of the disease and it returns normal with recovery. However, it should be concerned that the normal pressure values are different between different age groups. Minns *et al.* reported that RICP was found in 33 out of 35 infants with bacterial meningitis with a median pressure of 204 mmH$_2$O. They concluded that RICP is a frequent accompaniment of childhood meningitis and may need treatment in its own right and is an important factor influencing the course and outcome of childhood meningitis (Minns, Engleman et al., 1989).

At the time of first LP in bacterial meningitis, the cell count of CSF is almost always between 1,000 to 10,000 WBC/mm^3; and rarely is less than 100 or greater than 20,000 WBC/mm^3. Findings are remarkably the same, regardless of the type of causative organism. A recent study in Alberta, Canada revealed that the cellular abnormality in the CSF did not change over the last fifty years (Hussein et al., 2000). In 90-95% of patients PMN accounts for the total WBC count of the CSF and in less than one quarter of cases do PMNs comprise less than 80% of the total leukocyte count (Venkatesan and Griffin, 2009). However, the CSF leukocyte count may be changed during the antibiotic therapy.

The basics for CSF diagnostic studies for meningitis include cell count with differentiation, measuring protein and glucose concentration, Veneral Disease Research Laboratories (VDRL) slide flocculation test, Gram stain and culture for bacterial pathogens. Hypoglycorrhachia in the presence of pleocytosis is usually diagnostic for pyogenic, tuberculous or fungal meningitis. Other studies are not routinely done in many centers especially in countries with poor resources such as latex agglutination for bacterial pathogens involving in the pathogenesis of bacterial meningitis, India ink for Cryptococcal surface antigen, and other fungal culture, Histoplasma polysacharride antigen, viral specific IgG and IgM for mosquito borne viral encephalitis, polymerase chain reaction (PCR) for HIV, Herpes viruses and enteroviruses. Smear for acid fast bacilli and culture for *Mycobacterium tuberculosis* are especially important diagnostic procedures to be done in countries with high incidence of tuberculosis. *Borrelia burgdorferi* antibodies for Lyme disease in endemic region should also be considered.

The CSF glucose content at first LP is usually moderately to severely reduced. In 75% of patients it is less than 50 mg/dL and in 25% of cases it is less than 10 mg/dL (Hussein and Shafran, 2000). For a long time it was assumed that bacteria use glucose in the CSF of patients with bacterial meningitis but the CSF glucose level stays at a subnormal level two weeks after effective treatment of bacterial meningitis. It suggests that polymorphonuclear leukocytes and cells of the adjacent brain tissue may consume glucose in anaerobic way increasing the lactate level of the CSF. Probably an inhibition entry mechanism of glucose into the CSF may be operative. The CSF glucose level may spuriously low, if CSF remains for a long time in room temperature. The normal range for CSF/serum glucose ratio is >0.6 however in another study of 217 patients with confirmed bacterial meningitis, the ratio was less than 0.23 (Spanos et al., 1989). Low glucose values in the CSF have been reported in patients with viral infections such as herpes simplex, zoster and mumps meningoencephalitis (Ropper and Samuels, 2009).

The CSF protein concentration is almost always increased. In more than 80% of patients the absolute value is more than 80mg/dL (Spanos, Harrell et al., 1989). In less than 8% of cases the protein concentration is greater than 1000 mg/dL, is often associated with subarachnoid block (Venkatesan and Griffin, 2009). Schutte *et al.* (Schutte et al., 1998) reported a good correlation between both the GCS and CSF-protein level on admission and the outcome of patients with meningitis was found, with the GCS value being a better prognostic indicator than high CSF protein levels. In their study CSF protein content was five times higher in patients with severe neurological deficit comparing to patients without any detectable deficit. The protein content of CSF in this situation often reaches to 500 mg/dL or more but viral infection with lymphocytic pleocytosis has lesser elevation of protein usually between 50-100 mg/dL; sometimes normal. In patients with meningeal irritation due to parameningeal infections (meningismus) protein value of the CSF is low. Values more than 1000 mg/dL is deeply yellow in color and may clot in the tube because of high content of fibrinogen which is called Froin syndrome.

13. Conclusions

Although collecting and analyzing CSF is an important part of diagnostic and sometimes therapeutic process in the management of various diseases but it needs careful search for contraindications and problems associated with the procedure. A complete description of the procedure and its possible complications to the patient is mandatory and legally important. The experienced physician also estimates how much sample must be obtained and which kind of especial laboratory analysis should be done before starting the procedure. Therefore, prompt delivery of samples to laboratory may reduce the risk of spurious reports.

14. References

Archer, B. D. (1993). "Computed tomography before lumbar puncture in acute meningitis: a review of the risks and benefits." *CMAJ* 148(6): 961-965, ISSN 0820-3946

Bart, A. J. and A. S. Wheeler (1978). "Comparison of epidural saline placement and epidural blood placement in the treatment of post-lumbar-puncture headache." *Anesthesiology* 48(3): 221-223, ISSN 0003-3022.

Baxter, A. L., J. C. Welch, B. L. Burke and D. J. Isaacman (2004). "Pain, position, and stylet styles: infant lumbar puncture practices of pediatric emergency attending physicians." *Pediatr Emerg Care* 20(12): 816-820, ISSN 1535-1815

Baysinger, C. L., E. J. Menk, E. Harte and R. Middaugh (1986). "The successful treatment of dural puncture headache after failed epidural blood patch." *Anesth Analg* 65(11): 1242-1244, ISSN 0003-2999

Benham, M. (1996). "Spinal needle damage during routine clinical practice." *Anaesthesia* 51(9): 843-845, ISSN 0003-2409

Berrettini, W. H., S. Simmons-Alling and J. I. Nurnberger, Jr. (1987). "Epidural blood patch does not prevent headache after lumbar puncture." *Lancet* 1(8537): 856-857, ISSN 0140-6736

Bhatoe, H. S., H. S. Gill, N. Kumar and S. Biswas (1994). "Post lumbar puncture discitis and vertebral collapse." *Postgrad Med J* 70(830): 882-884, ISSN 0032-5473

Bier, A. (1899). "Versuche uber Cocainisirung des Ruckenmarkes." *Deutsche Zeitschrift fur Chirurgie* 51: 361-369.

Bigner, S. H. (1992). "Cerebrospinal fluid (CSF) cytology: current status and diagnostic applications." *J Neuropathol Exp Neurol* 51(3): 235-245, ISSN 0022-3069

Bolder, P. M. (1986). "Postlumbar puncture headache in pediatric oncology patients." *Anesthesiology* 65(6): 696-698, ISSN 0003-3022

Boon, J. M., P. H. Abrahams, J. H. Meiring and T. Welch (2004). "Lumbar puncture: anatomical review of a clinical skill." *Clin Anat* 17(7): 544-553, ISSN 0897-3806

Broome, I. J. (1993). "Hearing loss and dural puncture." *Lancet* 341(8846): 667-668, ISSN 0140-6736

Carson, D. and M. Serpell (1996). "Choosing the best needle for diagnostic lumbar puncture." *Neurology* 47(1): 33-37, ISSN 0028-3878

Corbett, J. J. and M. P. Mehta (1983). "Cerebrospinal fluid pressure in normal obese subjects and patients with pseudotumor cerebri." *Neurology* 33(10): 1386-1388, ISSN 0028-3878

Dahlgren, N. and K. Tornebrandt (1995). "Neurological complications after anaesthesia. A follow-up of 18,000 spinal and epidural anaesthetics performed over three years." *Acta Anaesthesiol Scand* 39(7): 872-880, ISSN 0001-5172

Dakka, Y., N. Warra, R. J. Albadareen, M. Jankowski, et al. (2011). "Headache rate and cost of care following lumbar puncture at a single tertiary care hospital." *Neurology* 77(1): 71-74, ISSN 1526-632X

Domingo, P., J. Mancebo, L. Blanch, P. Coll, et al. (1994). "Iatrogenic streptococcal meningitis." *Clin Infect Dis* 19(2): 356-357, ISSN 1058-4838

Dripps, R. D. and L. D. Vandam (1951). "Hazards of lumbar puncture." *J Am Med Assoc* 147(12): 1118-1121, ISSN 0002-9955

Durand, M. L., S. B. Calderwood, D. J. Weber, S. I. Miller, et al. (1993). "Acute bacterial meningitis in adults. A review of 493 episodes." *N Engl J Med* 328(1): 21-28, ISSN 0028-4793

Edelson, R. N., N. L. Chernik and J. B. Posner (1974). "Spinal subdural hematomas complicating lumbar puncture." *Arch Neurol* 31(2): 134-137, ISSN 0003-9942

Eskey, C. J. and C. S. Ogilvy (2001). "Fluoroscopy-guided lumbar puncture: decreased frequency of traumatic tap and implications for the assessment of CT-negative acute subarachnoid hemorrhage." *AJNR Am J Neuroradiol* 22(3): 571-576, ISSN 0195-6108

Evans, R. W. (1998). "Complications of lumbar puncture." *Neurol Clin* 16(1): 83-105, ISSN 0733-8619

Evans, R. W., C. Armon, E. M. Frohman and D. S. Goodin (2000). "Assessment: prevention of post-lumbar puncture headaches: report of the therapeutics and technology assessment subcommittee of the american academy of neurology." *Neurology* 55(7): 909-914, ISSN 0028-3878

Fishman, R. A. (1992a). Composition of the cerebrospinal fluid. In: *Fishman RA, ed. Cerebrospinal Fluid in Diseases of the Nervous System.* WB Saunders, ISBN 07216-35571. Philadelphia: 183-252.

Fishman, R. A. (1992b). Examination of the cerebrospinal fluid: techniques and complications. In: *Fishman RA, ed. Cerebrospinal Fluid in Diseases of the Nervous System.* WB Saunders, ISBN 07216-35571. Philadelphia: 157-182.

Flaatten, H., T. Thorsen, B. Askeland, M. Finne, et al. (1998). "Puncture technique and postural postdural puncture headache. A randomised, double-blind study comparing transverse and parallel puncture." *Acta Anaesthesiol Scand* 42(10): 1209-1214, ISSN 0001-5172

Frederiks, J. A. and P. J. Koehler (1997). "The first lumbar puncture." *J Hist Neurosci* 6(2): 147-153, ISSN 0964-704X

Gower, D. J., A. L. Baker, W. O. Bell and M. R. Ball (1987). "Contraindications to lumbar puncture as defined by computed cranial tomography." *J Neurol Neurosurg Psychiatry* 50(8): 1071-1074, ISSN 0022-3050

Gurkanlar, D., C. Acikbas, G. K. Cengiz and R. Tuncer (2007). "Lumbar epidural hematoma following lumbar puncture: the role of high dose LMWH and late surgery. A case report." *Neurocirugia (Astur)* 18(1): 52-55, ISSN 1130-1473

Halpern, S. and R. Preston (1994). "Postdural puncture headache and spinal needle design. Metaanalyses." *Anesthesiology* 81(6): 1376-1383, ISSN 0003-3022.

Hart, J. R. and R. J. Whitacre (1951). "Pencil-point needle in prevention of postspinal headache." *JAMA* 147(7): 657-658, ISSN 0002-9955

Hasbun, R., J. Abrahams, J. Jekel and V. J. Quagliarello (2001). "Computed tomography of the head before lumbar puncture in adults with suspected meningitis." *N Engl J Med* 345(24): 1727-1733, ISSN 0028-4793

Hussein, A. S. and S. D. Shafran (2000). "Acute bacterial meningitis in adults. A 12-year review." *Medicine (Baltimore)* 79(6): 360-368, ISSN 0025-7974

Jager, H., M. Krane and K. Schimrigk (1993). "[Lumbar puncture--the post-puncture syndrome. Prevention with an "atraumatic" puncture needle, clinical observations]." *Schweiz Med Wochenschr* 123(42): 1985-1990, ISSN 0036-7672

Joffe, A. R. (2007). "Lumbar puncture and brain herniation in acute bacterial meningitis: a review." *J Intensive Care Med* 22(4): 194-207, ISSN 0885-0666

Kamiyama, Y. (2006). "Two cases of spinal epidural abscess with granulation tissue associated with epidural catheterization." *J Anesth* 20(2): 102-105, ISSN 0913-8668

Kastenbauer, S., F. Winkler and H. W. Pfister (2002). "Cranial CT before lumbar puncture in suspected meningitis." *N Engl J Med* 346(16): 1248-1251, ISSN 1533-4406

Korein, J., H. Cravioto and M. Leicach (1959). "Reevaluation of lumbar puncture; a study of 129 patients with papilledema or intracranial hypertension." *Neurology* 9(4): 290-297, ISSN 0028-3878.

Kuntz, K. M., E. Kokmen, J. C. Stevens, P. Miller, et al. (1992). "Post-lumbar puncture headaches: experience in 501 consecutive procedures." *Neurology* 42(10): 1884-1887, ISSN 0028-3878.

Lee, S. J., Y. Y. Lin, C. W. Hsu, S. J. Chu, et al. (2009). "Intraventricular hematoma, subarachnoid hematoma and spinal epidural hematoma caused by lumbar puncture: an unusual complication." *Am J Med Sci* 337(2): 143-145, ISSN 0002-9629

Levine, J. F., E. M. Hiesiger, M. A. Whelan, A. A. Pollock, et al. (1982). "Pneumococcal meningitis associated with retroperitoneal abscess. A rare complication of lumbar puncture." *JAMA* 248(18): 2308-2309, ISSN 0098-7484

Lybecker, H. and T. Andersen (1995a). "Repetitive hearing loss following dural puncture treated with autologous epidural blood patch." *Acta Anaesthesiol Scand* 39(7): 987-989, ISSN 0001-5172

Lybecker, H., M. Djernes and J. F. Schmidt (1995b). "Postdural puncture headache (PDPH): onset, duration, severity, and associated symptoms. An analysis of 75 consecutive patients with PDPH." *Acta Anaesthesiol Scand* 39(5): 605-612, ISSN 0001-5172

Lybecker, H., J. T. Moller, O. May and H. K. Nielsen (1990). "Incidence and prediction of postdural puncture headache. A prospective study of 1021 spinal anesthesias." *Anesth Analg* 70(4): 389-394, ISSN 0003-2999.

Minns, R. A., H. M. Engleman and H. Stirling (1989). "Cerebrospinal fluid pressure in pyogenic meningitis." *Arch Dis Child* 64(6): 814-820, ISSN 1468-2044

Muller, B., K. Adelt, H. Reichmann and K. Toyka (1994). "Atraumatic needle reduces the incidence of post-lumbar puncture syndrome." *J Neurol* 241(6): 376-380, ISSN 0340-5354

Norris, M. C., B. L. Leighton and C. A. DeSimone (1989). "Needle bevel direction and headache after inadvertent dural puncture." *Anesthesiology* 70(5): 729-731, ISSN 0003-3022

Peterson, M. A. and J. Abele (2005). "Bedside ultrasound for difficult lumbar puncture." *J Emerg Med* 28(2): 197-200, ISSN 0736-4679

Phillips, J. M., J. C. Stedeford, E. Hartsilver and C. Roberts (2002). "Epidural abscess complicating insertion of epidural catheters." *Br J Anaesth* 89(5): 778-782, ISSN 0007-0912

Raskin, N. H. (1990). "Lumbar puncture headache: a review." *Headache* 30(4): 197-200, ISSN 0017-8748

Rebaud, P., J. C. Berthier, E. Hartemann and D. Floret (1988). "Intracranial pressure in childhood central nervous system infections." *Intensive Care Med* 14(5): 522-525, ISSN 0342-4642

Rennick, G., F. Shann and J. de Campo (1993). "Cerebral herniation during bacterial meningitis in children." *BMJ* 306(6883): 953-955, ISSN 0959-8138

Roos, K. (2003). "Lumbar puncture." *Semin Neurol* 23(1): 105-114.

Ropper, A. H. and M. A. Samuels (2009). Special techniques for neurologic diagnosis: Introduction. In: *Adams and victor's principles of neurology*. McGraw-Hill, ISBN 0071-469710. New York: 11-32.

Saez-Llorens, X. and G. H. McCracken, Jr. (2003). "Bacterial meningitis in children." *Lancet* 361(9375): 2139-2148, ISSN 1474-547X

Schutte, C. M. and C. H. van der Meyden (1998). "A prospective study of Glasgow Coma Scale (GCS), age, CSF-neutrophil count, and CSF-protein and glucose levels as prognostic indicators in 100 adult patients with meningitis." *J Infect* 37(2): 112-115, 0163-4453

Scott, E. W., C. R. Cazenave and C. Virapongse (1989). "Spinal subarachnoid hematoma complicating lumbar puncture: diagnosis and management." *Neurosurgery* 25(2): 287-292; discussion 292-283, 0148-396X

Spanos, A., F. E. Harrell, Jr. and D. T. Durack (1989). "Differential diagnosis of acute meningitis. An analysis of the predictive value of initial observations." *JAMA* 262(19): 2700-2707, 0098-7484

Spriggs, D. A., D. J. Burn, J. French, N. E. Cartlidge, et al. (1992). "Is bed rest useful after diagnostic lumbar puncture?" *Postgrad Med J* 68(801): 581-583, 0032-5473

Sprotte, G., R. Schedel and H. Pajunk (1987). "[An "atraumatic" universal needle for single-shot regional anesthesia: clinical results and a 6 year trial in over 30,000 regional anesthesias]." *Reg Anaesth* 10(3): 104-108, ISSN 0171-1946

Strupp, M., T. Brandt and A. Muller (1998). "Incidence of post-lumbar puncture syndrome reduced by reinserting the stylet: a randomized prospective study of 600 patients." *J Neurol* 245(9): 589-592, ISSN 0340-5354

Sweasey, T. A., H. C. Coester, H. Rawal, M. Blaivas, et al. (1992). "Ligamentum flavum hematoma. Report of two cases." *J Neurosurg* 76(3): 534-537, ISSN 0022-3085

Tarkkila, P. J., J. A. Miralles and E. A. Palomaki (1989). "The subjective complications and efficiency of the epidural blood patch in the treatment of postdural puncture headache." *Reg Anesth* 14(5): 247-250, ISSN 0146-521X

Tourtellotte, W. W., W. G. Henderson, R. P. Tucker, O. Gilland, et al. (1972). "A randomized, double-blind clinical trial comparing the 22 versus 26 gauge needle in the production of the post-lumbar puncture syndrome in normal individuals." *Headache* 12(2): 73-78, ISSN 0017-8748 van Crevel, H., A. Hijdra and J. de Gans (2002). "Lumbar puncture and the risk of herniation: when should we first perform CT?" *J Neurol* 249(2): 129-137, ISSN 0340-5354

Venkatesan, A. and D. E. Griffin (2009). Bacterial infections. In: *Cerebrospinal fluid in clinical practice.* Saunders-Elsevier, ISBN 978-1-4160-2908-3. Philadelphia: 167-175.

Vilming, S. T. and R. Kloster (1998). "Pain location and associated symptoms in post-lumbar puncture headache." *Cephalalgia* 18(10): 697-703, ISSN 0333-1024

Vos, P. E., W. A. de Boer, J. A. Wurzer and J. van Gijn (1991). "Subdural hematoma after lumbar puncture: two case reports and review of the literature." *Clin Neurol Neurosurg* 93(2): 127-132, ISSN 0303-8467

Weisman, L. E., G. B. Merenstein and J. R. Steenbarger (1983). "The effect of lumbar puncture position in sick neonates." *Am J Dis Child* 137(11): 1077-1079, ISSN 0002-922X

4

Emergent Procedure Training in the 21st Century

Ernest E. Wang

NorthShore University HealthSystem,University of Chicago Pritzker School of Medicine
USA

1. Introduction

Procedural competency is a substantial part of the emergency physician's (EP) skill set. Emergency Medicine (EM) is unique in that the practicing EP must be comfortable with a wide array of procedures that have the following features: 1) They span the entire human body and cross many disciplines in medicine and surgery; 2) There are both invasive and non-invasive procedures; 3) They occur at unpredictable frequencies and never on a schedule; 4) They often need to performed under significant time-pressure; and 5) The patients they need to be performed on are often critically ill and unstable.

The Model of the Clinical Practice of Emergency Medicine (EM Model) serves as the guide for the content expertise that EPs are expected to have as active practitioners in the specialty. The EM Model was first developed in 2001 by the Core Content Task Force II and involved the collaboration of six EM organizations: the American Board of Emergency Medicine (ABEM), the American College of Emergency Physicians (ACEP), the Council of Emergency Medicine Residency Directors (CORD), the Emergency Medicine Residents' Association (EMRA), the Residency Review Committee for Emergency Medicine (RRC-EM), and the Society for Academic Emergency Medicine (SAEM).(1) It has undergone biannual revisions with the most recent revision in 2009. The EM Model specifies the types of procedures representative of the domain of emergency medicine (Table 1).(2) These include procedures such as: airway techniques, anesthetic techniques, bedside and procedural ultrasonography, obstetrics, resuscitation, head and neck procedures, thoracic procedures, skeletal procedures, vascular access, wound management, genitourinary procedures, gastrointestinal procedures, lumbar puncture, and others.

The procedures in the EM Model can be roughly divided into two groups, high and low frequency, and two types, higher and lower risk (Table 2). EPs need to be able to perform high frequency procedures precisely and reliably so as to minimize complications and morbidity. EPs need to be able to be proficient with infrequent high risk procedures so that when the situation arises (usually unpredictably and under significant time pressure), they have the greatest chance to complete the procedure successfully.

Prior to the advent of simulation-based trainers, traditional training opportunities consisted of cadaveric experience or through the apprenticeship model, succinctly described by the ubiquitous medical adage "See one, do one, teach one." These methods provided limited training opportunities due to expense and scarcity (cadavers) or due to unpredictable

Airway Techniques
  Airway adjuncts
  Cricothyrotomy
  Foreign body removal
  Intubation
  Mechanical ventilation
  Percutaneous transtracheal ventilation
  Capnometry
  Non-invasive ventilatory management

Anesthesia
  Local
  Regional nerve block
  Sedation - analgesia for procedures

Blood, Fluid, and Component Therapy Administration

Diagnostic Procedures
  Anoscopy
  Arthrocentesis
  Bedside ultrasonography
  Cystourethrogram
  Lumbar puncture
  Nasogastric tube
  Paracentesis
  Pericardiocentesis
  Slit lamp examination
  Thoracentesis
  Tonometry
  Compartment pressure measurement

Genital/Urinary
  Bladder catheterization
    o Foley catheter
    o Suprapubic
  Testicular detorsion

Head and Neck
  Control of epistaxis
    Laryngoscopy
  Drainage of peritonsillar abscess
  Removal of rust ring
  Tooth stabilization
  Lateral canthotomy

Hemodynamic Techniques
  Arterial catheter insertion

Central venous access
Intraosseous infusion
Peripheral venous cutdown

Obstetrics
  Delivery of newborn

Other Techniques
  Excision of thrombosed hemorrhoids
  Foreign body removal
  Gastric lavage
  Gastrostomy tube replacement
  Incision/Drainage
  Pain management
  Violent patient management/restraint
  Sexual assault examination
  Trephination, nails
  Wound closure techniques
  Wound management
  Procedural ultrasonography
  Escharotomy

Resuscitation
  Cardiopulmonary resuscitation (CPR)
  Neonatal resuscitation

Skeletal Procedures
  Fracture/Dislocation immobilization techniques
  Fracture/Dislocation reduction techniques
  Spine immobilization techniques

Thoracic
  Cardiac pacing
    o Cutaneous
    o Transvenous
  Defibrillation/Cardioversion
  Thoracostomy
  Thoracotomy

Exposure Management
  Personal Protection (equipment and techniques)
  Decontamination

* Adapted from the 2009 Model of the Clinical Practice of Emergency Medicine

Table 1. Procedures and Skills Integral to the Practice of Emergency Medicine*.

	Higher frequency	Lower frequency
Higher risk	• Airway adjuncts (nasopharyngeal airway, oropharyngeal airway) • Intubation • Mechanical ventilation • Capnometry • Non-invasive ventilatory management • Sedation – analgesia for procedures • Blood, Fluid, and Component Therapy Administration • Lumbar puncture • Control of epistaxis (posterior) • Arterial catheter insertion • Central venous access • Cardiopulmonary resuscitation • Fracture/dislocation reduction techniques • Thoracostomy	• Cricothyrotomy • Foreign body removal (Airway) • Percutaneous transtracheal ventilation • Cystourethrogram • Pericardiocentesis • Thoracentesis • Compartment pressure measurement • Bladder catheterization (Suprapubic) • Drainage of peritonsillar abscess • Removal of rust ring • Lateral canthotomy • Peripheral venous cutdown • Delivery of newborn • Gastric lavage • Escharotomy • Neonatal resuscitation • Cutaneous cardiac pacing • Transvenous cardiac pacing • Thoracotomy
Lower risk	• Local anesthesia • Anoscopy • Arthrocentesis • Bedside Ultrasound • Procedural Ultrasound • Nasogastric tube • Slit lamp examination • Tonometry • Bladder catheterization (Foley) • Control of epistaxis (anterior) • Laryngoscopy • Intraosseous infusion • Incision and drainage • Nail trephination • Wound closure techniques • Fracture/dislocation immobilization techniques	• Regional anesthesia • Paracentesis • Tooth stabilization • Excision of thrombosed hemorrhoid • Foreign body removal (ear, nose, skin) • Gastrostomy tube replacement

** Categorization of the procedures in this table recognizes that local variations in procedural frequency exist and relative risk is dictated by patient co-morbidities and clinical presentation.

Table 2. Categorization of EM Model Procedures by frequency and risk**.

chance presentations (clinical patient care). As a result, it was not uncommon for residency-trained graduates to have little or no experience with rarely performed procedures. It also resulted in the potential for incomplete or unrefined command of the necessary steps for successful completion of complex or high stress procedures. Recent changes in residency work hour restrictions may also lead to limitations in clinical patient contact. The RRC-EM has recommended that residency graduates be exposed to a core group of procedures and resuscitations during residency training (Table 3).(3) The guidelines specify that these experiences may occur during patient care or in simulations.

Adult medical resuscitation	45
Adult trauma resuscitation	35
ED Bedside ultrasound	*
Cardiac pacing	06
Central venous access	20
Chest tubes	10
Procedural sedation	15
Cricothyrotomy	03
Disclocation reduction	10
Intubations	35
Lumbar Puncture	15
Pediatric medical resuscitation	15
Pediatric trauma resuscitation	10
Pericardiocentesis	03
Vaginal delivery	10

* Covered in separate Procedural Competency Guideline recommendations in the RRC-EM guidelines

Table 3. RRC-EM Recommended Guidelines for Procedures and Resuscitations.

2. Procedural skill acquisition

In the 21st century, the "See one, do one, teach one" model has been rendered outmoded by the several factors. The general patient public is growing intolerant of being used as a training vehicle for novices and will often decline procedures from physicians with little experience. The Institute of Medicine's 1999 report, "To Err is Human" has propelled the patient safety movement in health care so that practitioners are have become more aware of there responsibilities to patients to first do no harm. Finally, the emergence of realistic procedural task trainers have brought simulation-based training to the forefront of medicine as a way to bridge the experiential gap between the novice and the expert.

Ziv et al. described physicians' moral imperative to use simulation-based training as this: "The use of simulation wherever feasible conveys a critical educational and ethical message to all: patients are to be protected whenever possible and they are not commodities to be used as conveniences of training."(4) Studies have shown that patients are more willing to have procedure performed on them by physicians who have undergone simulation training first. (5-7)

The guiding principle behind the efficacy of simulation-based procedural training is the concept of "deliberate practice" (DP). According to Dr. K Anders Ericsson, "Expert performance can be traced to active engagement in deliberate practice (DP), where training (often designed and arranged by their teachers and coaches) is focused on improving particular tasks. DP also involves the provision of immediate feedback, time for problem-solving and evaluation, and opportunities for repeated performance to refine behavior."(8) McGaghie et al. have further defined the necessary conditions for DP to be effective (Table 4).(9-10) These features are listed in order of reported frequency (percent) among the final BEME pool of 109 articles.These include immediate feedback, repetition, increasing levels of difficulty, clinical variation, simulation providing valid representation of clinical practice, and a controlled environment.(9-10)

1. Feedback is provided during learning experiences	(47%)
2. Learners engage in repetitive practice	(39%)
3. Simulation is integrated into an overall curriculum	(25%)
4. Learners practice tasks with increasing levels of difficulty	(14%)
5. Simulation is adaptable to multiple learning strategies	(10%)
6. Clinical variation is built into simulation experiences	(10%)
7. Simulation events occur in a controlled environment	(9%)
8. Individualized learning is an option	(9%)
9. Outcomes or benchmarks are clearly defined or measured	(6%)
10. The simulation is a valid representation of clinical practice	(3%)

*Adapted from McGaghie et al. Lessons for continuing medical education from simulation research in undergraduate and graduate medical education: effectiveness of continuing medical education: American College of Chest Physicians Evidence-Based Educational Guidelines. Chest. 2009 Mar;135(3 Suppl):62S-68S.

Table 4. The Ten Conditions Necessary for Effective Deliberate Practice*.

Literature across multiple medical disciplines supports the efficacy of simulation based procedural training with deliberate practice. Wong et al. demonstrated that repetitive practice of cricothyroidotomy on mannequins leads to reductions in procedural performance times and improvement in success rates.(11) Barsuk et al. demonstrated improved safety and decreased central line infections after simulation-based central venous catheter insertions.(12) Draycott et al. demonstrated improved neonatal outcomes after shoulder dystocia training.(13) Andreatta et al. reported that simulation-based mock code training significantly correlated with improved pediatric patient cardiopulmonary arrest survival rates.(14) A meta-analysis performed by McGaghie et al. reported that simulation-based training with DP is superior to traditional clinical medical education in achieving specific clinical skill acquisition goals.(15)

Additionally, Weinger argues that, in order to achieve the maximal desired effect, procedural skills acquisition and retention likely occur in a dose-response relationship, similar to drug pharmacology, with the best retention achieved using intermittent regular repetition over time rather than in single-day course training.(16) Interval simulation training over time makes intuitive sense, allowing for consolidation of training lessons and refining of muscle memory. Learners can break down procedures into their basic steps and focus on those particular steps that they have more difficulty with or feel they need to work on. These concepts are familiar to anyone who has ever learned to play a musical instrument. The argument of the dose-response relationship of simulation was supported by Conroy et al. in a recent study demonstrating competence and retention of lumbar puncture training skills using interval reinforcement.(17)

Another consideration in simulation procedural training is the "first cut" experience. Prior to simulation task trainers, procedures such as cricothytomy were performed on cadavers and the initial incision through the cricothyroid membrane could only be performed "natively" once. After that, subsequent learners could not experience the first cut sensation. With the development of procedural simulators, each learner can not only experience the first cut experience, but they can experience it over and over again.

3. Available procedural simulation

In recent years, the commercial availability of procedure specific task trainers has significantly increased. Additionally, the fidelity (or realism) has improved as well. These improvements allow medical professionals who teach using simulation modalities, otherwise known as "simulationists," to provide better procedural training for their students.

There are commercially available simulators for just about every procedure listed in Table 2. Central line simulators such as those shown in Figure 1 (Simulab Corporation, Seattle, WA. www.simulab.com; Blue Phantom, Redmond, WA. www.bluephantom.com) allow for ultrasound guided vascular access practice where the learner can repeated perform the vessel cannulation and insert the entire central line as many times as necessary until proficiency is reached. In addition to vascular access, certain models can also provide simulated regional anesthesia training (Figure 2).

Common procedures such as lumbar puncture can be practiced using task trainers such as that shown in Figures 3 (Limbs and Things, LTD, Savannah, GA. www.limbsandthings.com). These models have the added ability to simulate obese and elderly patient lumbar anatomy using "obesity" and "senior" lumbar blocks (Figure 3B). These add to the difficulty levels that can be simulated. Infant lumbar puncture simulators (Figure 4) can be used to teach the procedure on an age- and size-appropriate model (Limbs and Things, LTD, Savannah, GA. www.limbsandthings.com).

Trauma procedures such as tube thoracostomy and surgical cricothyrotomy using systems such as TraumaMan® (Simulab Corporation, Seattle, WA. www.simulab.com) have become viable alternatives to cadaver based training because the skin on the trainer can be replaced (Figure 5). This allows for the very important "first cut" visual and tactile experience that is necessary for developing the cognitive and manual skills necessary for these procedures.

Focused Assessment with Sonography for Trauma (FAST) can be performed with varying levels of difficulty (Figure 6). The Blue Phantom FAST Exam Real Time Ultrasound Training Model (Blue Phantom, Redmond, WA. www.bluephantom.com) is one of the few ultrasound simulators that has adjustable internal bleeding levels to increase or decrease the level of difficulty. "Realistic internal bleeding in each organ space that can be adjusted by the user to simulate a wide variety of effusion states including: small, medium and large effusions or no effusions at all around the liver, spleen, heart, and bladder."

Table 5 provides a partial listing of commercially available procedural task trainers for emergency medicine relevant procedures.

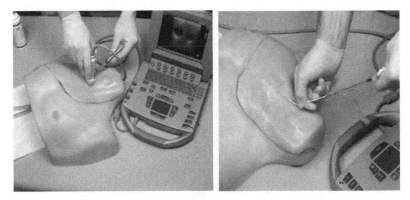

http://www.simulab.com/product/ultrasound-trainers/centralineman-system

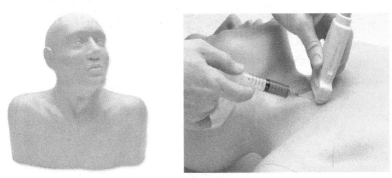

http://www.bluephantom.com/details.aspx?pid=51&cid=

Fig. 1. Central Line Trainers.

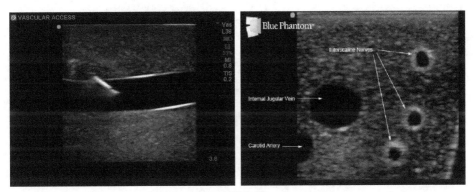

http://www.bluephantom.com/details.aspx?pid=51&cid=

Fig. 2. Ultrasound guided simulator for vascular access and regional anesthesia.

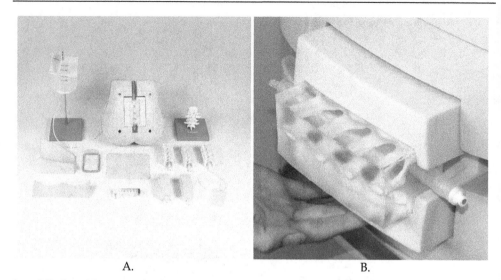

A.   B.

http://limbsandthings.com/us/products/lumbar-puncture-epidural-simulator-mk-2/

Fig. 3. Adult lumbar puncture simulator.

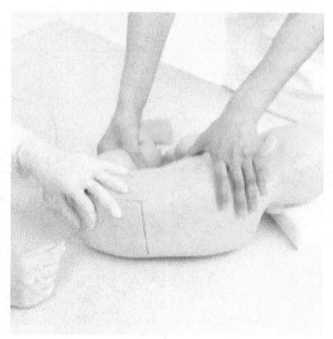

http://limbsandthings.com/us/products/pediatric-lumbar-puncture-simulator/

Fig. 4. Pediatric lumbar puncture simulator.

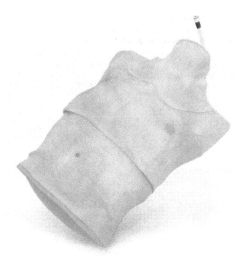

http://www.simulab.com/product/surgery/open/traumaman-system

Fig. 5. TraumaMan® System for tube thoracostomy and surgical cricothyrotomy.

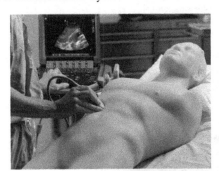 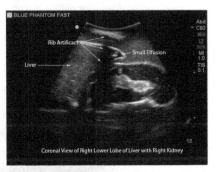

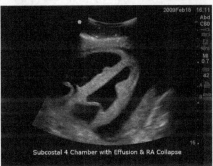

http://www.bluephantom.com/product/FAST-Exam-Real-Time-Ultrasound-Training-Model.aspx?cid=532

Fig. 6. FAST scan simulator.

Airway adjuncts
http://www.simulaids.com/SB32893.htm
http://www.trucorp.co.uk/sections/default.asp?secid=4&cms=
AirSim_AirSim+Advance+Crico&cmsid=4_53&id=53

Cricothyrotomy simulator
http://www.simulaids.com/LF01082U.htm

IV arm
http://www.simulaids.com/120.htm
http://www.kyotokagaku.com/products/detail01/m50b.html
http://limbsandthings.com/us/products/standard-venepuncture-arm/

Regional anesthesia
http://www.bluephantom.com/product/Femoral-Regional-Anesthesia-AND-
Vascular-Access-with-DVT-Option.aspx?cid=394
http://www.bluephantom.com/product/Regional-Anesthesia-and-Central-
Venous-Access-Ultrasound-Training-Model.aspx?cid=414

Joint aspiration
http://limbsandthings.com/us/products/knee-for-aspiration-mk-2/
http://limbsandthings.com/us/products/shoulder-for-joint-injection/
http://limbsandthings.com/us/products/foot-ankle-for-joint-injection/
http://limbsandthings.com/us/products/elbow-for-joint-injection/

Nasogastric tube
http://limbsandthings.com/us/products/ng-tube-tracheostomy-care/
http://www.enasco.com/product/LF01174U

Paracentesis
http://bluephantom.com/details.aspx?pid=55&cid=

Thoracentesis
http://bluephantom.com/category/Shop-By-Specialty_Emergency-
Medicine_Thoracentesis.aspx

Pericardiocentesis
http://bluephantom.com/details.aspx?pid=43&cid=

Pediatric Trauma
http://www.simulab.com/product/surgery/open/traumachild-system

Tube Thoracostomy
http://www.simulab.com/product/surgery/open/traumaman-system

Wound closure
http://limbsandthings.com/us/products/wound-closure-pad-light/
http://www.simulab.com/product/packaged-savings/deluxe-boss-starter-package

Table 5. Commercially available procedural task trainers.

While these trainers are continuously improving with each model generation, most current task trainers are not yet able to provide simulated training with increasing levels of difficulty, providing significant clinical variation, and providing a valid representation of *clinical practice*. These three deficiencies with respect to the ten conditions required for deliberate practice described earlier still need to be addressed before procedural simulation will be able to adequately simulate human tissue. *Until then, there will still be a gap between simulated practice and performance in patient care.*

4. Future of procedural simulation

As we move further away from organic (cadaveric and animal) models, new areas are emerging to provide EM trainees and practitioners with alternative methods for experiential practice and maintenance of skills.

In addition to the features of current simulators, improvements to current simulators are being developed both commercially and by simulationists who desire to bridge the gap between what is currently available and what can be possible. Examples include modification of a Laerdal SimBaby to include an integrated umbilical cannulation task trainer,[18] homegrown hybrid cricothyrotomy simulators using synthetic skin and sheep larynx/trachea,[19] and homegrown epistaxis task trainer simulators.[20]

The future of procedural simulation will likely lie in the development and convergence of haptic technology and virtual reality. Haptics is a type of tactile feedback technology that allows the reporting of a learner's touch pressure forces through a virtual interface. Haptics development has been led by the surgical disciplines where its use in laparoscopy, gynecology, urology, endoscopy, ophthalmology, dentistry, ENT, and robotic surgery have advanced training and technical skills. Simbionix (Simbionix USA Corporation, Cleveland, OH. www.simbionix.com) has created a Mentor Series of VR simulators for laparoscopy, angiography, bronchoscopy, endoscopy, endourology and TURP, percutaneous access, hysteroscopy, and pelvic examination.

For EM skills, a haptic-based VR trainer is now commercially available for IV insertion (Figure 6 - Laerdal Medical, Wappingers Falls, NY. www.laerdal.com). Work by Loukas et al. reported that this simulation model enhanced the skills of inexperienced subjects significantly and that "The VR simulator demonstrated construct validity for three different levels of experience. The number of attempts over a series of equal difficulty scenarios provides a valuable alternative to the traditional measures of the learning curve."[21] Investigations in cardiology-based simulation also support the utility of a VR-enhanced experience. [22-23]

Investigational trainers are being developed for endotracheal intubation,[24] lumbar punctures,[25] and cricothyrotomy,[26] with other haptic-enhanced physical models or VR procedural trainers likely to follow. Other opportunities for enhancing EM procedural training include improved seldinger technique simulation[27] and ultrasound practice[28-9] to improve hand-eye coordination.

Virtual reality integration with remote learning opportunities will likely be available in the future as well. Alverson et al. have reported the feasibility and acceptability by students in the use of VR simulation integrated into a Problem Based Learning (PBL) session, "... as well as multipoint distance technologies that allowed interaction between students and tutors in different locations."[30] The authors believe this method of interactive experiential learning can be widely applied in a distributed network or on site.

One can imagine that, in the future, web-based VR simulation learning network will be widely available. In this type of learning system, instructors around the world, using a shared VR learning platform, upload metadata for a specific procedural task (i.e. difficulty airway scenarios using a haptic-enhanced VR intubation program) to a central server. These cases can then be accessed at any local training center for training and validation purposes.

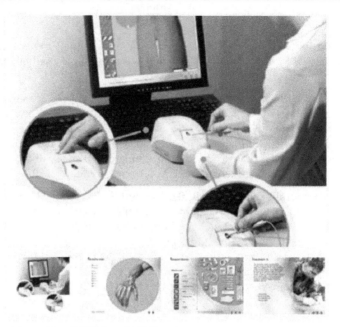

http://www.laerdal.com/doc/245/Virtual-I-V-Simulator

Fig. 7. Virtual I.V.™ Simulator.

5. Summary

Whatever form that emergency medicine procedural training takes in the future, one thing is clear – simulated training will be the mainstay for the initial introduction to the steps and mechanics involved in performing a procedure, for accelerating the technical skill acquisition learning curve for the procedure, and for the maintenance of competency of the skills once developed. The end result will be the delivery of higher quality, more uniform, and safer care at the bedside.

6. References

[1] American Board of Emergency Medicine. EM Model History.
    https://www.abem.org/PUBLIC/portal/alias__Rainbow/lang__en-
    US/tabID__4224/DesktopDefault.aspx. Accessed October 10, 2011.
[2] American Board of Emergency Medicine. EM Model.
    https://www.abem.org/PUBLIC/portal/alias__Rainbow/lang__en-
    US/tabID__4223/DesktopDefault.aspx. Accessed October 10, 2011.
[3] Accreditation Council for Graduate Medical Education. Emergency Medicine Guidelines.
    http://acgme.org/acWebsite/RRC_110/110_guidelines.asp. Accessed October 10, 2011.
[4] Ziv A, Wolpe PR, Small SD, Glick S. Simulation-Based Medical Education: An Ethical Imperative. Acad. Med. 2003;78:783–788.

[5] Mourad M, Auerbach AD, Maselli J, Sliwka D. Patient satisfaction with a hospitalist procedure service: is bedside procedure teaching reassuring to patients? J Hosp Med. 2011 Apr;6(4):219-24. doi: 10.1002/jhm.856.

[6] Graber MA, Wyatt C, Kasparek L, Xu Y.Does simulator training for medical students change patient opinions and attitudes toward medical student procedures in the emergency department? Acad Emerg Med. 2005 Jul;12(7):635-9.

[7] Lammers RL, Temple KJ, Wagner MJ, Ray D. Competence of new emergency medicine residents in the performance of lumbar punctures. Acad Emerg Med. 2005 Jul;12(7):622-8.

[8] Anders Ericsson, K. (2008), Deliberate Practice and Acquisition of Expert Performance: A General Overview. Acad Emerg Med. 2008 Nov;15(11):988–994.

[9] McGaghie WC, Siddall VJ, Mazmanian PE, Myers J; American College of Chest Physicians Health and Science Policy Committee. Lessons for continuing medical education from simulation research in undergraduate and graduate medical education: effectiveness of continuing medical education: American College of Chest Physicians Evidence-Based Educational Guidelines. Chest. 2009 Mar;135(3 Suppl):62S-68S.

[10] Issenberg SB, McGaghie WC, Petrusa ER, et al. Features and uses of high-fidelity medical simulations that lead to effective learning: a BEME systematic review. Med Teach. 2005; 27:10–28.

[11] Wong DT, Prabhu AJ, Coloma M, Imasogie N, Chung FF. What is the minimum training required for successful cricothyroidotomy?: a study in mannequins. Anesthesiology. 2003 Feb;98(2):349-53.

[12] Barsuk JH, McGaghie WC, Cohen ER, O'Leary KJ, Wayne DB. Simulation-based mastery learning reduces complications during central venous catheter insertion in a medical intensive care unit. Crit Care Med. 2009 Oct;37(10):2697-701.

[13] Draycott TJ, Crofts JF, Ash JP, Wilson LV, Yard E, Sibanda T, Whitelaw A. Improving neonatal outcome through practical shoulder dystocia training. Obstet Gynecol. 2008 Jul;112(1):14-20.

[14] Andreatta P, Saxton E, Thompson M, Annich G. Simulation-based mock codes significantly correlate with improved pediatric patient cardiopulmonary arrest survival rates. Pediatr Crit Care Med. 2011 Jan;12(1):33-8.

[15] McGaghie WC, Issenberg SB, Cohen ER, Barsuk JH, Wayne DB. Does simulation-based medical education with deliberate practice yield better results than traditional clinical education? A meta-analytic comparative review of the evidence. Acad Med. 2011 Jun;86(6):706-11.

[16] Weinger MB. The pharmacology of simulation: a conceptual framework to inform progress in simulation research. Simul Healthc. 2010 Feb;5(1):8-15.

[17] Conroy SM, Bond WF, Pheasant KS, Ceccacci N. Competence and retention in performance of the lumbar puncture procedure in a task trainer model. Simul Healthc. 2010 Jun;5(3):133-8.

[18] Sawyer T, Hara K, Thompson MW, Chan DS, Berg B. Modification of the Laerdal SimBaby to include an integrated umbilical cannulation task trainer. Simul Healthc. 2009 Fall;4(3):174-8.

[19] Pettineo CM, Vozenilek JA, Wang E, Flaherty J, Kharasch M, Aitchison P. Simulated emergency department procedures with minimal monetary investment: cricothyrotomy simulator. Simul Healthc. 2009 Spring;4(1):60-4.

[20] Pettineo CM, Vozenilek JA, Kharasch M, Wang E, Aitchison P. Epistaxis simulator: an innovative design. Simul Healthc. 2008 Winter;3(4):239-41.

[21] Loukas C, Nikiteas N, Kanakis M, Georgiou E. Evaluating the effectiveness of virtual reality simulation training in intravenous cannulation. Simul Healthc. 2011 Aug;6(4):213-7.

[22] Aloisio G, Barone L, Bergamasco M, Avizzano CA, De Paolis LT, Franceschini M, Mongelli A, Pantile G, Provenzano L, Raspolli M. Computer-based simulator for catheter insertion training. Stud Health Technol Inform. 2004;98:4-6.

[23] Schuetz M, Moenk S, Vollmer J, Kurz S, Mollnau H, Post F, Heinrichs W. High degree of realism in teaching percutaneous coronary interventions by combining a virtual reality trainer with a full scale patient simulator. Simul Healthc. 2008 Winter;3(4):242-6.

[24] Mayrose J, Myers JW. Endotracheal intubation: application of virtual reality to emergency medical services education. Simul Healthc. 2007 Winter;2(4):231-4.

[25] Färber M, Hummel F, Gerloff C, Handels H. Virtual reality simulator for the training of lumbar punctures. Methods Inf Med. 2009;48(5):493-501.

[26] Liu A, Bhasin Y, Bowyer M. A haptic-enabled simulator for cricothyroidotomy. Stud Health Technol Inform. 2005;111:308-13.

[27] Luboz V, Hughes C, Gould D, John N, Bello F. Real-time Seldinger technique simulation in complex vascular models. Int J Comput Assist Radiol Surg. 2009 Nov;4(6):589-96.

[28] Nicolau SA, Vemuri A, Wu HS, Huang MH, Ho Y, Charnoz A, Hostettler A, Forest C, Soler L, Marescaux J. A cost effective simulator for education of ultrasound image interpretation and probe manipulation. Stud Health Technol Inform. 2011;163:403-7.

[29] Samosky JT, Allen P, Boronyak S, Branstetter B, Hein S, Juhas M, Nelson DA, Orebaugh S, Pinto R, Smelko A, Thompson M, Weaver RA. Toward a comprehensive hybrid physical-virtual reality simulator of peripheral anesthesia with ultrasound and neurostimulator guidance. Stud Health Technol Inform. 2011;163:552-4.

[30] Alverson DC, Saiki SM Jr, Kalishman S, Lindberg M, Mennin S, Mines J, Serna L, Summers K, Jacobs J, Lozanoff S, Lozanoff B, Saland L, Mitchell S, Umland B, Greene G, Buchanan HS, Keep M, Wilks D, Wax DS, Coulter R, Goldsmith TE, Caudell TP. Medical students learn over distance using virtual reality simulation. Simul Healthc. 2008 Spring;3(1):10-5.

5

Delays in the Diagnosis of Pulmonary Thromboembolism and Risk Factors

Savas Ozsu

Karadeniz Technical University

Department of Chest Diseases School of Medicine, Trabzon,

Turkey

1. Introduction

Pulmonary thromboembolism (PE) is a relatively common cardiovascular emergency and it is healthy important issue. Overall, VTE occurs for the first time in approximately 1 case per 1000 each year. PE has been estimated to occur in 600,000 patients annually in the United States and is reported to cause or attribute to 50,000 to 200,000 deaths (Wood, 2002). PE is a difficult diagnosis that may be missed because of non-specific clinical presentation. Clinical scoring systems have been widely used to determine the risk of PE (Table 1). These scoring systems include age and cancer which can be risk factors causing PE. However specificity and sensitivity of these scoring systems range from 60-85% to 50-80% in a current metaanalysis(Lucassen, 2011). An increased prevalence of PE was found associated with higher sensitivity and lower specificity. Thus lower specificity of these scoring systems cause the unnecessary diagnostic workup. Diagnosis of PE by pulmonary computerized tomography angiography has been increasing in the last 10 years. Actually, Pulmonary CTA confirmed PE in only a minority of patients and may be overused. A retrospective study demonstrated that pulmonary CTA was positive for PE in only 39 (14.9%) of 261 patients. (Haap, 2011)

In addition, during the past 2 decades, prevention of venous thromboembolism (VTE) has become widely accepted as an effective and worthwhile strategy. North American and European guidelines have provided detailed recommendations for prophylaxis among virtually all groups of hospitalized patients, especially in those with heart failure, active cancer, or sepsis.

However, despite advances in prophylaxis and newer diagnostic methods delays in the diagnosis of PE is stil common. Pulmonary embolism has been determined in 15% of the autopsy series, whereas the antemortem diagnosis of fatal PE has not changed appreciably over time, remaining fixed at approximately 30% [Wood,2002]. Most patients who die of PE do so within hours of the event (Dalen,2002). 30% of all hospital deaths are also caused by pulmonary embolism. Whereas, earlier diagnoses of DVT and PE will reduce the morbidity and mortality associated with venous thromboembolism.

In several studies, 16% to 30.4% of the patients with acute PE were diagnosed one week or longer after the symptom onset, and the mean time to diagnosis was 4.8 to 8.4 days. It has

Revised Geneva score		Wells score	
Variable	**Points**	**Variable**	**Points**
Predisposing factors		Predisposing factors	
Age > 65 years	+1		
Previous DVT or PE	+3	Previous DVT or PE	+1.5
Surgery or fracture within 1 month	+2	Recent surgery or immobilization	+1.5
Active malignancy	+2	Cancer	+1
Symptoms		Symptoms	
Unilateral lower limb pain	+3		
Haemoptysis	+2	Haemoptysis	+1
Clinical signs		Clinical signs	
Heart rate		Heart rate	
75–94 beats/min	+3	> 100 beats/min	+1.5
≥ 95 beats/min	+5		
Pain on lower limb deep vein at palpation and unilateral oedema	+4	Clinical signs of DVT	+3
		Clinical judgement	
		Alternative diagnosis less likely than PE	+3
Clinical probability	**Total**	**Clinical probability**	**Total**
Low	0–3	Low	0–1
Intermediate	4–10	Intermediate	2–6
High	≥ 11	High	≥7
		Clinical probability	
		PE unlikely	0–4
		PE likely	>4

Table 1. Clinical probability rules for PE: revised Geneva score and Wells score.

been reported that 31.6% to 50% of the patients presented within 24 hours of symptom onset [Bulbul 2009,Castro,2007, Elliott 2005,Timmons 2003]. In our study, 29.6% of the patients had presented within the first 24 hours and 72.3% within the first week, with an average of 6.9 days between onset of symptoms and diagnosis. In the two previous studies, delays from first medical attention to diagnosis were determined to range from 0.9 to 2 days [Bulbul 2009, Elliott 2005]. In another study, PE was diagnosed in 12% of the patients more than 48 hours after admission to the ED [Kline,2007]. In our study, the mean time to diagnosis was found as 2.4 days. As a result, the majority of patients that die from PE do so within hours of the event. Therefore, early diagnosis is fundamental, since immediate treatment is highly life-saving.

The most important factor in the delayed diagnosis of PE is lack of suspicion for the PE disease itself. In addition to this, accompanying comorbidities and risk factors may affect the time to diagnosis. The presence of a risk factor in PE is important step in the diagnosis of PE and it should be questioned. Although PE can occur in patients without any identifiable risk factors, one or more of these factors are usually determined (secondary PE). Symptoms are often attributed to these diseases because of risk factors and associated comorbidities. Therefore it is inevitable to cause diagnostic delay. The proportion of patients with idiopathic or unprovoked PE was about 20% in the literature. Actually it seems to be a important factor to cause delays in diagnosis of pulmonary embolism.

In this section, we will investigated the effect of risk factors on delay to diagnosis in acute PE and also the relationship between delays and outcome of the disease.

2. Definitions

The time from the onset of symptoms to diagnosis was defined as *"time to diagnosis"* and delay from the first medical attention to diagnosis *"presentation to diagnosis"*. Especially, diagnostic delay was determined as diagnosis of PE more than 5-10 days after symptom onset in different studies. But delay in the diagnosis of PE was defined as shorter that was 12-24 hours in 2 different studies. Actually the time for delayed diagnosis of PE patients who have no diagnosis is an obscure area and therefore there is no known answer yet for answering the optimal time fort he diagnosis of PE.

3. Diagnostic delays in PE and risk factors

There is a limited data about the effect of risk factors on time to diagnosis of PE. PE is still a major cause of death in hospital patients, in medical service especially. Therefore medical risk factors are one of the important reasons leading to the diagnostic delay in PE. It is thought that previous hospitalization history may lead an idea of an inadequate prophylaxis or underestimation the diagnosis of PE.

We retrospectively evaluated the records of 408 diagnosed with PE. The mean time to diagnosis was 4.39 ± 7.6 days (median, 2 days; range, 0-45 days) in the surgical group and 8.0 ± 8.6 days (median, 4 days; range, 0-45 days) in the medical group. The percentage of cases diagnosed within the first week (87.5% of the surgical group, 66% of the medical group) was significantly higher in the surgical group patients with acute PE. In our study, the mean time to diagnosis in the medical group was approximately four times greater than that of the surgical group on univariate analysis. In multivariate analysis surgery, presence of cancer, and stroke were found to be related with early diagnosis in PE. We think that presence of medical disease is a risk factor for PE and can also mask PE symptoms, thus delaying diagnosis. Bulbul et al. also reported that patients with a trauma or surgical risk factor were diagnosed earlier (Bulbul,2009).

In MASTER study, is an Italian, multicenter, observational study included 542 PE patients, was found by Ageno et al. the presence of transient risk factors (recent surgery, recent trauma, severe medical diseases, immobilization, pregnancy, puerperium, oral contraceptives, central venous catheters) for PE predicted earlier diagnosis of PE. As interesting, known thrombophilia, active cancer and previous PE or DVT was not predicted earlier diagnosis of PE in this study (Ageno, 2008).

Castro et al. prospectively was evaluated 397 consecutive patients with acute PE objectively diagnosed in an Emergency Department. Eighteen percent of patients had a diagnostic delay with symptoms beginning more than 1 week prior to the diagnosis of PE. Similarly Castro et al found that active cancer, immobility and presence of previous VTE does not predict the early diagnosis of PE (Castro,2007).

Berghaus et al. suggested that delay in diagnosis was significant greater in patients with recurrent than in patients with first PE (3.4 ± 2.3 vs. 2.2 ± 1.7 days) (Berghaus,2011).

A recent study, Smith et al. studied 400 patients with acute PE who were diagnosed either within 12 h or after 12 h from ED arrival. They found that patients with delayed diagnosis were morbid obesity, whereas patients with early diagnosis more frequently had recent immobility (Smith,2011). Obesity that was found to be associated with the delayed diagnosis of PE was composed of the 11.5% of the patients in this study. Immobility is important for obese patients so that delayed diagnosis is possibly related to the immobility.

Actually, in patients with previous PE must be associated with early diagnosis of PE. Up to now, it is unknown whether patients with recurrent PE are diagnosed earlier than those with their first episode. Surprisingly, Barghaus et al. were found that patients with recurrent PE was not diagnosed earlier but even later than those with their first episode, although all enrolled patients reported common clinical signs of PE. They reported that delay in diagnosis after symptom onset was significantly greater in patients with recurrent than in patients with their first PE (3.4 ± 2.3 vs. 2.2 ± 1.7 days) (Barghaus,2011).

In the light of the data above, effect of risk factors on the delayed diagnosis of PE seems to be contrversial. Especially in these mentioned studies, it has been seen that percentage of risk factors causing PE was various.

For example immobility has been found as a risk factor of 42% of the PE patients in the study by Stein et al. whereas this percentage was 17% in the study by Castro et al.

Threfore, it is diffucult to determine whether immobility causes early or late diagnosis of PE in this case.

Immobility was found to be related to early diagnosis of PE in the univariate analysis of our study. We are on side of the opinion that presence of immobility is an obvious clue in the patients with PE suspicion for the early diagnosis. Similarly, surgery was present as a risk factior in 30% of our study population of PE in our study but this percentage was only 9% in study by Castro et al.

Hospitalization of the most of the operated patients and development of PE after a short time of operation in these patients provides an easy way to diagnosis of PE.

Immobility and the presence of cancer alone constitutes a low risk for PE according to Wells criteria. A frequent complication is the occurrence of venous thromboembolism , for which cancer is one of the most relevant risk factors..However diagnosis of PE was found as difficult in cancer patients in 2 different studies.It was seen that suspicion of PE diagnosis was present in 6(75%) of 8 patients in an autopsy study by Pineda et al..It is possible that symptoms and signs of these patients were associated with the cancer and diagnostic work-up was not done. D-dimer positivity is an expected sign in cancer patients. Therefore presence of low risk with the D-dimer positivity needs CT pulmonary angiography in these patients. Moreover recently appeared VTE (pulmonary embolism or deep vein thrombosis) occurred in 12-32% of cases with the diagnosis of cancer during follow-up period (Goldhaber 2004,. Kroger 2006).

According to the recent data, asymptomatic DVT and PE was found in 8% and 3.3% of patients with the diagnosis of cancer during their screening workup by computerized tomography (Cronin 2006). These data showed that the diagnosis of PE was delayed in cancer patients. Therfore it is necessary to suspect the diagnosis of PE in cancer patients more than the others.

4. Diagnostic delays in PE and age

The incidences of venous thromboembolism and PE are known to increase with age The patients with the diagnosis of PE were mostly above the 65 years old. The annual incidence of PE is 1.3/1000 at age 65–69 years and 3.1/1000 at age 85–89 years of age [Kniffer, 1994]. With age is variable thrombotic/antithrombotic balance, fibrinogen levels increase and anti-thrombin 3 levels decline [Hager,1989], while reduced lower limb musculature and immobility may encourage venous stasis. Although these physiological changes may predispose eldery persons to thromboembolism, there is also a rise in specific risk factors for thromboembolism with aging, such as congestive heart failure, stroke and hip fracture, among many comorbid condition (eg. cancer)

An important factor leading to delay in PE diagnosis is age, but this contribution is also controversial. Several earlier studies found that the clinical presentation of older patients with acute PE may be atypical, potentially leading to a delay in diagnosis and initiation of treatment. Otherwise, in a recent study, Berghaus et al. found that delay in diagnosis had not was not significantly different in the younger and older age group(Berghaus, 2011). Contrary, in an autopsy studies was found that the post-mortem diagnosis of PE was significantly more frequent in older patients (Mangion, 1989)

In this section, we will discuss impact of risk factors in delays according to literature.

5. The impact of delay on outcome of embolism

Diagnostic delay and its impact on outcome of the disease were studied in seven studies. In this section, we will discuss and review the impact of delays on mortality and recurrence rates of pulmonary embolism.

5.1 Mortality

Although early diagnosis of PE is thought to reduce mortality, sufficient data on the subject are still limited. Mortality of PE has not been changed although the use of spiral BT increase rate of diagnosis in PE patients.

In the 1950s, the results of large-scale autopsy studies showed that only 11 to 12% of patients with PE received correct diagnoses before death (Uhland,1964). Pineda and colleagues reported a 45 % rate of correct antemortem diagnosis in a study that was done from 1991 to 1996 (Pineda,2001). Actually it has been seen that the mortality decrease according to the years.

Two different study suggest that early or late diagnosis did not change PE mortality.

There were no statistical differences between the 2 groups in terms of mortality in our study. Delay in diagnosis was not different between those who died and those who survived. The mean time to diagnosis in the 40 patients who died was 5.7 ± 6.7 days (median, 3 days; range, 0-30 days) and 7.1 ± 8.7 days (median, 3 days; range, 0-45 days) in those who survived. We found that earlier diagnosis had no impact on mortality (Ozsu,2011).

Kline et al. found inhospital adverse outcomes (Death, circulatory shock, or endotracheal intubation for respiratory distress) of patients with delayed diagnosis were worse than those of patients with PE diagnosed in the emergency department. Advers events were seen in 30% of the patients who have delayed diagnosis compared to the advers events seen in 8.5% of the patients who have no delayed diagnosis of PE (Kline,2007).

Approximately 30% of PE patients are died from PE without having any diagnosis.

Patients presenting with PE who are immediately treated with anticoagulation have a lower rate of in-hospital death (1.5%) compared with those who are not treated (5-23%) (Douketis,1998).

Smith et al. compared that patients receiving heparin either in the emergency department or after admission. They found patients who received heparin in the ED had lower in-hospital (1.4% vs 6.7%) and 30-day (4.4% vs 15.3%) mortality rates as compared with patients given heparin after admission. Patients who achieved a therapeutic aPTT within 24 h had lower in-hospital (1.5% vs 5.6%) and 30-day (5.6% vs 14.8%) mortality rates as compared with patients who achieved a therapeutic aPTT after 24 h. In multiple logistic regression models, receiving heparin in the ED was remained predictive of reduced mortality, and ICU admission was remained predictive of increased mortality in the same study (Smith,2010).

Studies concerning with the relationship between mortality and diagnostic delay of PE was done in patients already having the PE diagnosis. These patients have PE diagnosis and survived anyway. However many patients are died from PE without having the antemortem PE diagnosis in postmortem studies. Delayed diagnosis of PE can be fatal according to these data.

The main problem is to diagnose these PE patients who can be fatal early and to start their treatment. The patients were classified as high risk and non-high risk patients according to risk groups. This can affect the results. Because, hours or even minutes are important for these high risk patients. Moreover it is necessary to investigate the mortality of the high risk patients whose diagnosis was made within 6-12 hours

Because there is no sufficient data about this subject. Thus effect of mortality on delayed diagnosis of PE may be understood more easily. Early diagnosis and treatment in PE is life-saving. Guidelines recommend initiation of anticoagulation if clinical suspicion for PE is high, even prior to confirmatory testing.

5.2 Re-embolism

The most important long-term complication of PTE is re-embolism that is associated with considerable morbidity and mortality. Delay in diagnosis of PE may be associated with chronic thrombo-embolic pulmonary hypertension rather than re-embolism. However, there is well not documented this issue.

Castro et al. did not detect an association between a delay in diagnosis and an PE recurrence during the ensuing 3 months of treatment. They found that recurrent VTE in 3 (4.2%) of 72 patients with diagnostic delay and in 15 (4.6%) of 325 patients without diagnostic delay (Castro,2007)

6. Recommendations

Late diagnosis also depends on patients delay in seeking medical awareness. In the North American study, 80%of the delay in diagnosis of DVT found before medical evaluation, whereas delays in the diagnosis of PE represented both delays in seeking medical attention and delays from medical assessment to proper objective testing [Elliott,2005]. It has been seen that many patients who had delayed diagnosis had admitted to a physcian before.

Bulbul et al. showed that previous hospital or doctor visits were associated with an approximately 11 times longer diagnostic delay than the patients who did not visit a doctor or a hospital in univariate logistic regression analysis (Bulbul,2011). Data has been shown that there is no sufficient suspicion effort he diagnosis of PE..

Suspicion for PE is first step for the diagnosis of PE then it is necessary to perform rapid tests for the diagnosis. Bolus heparin should be done especially in high risk patients Clinical presentation is non-spesific for PTE and most important point in diagnosis is suspicion for PTE. Therefore more efforts are needed by experts effort he diagnosis of PE.

In addition it has been known that there is no spesific marker for PE yet. Although negative predictive value of D-dimer is high, most of the patients admitted to the hospital have positive D-dimer level. Therefore advanced studies are needed for this issue. Another important point is that there is need for more spesific scoring systems of the PE diagnosis.

Because history of previous VTE alone is classified as intermediate ris for the PE according to the Well's criteria. However diagnosis is delayed in patients having VTE in studies. This is a obvious contraversion. Perhaps physicians do not use clinical scoring systems efficienly for the diagnosis of PE.

Moreover it is known that both history given by patients and taken by physician is not sufficient for the diagnosis of PE. Also patients should be stratified for the diagnosis of PE. It was shown that level of patients' education was related to the delayed diagnosis of PE (Bulbul, 2011). Because it was shown that even the patients having previous PE diagnosis had also delayed diagnosis of PE.

Finally, public and professional education represents a critical step for the early diagnosis and treatment in this patients, especially. My opinion, earlier diagnoses of PE will reduce the morbidity and mortality associated with PE.

Late presentation	early presentation
*Immobility	Recent surgery/ trauma
Idiopathic	Severe medical diseases
*Elderly	Pregnancy/ puerperium
*Cancer	Oral contraceptives,
Previous VTE	central venous catheter

*There are studies showed that these risk factors were related to the early presentation

Table 2. Risk factors relation to early/late presentation.

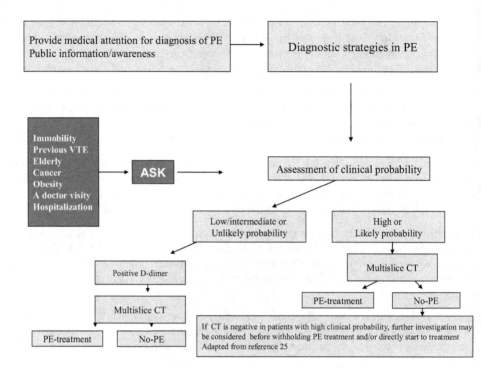

Table 3. Approach to diagnosis of PE.

7. References

[1] Kenneth E. Wood. Review of a Pathophysiologic Approach to the Golden Hour of Hemodynamically Significant Pulmonary Embolism Chest 2002;121;877-905

[2] Lucassen W, Geersing GJ, Erkens PM, Reitsma JB, Moons KG, Büller H, van Weert HC. Clinical Decision Rules for Excluding Pulmonary Embolism: A Meta-analysis. Ann Intern Med. 2011 Oct 4;155(7):448-60.

[3] Haap MM, Gatidis S, Horger M, et al. .Computed tomography angiography in patients with suspected pulmonary embolism—too often considered. Am J Emerg Med. 2011 Jan 27. [Epub ahead of print]

[4] Dalen JE. Pulmonary embolism: what have we learned since Virchow? Chest 2002;122:1440-6.

[5] Bulbul Y, Ozsu S, Kosucu P, Oztuna F, Ozlu T, Topbas, M. Time delay between onset of symptoms and diagnosis in pulmonary thromboembolism. Respiration. 2009;78:36–41.

[6] Jiménez Castro D, Sueiro A, Díaz G, Escobar C, García-Rull S, Picher J, Taboada D, Yusen RD. Prognostic significance of delays in diagnosis of pulmonary embolism. Thromb Res. 2007;121(2):153-8.

[7] Elliott CG, Goldhaber SZ, Jensen RL. Delays in diagnosis of deep vein thrombosis and pulmonary embolism. Chest. 2005; 128:3372-6.

[8] Timmons S, Kingston M, Hussain M, Kelly H, Liston R. Pulmonary embolism: differences in presentation between older and younger patients. Age Ageing 2003;32(6):601-5.

[9] Kline JA, Hernandez-Nino J, Jones AE, et al. Prospective study of the clinical features and outcomes of emergency department patients with delayed diagnosis of pulmonary embolism. Acad Emerg Med 2007;14: 592-8.

[10] Ozsu S, Oztuna F, Bulbul Y, Topbas M, Ozlu T, Kosucu P, et al. The role of risk factors in delayed diagnosis of pulmonary embolism. Am J Emerg Med. 2010;29(1):26-32

[11] Ageno W, Agnelli G, Imberti D, Moia M, Palareti G, Pistelli R, et al. Factors associated with the timing of diagnosis of venous thromboembolism: Results from the MASTER registry. Thromb Res. 2008;121:751-6.

[12] Berghaus TM, von Scheidt W, Schwaiblmair M. Time between first symptoms and diagnosis in patients with acute pulmonary embolism: are patients with recurrent episodes diagnosed earlier? Clin Res Cardiol. 2011;100(2):117-119

[13] Berghaus TM, Thilo C, von Scheidt W, Schwaiblmair M. The Impact of Age on the Delay in Diagnosis in Patients With Acute Pulmonary Embolism. Clin Appl Thromb Hemost. 2011 May 17. [Epub ahead of print]

[14] Mangion DM. Pulmonary embolism — incidence and prognosis in hospitalized elderly. Postgrad Med J. 1989;65(769):814-817.

[15] Goldhaber SZ, Dunn K, MacDougall .New onset of venous thromboembolism among hospitalized patients at Brigham and Women's Hospital is caused more often by prophylaxis failure than by withholding treatment. Chest 2000;118; 1680-1684

[16] Douketis JD, Kearon C, Bates S, Duku EK, Ginsberg JS. Risk of fatal pulmonary embolism in patients with treated venous thromboembolism. JAMA 1998;279:458-62.

[17] Goldhaber SZ, Tapson VF. DVT FREE Steering Committee. A prospective registry of 5,451 patients with ultrasound-confirmed deep vein thrombosis. Am J Cardiol 2004; 93: 259-62.

[18] Kroger K,Weiland D,Ose C,et al. Risk factors for venous thromboembolic events in cancer patients. Annals of Oncology 2006;17: 297-303.

[19] Cronin CG, Lohan DG, Keane M. Prevalence and Significance of Asymptomatic Venous Thromboembolic Disease Found on Oncologic Staging CT. AJR 2007; 189:162-70.

[20] Kniffin WD, Baron JA, Barrett J et al. The epidemiology of diagnosed pulmonary embolism and deep venous thrombosis in the elderly. Arch Intern Med 1994; 154: 861-6.

[21] Hager K, Setzer J, Vogl T et al. Blood coagulation factors in the elderly. Arch Gerontol Geriatr 1989; 9: 277-82.

[22] Bulbul Y, Ayik S, Oztuna F, Ozlu T, Sahin S. The relationship between socio-demographic characteristics of patients and diagnostic delay in acute pulmonary thromboembolism. Ups J Med Sci. 2011;116(1):72-6.

[23] Uhland H, Goldberg LM. Pulmonary embolism: a commonly missed clinical entity. Dis Chest 1964; 45:533-536

[24] Pineda LA, Hathwar VS, Grant BJ. Clinical Suspicion of Fatal Pulmonary Embolism. Chest. 2001 Sep;120(3):791-5.

[25] Guidelines on the diagnosis and management of acute pulmonary embolism. Eur Heart J 2008;29:2276–315.

6

Prehospital Airway Management

Flavia Petrini[1], Maurizio Menarini[2] and Elena Bigi[2]
¹University of Chieti–Pescara
²AUSL di Bologna
Italy

1. Introduction

Correct airway management and the maintenance of its patency is an essential skill of the health-care team which intervenes at the prehospital scene of emergencies. Airway patency is crucial in ensuring valid oxygenation and good ventilation in critical patients. Up until now, there has been a general consensus in the scientific world on this.

Recently, however, various different works have been published which have cast doubt on the real efficacy of tracheal intubation, a maneuver which is considered to be the gold standard in airway management. In some cases the management of prehospital tracheal intubation has been attributed to potentially worsening the critical patient's final outcome. Unfortunately, an analysis of prehospital airway management studies, especially the more recently published articles, has created more questions than answers.

Significant difficulties have been recorded in the collecting of high quality data in the prehospital setting. This has been mainly due to the fact that it is a notoriously complicated field and often impossible, for ethical reasons, to design randomized surveys which can be controlled in double blind studies. To this we can also add that it is often necessary to recruit a large number of patients in order to obtain sufficient statistical power to demonstrate the effect on the outcome.

Nevertheless, here we will try to provide some answers to the open questions regarding prehospital airway management and propose a rational approach method.

2. Prehospital airway management: open questions

Tracheal intubation is universally accepted as being the gold standard in ensuring airway patency.

There are several advantages:

1. it provides the best ventilation
2. it protects against pulmonary aspiration
3. it permits the aspiration of secretions

In terms of efficacy, however, the question we should ask is: does successful prehospital endotracheal intubation improve survival in critically ill patients? We can try to provide answers to this question by introducing some key elements.

2.1 Useful definitions

We report some definitions used by Italian Society of Anaesthesiologists (Petrini et al, 2005).

a.   Difficult airway control

Airway control difficulty is defined as ventilation difficulty (using either face mask or extraglottic devices) and/or intubation difficulty with standard equipment (curve blade laryngoscope and simple endotracheal tube.

b.   Difficult ventilation

Difficult mask ventilation occurs whenever the required tidal volume cannot be administered to the patient without any airway device or external help (i.e. airway or three-hand face mask ventilation), standard procedure withdrawal (i.e. face mask switched for any extraglottic device) or intubation (i.e. failure of the extraglottic device).

c.   Difficult intubation

Difficult and/or impossible intubation is defined as a maneuver performed with a correct head position and external laryngeal manipulation resulting in: a) difficult laryngoscopy (in a wide definition); b) necessity of repeated attempts; c) necessity of no standard devices and/or procedures; d) withdrawal and procedure replanning.

d.   Difficult laryngoscopy

Difficult laryngoscopy is defined as the impossibility of obtaining a view of the vocal cords even after the best external laryngeal manipulation.

2.2 Critically ill patients continuity of care

The general objective of an "emergency system" is to guarantee a diagnostic-therapeutic pathway from the scene of the event, where the prehospital team ensures qualified treatment, to the Emergency Room. When we talk about continuity of care, this is precisely what we mean. The conditions necessary for appropriate treatment at the scene of the event, in relation to the complexity of the situation which the emergency team is faced with, is an effective, multi-professional and multi-disciplinary collaboration. It is necessary to consider that different elements can condition the strategy of the intervention and the quality of the treatment administered in the prehospital setting.

In particular, we must bear in mind:

-   the clinical competence and the experience of the health-care team (Timmermann et al, 2006; Sollid et al. 2008)
-   their technical abilities
-   the non-technical skills of the emergency team (teamwork)

Despite its accepted role in clinical practice for more than 25 years, a growing body of evidence suggests that prehospital endotracheal intubation is not achieving its intended, overarching goal. In selected cases the intervention may actually be causing more harm than good (Wang & Yealy, 2006; Klemen & Grimec, 2006; Wang et al, 2004; Davis et al, 2003, 2005). The Cochrane Review (Lecky et al, 2008) has recently analyzed this issue to determine whether emergency endotracheal intubation in seriously ill and injured patients improves their outcome in terms of survival and degree of disability. They conclude that:

"This review found no differences between endotracheal intubation and other airway securing strategies in reducing deaths after acute illness or injury; however, better studies are needed".

This review also concludes that:

- clinicians need to establish safe airways and adequate ventilation for patients in emergency situations
- the skill level of the operator may be key in determining efficacy
- in pediatric and trauma patients the current evidence base provides no imperative to extend the practice of prehospital intubation to urban and short transit time systems.

Some important considerations have therefore emerged from what has been reported. Airway obstructions are common in numerous pathological emergency conditions, with consequent alterations in ventilation and oxygenation. The presence of important pathophysiological alterations (severe hypoxia, hypoperfusion and states of shock) can compromise the vital functions which, on the one hand, render the immediate execution of the intervention necessary and, on the other, can make airway management even more difficult (physiologically difficult airway).

In all probability, due to methodological and ethical issues, we must make do with studies based on low levels of evidence. Moreover, an analysis of the literature shows an extreme non-homogeneity between the quality of the studies, making it impossible to compare data. In particular, patients suffering from cranial trauma or cardiac arrest are often compared with those who are not and EMS systems are often very different (medical personnel or not, paramedics and technicians) (Herff et al, 2009).

2.3 Quality in prehospital airway management

Is successful prehospital endotracheal intubation are data itself enough to describe the quality of airway management? Unfortunately, the answer is no. It can never be stressed enough that it is not the mere positioning of the maneuver (in this case, the positioning of the tube in the trachea) which correlates with the outcome, but the total quality of the intervention on the scene and during transportation. It is evident that suboptimal airway management can create an increased risk in patients.

The so called "*inverse care law*" (Boylan & Cavanagh, 2008) states that, in the prehospital setting, the most critically ill patients are not always treated by those who are the most competent and expert. Operators and teams which are not competent and experienced enough do not guarantee a prehospital airway management in line with the established standards. This has obvious negative outcomes for the patients themselves, whether they are traumatized or not (Deakin et al., 2009; Warner et al, 2010, Timmermann et al, 2006; Fakhry et al, 2006).

For example, the indicators of insufficient quality in prehospital airway management are: a laryngoscopy and intubation performed without pharmacological help in reactive patients, repeated intubation attempts with resulting airway trauma, extended periods of time on the scene due to patient instability, and the estimated control of the correct positioning of the tube in the trachea (Donald & Paterson 2008; Timmermann et al, 2007; Bacon et al, 2001).

Major complications in patients, like esophageal intubation or misplaced endotracheal tubes, range from as little as 0.3% to as much as 25% (Wirtz et al, 2007; Katz & Falk 2001). However, retrospective studies of endotracheal intubation are likely to have underestimated the true complication rate. These studies have often relied on the paramedic's own reports regarding success and complications and often reviewed emergency department records after the fact. Indubitably, in this case the problem is not endotracheal intubation but the quality of airway management itself.

An interesting study was conducted to evaluate the effects of rapid sequence intubation (RSI) on patients with severe traumatic brain injury (Davis et al, 2003). It concluded that prehospital endotracheal intubation in patients with severe traumatic brain injury was associated with an increase in mortality and a decrease in positive outcomes. The problem is the lack of attention paid to airway management complications and to post-intubation ventilation.

For instance:

-   desaturation during the intubation attempt (especially in the case of very difficult airways)
-   too much time on the scene
-   post-intubation management (hyperventilation in head injured patients with increased risk of cerebral ischemia by hypocapnia)

How can we guarantee the best quality in prehospital airway management? First of all, we need to consider that airway patency is the best way of attaining our goals: oxygenation and ventilation. Far too often, the rescuers forget this and focus exclusively on the maneuver. Therefore, we need to consider that airway management (and more generally, prehospital care) is just a process and not a maneuver carried out by an individual rescuer. Teamwork is essential for successful airway management: the simultaneous intervention of expert rescuers assures the reduction of on-scene times, a better monitoring of vital signs and full cooperation with the principal operator ("intubator").

3. Prehospital airway management: an algorithm

Clear indications regarding treatment, what the priorities are and the availability of alternative plans allow the emergency team to intervene in a qualified, efficient fashion. On the basis of the best that has been published, it has been possible to create guidelines and a simple algorithm for prehospital airway management (Wang et al, 2005; Rich et al, 2004). The objective is to reduce errors during prehospital airway management, through rational, operative choices and in-depth patient evaluations. An algorithm must be simple to follow to allow operators to find a clear pathway in an emergency situation. This algorithm is the result of a collaboration between SIAARTI (the Italian Society of Anaesthesia, Analgesia, Reanimation, Intensive Care and emergency) and PAMIA (the Italian Association for Prehospital Airway Management).

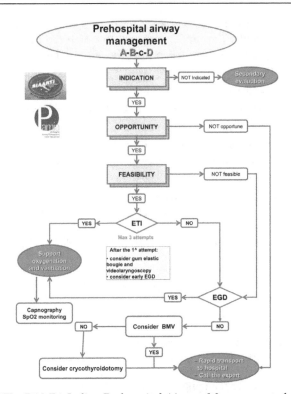

Fig. 1. The SIAARTI – PAMIA Italian Prehospital Airway Management algorithm.

The gold standard for airway management is tracheal intubation. The final decision to intubate the patient in the prehospital setting must always be the result of an extended evaluation. Although indication is only the first element, it is insufficient. In the algorithm, opportunity and feasibility have been added to the indication. In some cases the indication is clear. For example, an obstructed airway, severe hypoxemia with supplemental oxygen with mask and reservoir (high O2 concentration), a GCS < 9 associated with hypoxia/hypoventilation or if the patient is suffering from cardiac arrest or is required to ensure immediate airway patency. There are some cases in which the indicated intubation can be carried out in the more protected environment of the hospital. The concept of opportunity requires a detailed example.

A traumatized patient suffers a head injury after a car accident and has a neurological problem (GCS < 9) on the scene. Almost all guidelines report that a patient with GCS < 9 must be intubated. We agree with these guidelines, but the question is: does the rescuer always intubate the patient on the scene? The answer is that it depends.

If the patient is able to ventilate spontaneously, has good blood oxygenation (SpO2≥90) and intact gag reflexes and the Emergency Department (the right hospital) is nearby, it is inopportune to proceed with an endotracheal intubation. It is better to transfer the patient rapidly to the hospital where the emergency team can ensure an optimal airway management. This is especially true when the prehospital team does not have a lot of experience when it comes to difficult airways. However, if the same traumatized patient is unable to ventilate sufficiently (low SpO2) and/or has a high risk of pulmonary aspiration, it is opportune to assure the airway patency at the scene. The same is true if the right hospital is too far away.

When intubation is advisable, but not opportune, the algorithm indicates rapid transportation to the hospital and a call to the hospital emergency team. The aim is to guarantee continuity of care for the patient.

The third element in the decision to intubate regards its feasibility. Sometime an indicated and opportune prehospital endotracheal intubation is unfeasible. Unfeasible endotracheal intubation has been classified into three groups:

Operator/team dependent - Prehospital airway management is a team activity and an optimal performance requires the experience and competence of each and every member of the team. Generally speaking, all operators think that their personal experience is the main reason for an optimal airway management (Wang et al 2005, 2007). However, in many cases, if the operator has low levels of experience and carries out a small number of intubations per year, an endotracheal intubation might be unfeasible (Thomas et al, 2010). Airway skill maintenance is a real problem because many paramedics or physicians do not manage a sufficient number of cases to be able to manage complex situations. Airway management means teamwork and the team members must be properly trained. For this reason, it is important to perform simulations and to practice crisis resource management as often as possible. In general, paramedic and emergency physician training courses mainly emphasize airway management skills and techniques. Virtually no training is provided regarding the process of airway management; that is, how to assimilate and integrate airway assessment, management and procedural skills in response to changing conditions and non-technical skills.

Our algorithm provides a context for teaching this important concept.

Patient dependent – It is known that many anatomical features can prevent endotracheal intubation (for example, difficulty in opening the mouth and neck rigidity). Many traumatized patients can suffer from facial, or airway, traumas which render endotracheal intubation either difficult or impossible, even for the most competent and expert team. The ability to rapidly recognize the situations which can obstacle the coherent and correct carrying out of the maneuver allows us to avoid ulterior complications to the patient by using alternative plans.

Setting dependent –there are many difficulties (adverse lighting, the position of the patient, etc) which can lead to the unfeasibility of carrying out endotracheal intubation in the prehospital setting. If the patient is trapped in a car, for instance, a direct laryngoscopy is not feasible. If endotracheal intubation is unfeasible, the algorithm indicates the early use of extraglottic devices (EGDs)[1] to guarantee oxygenation and ventilation (Guyette et al, 2007; Kette et al., 2005; Frascone et al, 2008; Barata, 2008).

EGDs guarantee good oxygenation, adequate ventilation, and limit the risk of pulmonary aspiration. Several cases of EGDs being used on patients who are trapped in cars indicate

---

[1] In Italian Guidelines it is possible to read the definition of Extra-Glottic Device (EGD): literature indicates alternative devices as "supraglottic", while the GdS chose to group all ventilation devices that do not pass through the laryngeal aditus as "extraglottic " devices (Petrini et al, 2005).

that patients arrive in the Emergency Department with PaO2 and PaCO2 values within the limits of normality. The learning curve of EGDs is steeper if compared to the endotracheal intubation one.

If, at the end of an initial evaluation, endotracheal intubation is indicated, opportune and feasible, the operator and the team can proceed to intubate the patient. If the patient is not in cardiac arrest, the use of adjuvant drugs is indicated. Advanced airway management requires the selection of appropriate drugs for a particular clinical situation.

Correct drug selection:

- facilitates the laryngoscopy
- improves the likelihood of the quality and success of endotracheal intubation
- attenuates the physiologic response to intubation and reduces the risk of pulmonary aspiration and other intubation complications

However, drugs may cause side effects: for example, hypotension in patients with severe head injuries and hemorrhagic shock. Hypotension reduces cerebral perfusion and therefore increases the risk of ischemic cerebral damage.

When the team is preparing to intubate a patient, it must always bear in mind that the patient will suffer damage from hypoxia and not from the unsuccessful tracheal intubation. A simple laryngoscopy is considered to be "an attempt", even if the intubation is not actually performed. If endotracheal intubation is unsuccessful, we suggest to reassess the technique, the patient's position and the right dosage of drugs. The general rule is that the operator must not attempt to intubate the patient more than three times.

This is because if the tube cannot be positioned correctly after the second and third attempt, the rate of complications (hypoxia, regurgitation, airway trauma) increases dramatically and, in some cases, results in a "cannot ventilate cannot intubate (CVCI)" condition. A laryngeal manipulation technique can be useful; for example BURP - Backward, Upward, Right Pressure (Levitan et al, 2006).

The general rule is that three attempts should be made with alternative techniques and devices. After the first unsuccessful attempt, it is necessary consider an alternative plan.

In particular:

- the early use of EGDS: is, as mentioned previously, the best alternative in situations where it is too difficult to perform endotracheal intubation due to operator/team experience (unfeasible intubation)
- Gum elastic bougie: when the glottic view is limited (Cormack Lehane 2-e and 3) an introducer can be useful (Jabre et al., 2005). The gum elastic bougie technique is still used too little in the prehospital setting and therefore it is necessary to activate training courses to implement it.
- Videolaryngoscopy: in all probability, the future approach to airway management will be modified by the use of videolaryngoscopy in all settings. In the prehospital setting there are (Lim & Goh, 2009; Wayne & McDonnell, 2010) some situations which have demonstrated the usefulness of videolaryngoscopes, either as the instrument of first choice or as an alternative to a failed intubation attempt.

The possibility to train personnel in a different technique probably represents a favorable use of the videolaryngoscope. In any case, we should not forget the limitations of the videolargynoscope, for example when you have a good view of the glottis but find it difficult to position the tube. This can be caused by the curvature of the blade, which can make it difficult to guide the tube inside the trachea (Bjoernsen & Parquette, 2008)

We should also briefly mention the use of the Sellick maneuver. This is recommended in reducing the risk of pulmonary aspiration during advanced airway management. Several recently published studies have cast doubt on the efficacy of the maneuver in reducing the risk of pulmonary aspiration, and also underline how the it can worsen the visualization of the glottis and the positioning of a laryngeal mask (Ellis et al., 2007; Beavers et al. 2009).

A particularly delicate phase is represented by the control of the correct positioning of the tracheal tube. The literature reports various different ways of evaluating the correct position of the tracheal tube without encountering any particular problems, especially after a complicated, difficult laryngoscopy.

In this latter case it is not possible to visualize the passing of the tube through the vocal cords (an element which although useful, does not always guarantee that the tube is and, more importantly, remains correctly positioned). Moreover, auscultation and other indirect signs (expansion of the thorax) can be unreliable. For this reason, both instrumental and clinical evaluations are recommended.

In particular:

- capnography: it is evident that the capnographic curve (monitoring of end-tidal CO2) allows us to be certain that the tracheal tube (and the EGD) has been positioned correctly and highlights an eventual accidental extubation (the disappearance of the capnographic curve). When it comes to the respiratory and cardicirculatory state of the patient, capnographic monitoring is also recommended in the prehospital setting.
- oesophageal aspiration test (ODD) with self-expandable bulb or syringe: this is a very simple, inexpensive evaluation to perform and provides results which are extremely useful.

It will eventually be possible to identify tracheal rings or carina in the hospital with a fibrescope and, in some cases, identify the correct position of the tube by ultrasonography. The correct attachment of the tube is particularly important in the prehospital setting insofar as it is not uncommon for the tube to move (with the risk of positioning itself in the pharynx or in the esophagus) when the patient is being moved.

4. Prehospital intubation and drugs administration: rapid sequence intubation

If a patient is not experiencing a cardiac arrest and therefore present in one way or another, the tracheal intubation maneuver, as well as the positioning of a EGD, requires the administration of drugs.

The ideal conditions for advanced airway management are represented by the absence of the patient's muscle tone (it is facilitated by being able to open the mouth and, as a consequence, being able to visualize the glottides), the absence of induced responses (eg. vomit) and of endodynamic repercussions (tachycardia, hypertension and an increase in intracranial pressure).

Sedative-hypnotic drugs, analgesics, opiates, and other inductor medicines guarantee a significant efficacy, however, they are not without their dangerous side effects (which include the vasodilation effects of some sedatives-hypnotics which can cause severe hypotension in hypovolemic patients (especially in case of hemorraghic shock).

The knowledge of the pharmacokinetic and pharmacodynamic properties of the drugs being used is essential to obtain the benefits and reduce undesirable side effects. It is not uncommon for a tracheal intubation attempt to be unsuccessful because not enough drugs were administered (often for fear of the side effects) or because onset times had not been respected. Alongside the choice of drug, it is also important to know how the drug is administered. A general diagram follows below.

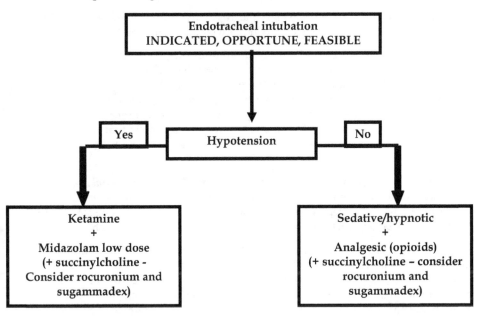

Fig. 2. The pharmacologic approach to endotracheal intubation in the prehospital setting.

An essential element in the choice of drug for tracheal intubation is represented by the patient's volemic state. It is recommended that hypovolemic patients use an inductor drug which guarantees hemodynamic stability and does not determine vasodilation or respiratory depression. Ketamine offers all of these advantages. Another excellent choice is etomidate, which has recently come under discussion for its corticosteroid synthesis suppression action.

Benzodiazepine (midazolam and opioid analgesics, in particular, fentanyl) are recommended for patients in a state of hemodynamic stability. An important element which needs to be considered is how to administer the drug.

The use of a combination of drugs is recommended increase their advantages, reducing their dosages and therefore their side effects. Moreover, when the patient's clinical conditions allow, (sufficient pulmonary exchange with SpO2 > 90), a titrated drug administration is indicated in order to obtain the desired result (sedation, muscular relaxation) with minimum dosages (less side effects).

Rapid Sequence Induction (RSI) was described over forty years ago (Stept & Safar, 1970). This technique was recommended in situations of anaesthesiological induction in patients with a full stomach in order to reduce the risk of regurgitation and successive pulmonary aspiration to a minimum. Over the years this technique has evolved into Rapid Sequence Intubation. RSI is defined as a series of steps, with the administration of sedative and paralytic agents, which facilitates rapid endotracheal intubation and minimize the complications. The paralytic agent of choice is succynilcholine. The recent availability of sugammadex might increase the use of rocuronium in the future.

An increasing body of evidence sustains the role played by sugammadex in the rapid reversal of neuromuscular blockade by rocuronium (at the maximum dosage, 16 mg/Kg.).

One of the advantages of administering rocuronium is that, if the patient is intubated, its considerable intubation dosage (0.6 – 1.2 mg/Kg) has a long-lasting effect and so facilitates mechanical ventilation. Succynilcholine has a short-lasting action and it is necessary to administer a long-acting neuromuscular blocking agent (i.e. vecuronium or rocuronium) after intubation. The paralytic agent can have significant side effects, the most important being apnea. If the operator/team is unable to ventilate and intubate the patient the consequences can be serious (CVCI with desaturation, bradycardia, cardiac arrest).

Some emergency medical services have introduced "*sedation facilitated intubation – SFI*": the rescuers use sedatives without any paralytic agents. The advantage of this is that it eliminates the risks associated with the use of muscle relaxants, but the side effect is that high dosages are required to obtain good, endotracheal intubation conditions.

A new technique, Rapid Sequence Airway (RSA) has recently been introduced (Braude & Richards, 2007) as an alternative to RSI. The pharmacological approach is the same as RSI: the operator can place an EGD immediately with the advantages of reducing the time necessary to obtain airway patency and thus reducing any side effects (i.e. hypoxia episodes during airway management). EGDs provide much more aspiration protection than many rescuers can believe.

The RSI steps are reported in the "9 Ps":

1. *Preparation* – The team verifies the availability of all that can be useful and mandatory for RSI. The SpO2, ECG and blood pressure monitoring are activated. A "*sure*" venous access is obtained.
2. *Preoxygenation* – The patient is preoxygenated through an oxygen mask with a reservoir (if he/she is able to breath spontaneously) or a bag-mask system. High concentrations of O2 are used to substitute the air in the lungs ("denitrogenation"). In this way the patient's oxygen reserves increase and desaturation during the apnea phase and the endotracheal intubation maneuver is less probable. If the patient is not breathing and is not ventilated, the desaturation progressively decreases, but if the lungs are rich in oxygen, the reduction is slow. The shape of the hemoglobin dissociation curve explains this. Serious problems can occur when the patient has a lung injury (contusion, laceration) or consolidation (pulmonary oedema, ARDS) which prevents good

pulmonary exchange and good blood saturation. In this case an immediate endotracheal intubation is necessary.

3. Pretreatment – the administration of drugs can be indicated to reduce the pathophysiological effects of laryngoscopy and intubation (for example, lidocaine 2 mg/Kg) or a defasciculating dose of non-depolarinzing muscle relaxants in case of the use of succynilcholine (for example vecuronium 0,01 mg/Kg).

4. *Paralysis and sedation* – The administration of sedatives and muscle relaxants is certainly useful when carrying out the tracheal intubation maneuver. Suggested dosages are:
   - Midazolam 0.2 – 0.3 mg/Kg.
   - Fentanyl 1.5 – 2 mcg/Kg.
   - Ketamine 1 – 2 mg/Kg.
   - Etomidate 0.3 mg/Kg.

   The administration of a sedative is followed by the administration of muscle relaxants. The suggested dosages are:

   - Succynilcholine 1.5 mg/Kg.
   - Rocuronium 0.6 – 1.2 mg/Kg.

5. *Protection* – After the drugs have been administered, the patient is not ventilated to prevent the risk of gastric insufflation and regurgitation due to the relaxation of the upper esophageal sphincter. A team member applies the Sellick maneuver (until the tube's cuff insufflation and the verification of endotracheal tube position have been performed). With trauma patients, a team member carries out manual in-line stabilization (MILS) of the head to limit neck movements during the laryngoscopy and intubation.

6. *Pass the tube* –the laringoscopy to ntroduction of the tube in trachea.

7. *Positioning* – this is an extremely important phase. The operator verifies the correct position of the tube in the trachea using clinical and instrumental methods.

8. *Postintubation management* – It is necessary to fix the tube firmly in the correct position because it can be displaced during transportation.

9. *Plan "B"* – An emergency plan (for example, early EGD) must be always considered.

5. Prehospital ventilation: brief considerations

An important study by Davis et al, 2003 raises some problems. In particular, it reports that significant, inadvertent hyperventilation after an endotracheal intubation on the scene in patients with severe head injuries (low $PaCO_2$) was associated with a decrease in good outcomes (together with more time on the scene and desaturation during intubation attempts). We need to ensure the quality of prehospital emergency care; this means considering the "*global*" treatment of the patient. Airway patency is the way to reach our goals: oxygenation and optimal ventilation.

How can we improve early ventilation in the prehospital setting? Many traumatized patients arrive at the hospital suffering from hypocapnia as a result of hyperventilation. Hypocapnia causes cerebral blood flow reduction and consequent ischemia (secondary brain damage). For example, in 122 traumatized patients (Helm et al., 2002) optimal oxygenation was achieved in 85.2% and adequate ventilation (normocapnia, $PaCO_2$ 35 – 45 mmHg) in 42.6% of patients upon admission to hospital. Optimal oxygenation, as well as adequate ventilation, was achieved in 37.7% of the study population.

Hypoxemia (PaO2 < 60 mmHg.) was observed in 2.5%, hypercapnia (PaCO2 > 45 mmHg.) in 16.4% and hypocapnia (PaCO2 < 35 mmHg.) in 40.9%. A high hypocapnia rate is not what we are looking for. An interesting conclusion of this study is that endotracheal intubation does not assure good ventilation *per se*. In all probability, the use of a capnography in the prehospital setting could guarantee better ventilation (Helm et al, 2003). It is necessary to consider the limitations of the capnography in unstable patients (the large difference between ETCO2 and PaCO2).

Setting ventilation at the tidal volume of 10 ml/Kg. is another important intervention in limiting inadvertent hyperventilation. The rescue team often uses manual ventilation, which has no controls on tidal volume and ventilatory frequency, and not portable ventilators.

We recommend the combined use of early, mechanical ventilation with controlled tidal volumes (*early* means immediately after the correct positioning of the verified tube) and continuous capnography (recommended for tube position control). Ideally, blood gas analysis could be helpful but its technical limitations reduce the use of this technique. The correct use of portable ventilators can reduce the incidence of the hemodynamic effects of positive pressure ventilation.

Positive intrathoracic pressure, which is determined by mechanical ventilation, causes a reduction in venous return and so reduces cardiac output and blood pressure (hypotension), especially in hypovolemic patients. The effect on blood pressure determined by positive pressure ventilation is important because it can cause severe secondary damage to patients (Pepe et al., 2003; Shafi & Gentilello 2005). The combination of hypotension and hypocapnia can be very dangerous for a traumatized brain.

6. Clinical cases

Here we report two clinical cases of difficult, prehospital intubation which consider the purposed algorithm as a pathway for the best patient treatment.

a. The patient was a middle-age woman who was riding her bike. A car hit her at high speed. When the rescuers arrived, she was on the ground, comatose (GCS = 7; E1, V,2, M4), had vomit and noisy breathing; SpO2 was 87% with high flow oxygen. The Trauma Center was far away: 50 minutes by ambulance. The physician evaluated the patient and decided to intubate because prehospital intubation was:
-   indicated: GCS < 9; airway partially obstructed; desaturation
-   opportune: the Trauma Center was far away
-   feasible: both the physician and the team were considered expert and there were no evident anatomic signs of difficulty

The team leader decided to apply the RSI. The heart rate was 82/ min. and blood pressure was 140/80 mmHg. The woman weighed 60 Kg. 12 mgs of Midazolam, 100 mcg of fentanyl. and 100 mg of succynilcholine were administered. The first intubation attempt was unsuccessful, and the patient desaturated rapidly during this attempt (SpO2 = 84%). The physician (team leader) thought that the problem was an incorrect technique (his incorrect position and difficulties due to excessive manual in-line stabilization of the head).

He re-ventilated the patient with a bag–mask and positioned her correctly while a team member applied correct manual in-line stabilization of the head. The second intubation attempt failed too. The glottic visualisation was classified Cormack-Lehane (modified) 3-e (3 extreme).

On the third attempt the physician used an introducer but failed to position the tube inside the trachea. The patient was desaturated and a Laryngeal Tube was positioned with good ventilation and oxygenation by a portable ventilator. The patient arrived in the Emergency Room an hour later: the SpO2 was 98%, and a blood gas analysis reported at PaO2 = 99 mmHg. and PaCO2 = 43 mmHg. She was intubated by the expert anesthesiologist with a laryngeal mask and fibrescope without any problem.

Comment: the physician probably did not evaluate the airway difficulty correctly, the patient remained on the scene too long and had severe complications (bad oxygenation). The choice of alternative device should have been the right choice to secure a valid oxygenation.

b. A 42 yr. old lorry/truck driver (male, weight 80 Kg.) had an accident: he fell asleep and his lorry ran into another one. The cab was restricted and the driver trapped. When the rescuers arrived he was comatose (GCS = 3; E1, V1, M1) and gasping. The prehospital intubation was:

- indicated: GCS < 9 and gasping
- opportune: the patient was entrapped
- unfeasible: a direct laryngoscopy was not feasible.

The physician (an expert emergency helicopter physician) and the team considered using a videolaryngoscope and a plan B (early EGD). In this case, due to the patient's clinical conditions, the administration of sedatives and muscle relaxants was unnecessary. The physician verified his personal safety and, assisted by a team member, approached the patient from the front through the windshield. First, he applied a basic maneuver to open the airway and then inserted an Airtraq™ (Prodol, Spain) into the mouth. He obtained a good glottic visualization and the tube was inserted into the trachea. The videolaryngoscope permitted the control of the correct position of the tube (anterior to the arythenoids cartilage) and the physician ventilated the patient with a portable ventilator during the complex intervention by the fire department. When the patient was removed, the physician controlled the tube position and then transported him to the Trauma Center.

Comment: in this case, the high levels of experience and competence permitted the team to ensure a good quality of airway management in an extremely difficult situation, both because of the patient's condition and the setting.

7. Conclusions

In this chapter we described a linear, simple way to manage airway in emergency prehospital settings. The application of this algorithm to the real world requires a complete evaluation of material, personnel resources and a professional control by EMS directors.

Prehospital airway management is a complicated field of emergency care but the data currently at our disposal regarding devices shows us that if emergency team personnel are adequately trained and follow a rational intervention procedure, high quality results will be obtained.

8. References

Bacon CL, Corriere C, Lavery RF, Livingston DH. (2001). The use of capnography in the air medical environment. *Air Med J*, Vol. 20, No. 5, (September-October 2001), pp. (27-29), ISSN 1067-991X

Barata I. (2008). The laryngeal mask airway: Prehospital and emergency department use. *Emerg Med Clin North Am*, Vol. 26, No. 4, (November 2008), pp. (1069-1083), ISSN 0733-8627

Beavers RA, Moos DD, Cudderford JD. (2009). Analysis of the application of cricoid pressure: Implications for the clinician. *J Perianesth Nurs*, Vol. 24, No. 2, (April 2009), pp. (92-102), ISSN 1089-9472

Bjoernsen LP, Parquette BT, Lindsay BM. (2008). Prehospital use of video laryngoscope by an air medical crew. *Air Med J*, Vol. 27, No. 5, (September 2008), pp. (242-244), ISSN 1067-991X

Boylan JF, Kavanagh BP. (2008). Emergency airway management: Competence vs expertise. *Anesthesiology*, Vol. 109, No. 6, (December 2008), pp. (945-947), ISSN 0003-3022

Braude D & Richards M. (2007). Rapid Sequence Airway (RSA) – A novel approach to prehospital airway management. *Prehospital Emergency Care*, Vol. 11, No. 2, (April/June 2007), pp. (250-2), ISSN 1545-0066

Davis DP, Hoyt DB, Ochs M, Fortlage D, Holbrook T, Marshall LW, Rosen P. (2003). The effect of paramedic rapid sequence intubation on outcome in patients with severe traumatic brain injury. *Journal of Trauma*, Vol. 54, No. 3 (March 2003), pp. (444-53), ISSN 0022-5282

Davis DP, Peay J, Sise MJ, Vilke GM, Kennedy F, Eastman BA, et al. (2005). The impact of prehospital endotracheal intubation on outcome in moderate to severe traumatic brain injury. *Journal of Trauma*, Vol. 58, No. 5, (May 2005), pp. (933-939), ISSN 0022-5282

Deakin CD, King P, Thompson F. (2009). Prehospital advanced airway management by ambulance technicians and paramedics: Is clinical practice sufficient to maintain skills?. *Emerg Med J*, Vol. 26, No. 12, (December 2009), pp. (888-891), ISSN 0736-4679

Donald MJ, Paterson B. (2006). End tidal carbon dioxide monitoring in prehospital and retrieval medicine: a review. *Emerg Med J*, Vol. 23, No. 9, (September 2006), pp. (728-730), ISSN 0736-4679

Ellis DY, Harris T, Zideman D. (2007). Cricoid pressure in emergency department rapid sequence tracheal intubations: A risk-benefit analysis. *Ann Emerg Med*, Vol. 50, No. 6, (December 2007), pp. (653-665), ISSN 0196-0644

Fakhry SM, Scanlon JM, Robinson L, Askari R, Watenpaugh RL, Fata P, et al. (2006). Prehospital rapid sequence intubation for head trauma: Conditions for a successful program. *Journal of Trauma*, Vol. 60, No. 5, (May 2006), pp. (997-1001), ISSN 0022-5282

Frascone RJ, Heegaard W, Pippert G, Dries D, Molinari P, Salzman J. (2008). Use of the intubating laryngeal mask airway in HEMS. *Air Med J*, Vol. 27, No. 4, (July-March 2008), pp. (182–184), ISSN 1067-991X

Guyette FX, Greenwood MJ, Neubecker D, Roth R, Wang HE. (2007). Alternate airways in the prehospital setting (resource document to NAEMSP position statement). *Prehosp Emerg Care*, Vol. 11, No. 1, (January-March 2007), pp. (56-61), ISSN 1545-0066

Helm M, Hauke J & Lampl L. (2002). A prospective study of the quality of prehospital emergency ventilation in patients with severe head injury. *Br J Anaesth*, Vol. 88, No. 3 (March 2002), pp. (345–9), ISSN 0007-0912

Helm M, Shuster R, Hauke J & Lampl L. (2003). Tight control of prehospital ventilation by capnography in major trauma victims. *Br J Anaesth*, Vol. 90, No. 3, (March 2003), pp. (327-32), ISSN 0007-0912

Herff H, Wenzel V, Lockey D. (2009). Prehospital intubation: The right tools in the right hands at the right time. *Anesth Analg*, Vol. 109, No. 2, (August 2009), pp. (303-305), ISSN 0003-2999

Jabre P, Combes X, Leroux B, Aaron E, Auger H, Margenet A, et al. (2005). Use of gum elastic bougie for prehospital difficult intubation. *Am J Emerg Med* , Vol. 23, No. 4, (July 2005), pp. (552–555), ISSN 0735-6757

Katz SH, Falk JL. (2001). Misplaced endotracheal tubes by paramedics in an urban emergency medical services system. *Ann Emerg Med*, Vol. 37, No. 1, (January 2001), pp. (32–37), ISSN 0196-0644

Kette F, Reffo L, Giordani G. (2005). The use of laryngeal tube by nurses in out-of-hospital emergencies: Preliminary experience. *Resuscitation*, Vol. 66, No.1, (July 2005), pp. (21–25), ISSN 0300-9572

Klemen P, Grmec S. (2006). Effect of prehospital advanced life support with rapid sequence intubation on outcome of severe traumatic brain injury. *Acta Anaesthesiol Scand*, Vol. 50, No. 10, (November 2006), pp. (1250-1254), ISSN 1399-6576

Lecky F, Bryden D, Little R, Tong N, Moulton C. (2008). Emergency intubation for acutely ill and injured patients (Review), In: *The Cochrane Library*, 2008, Issue 2, http://www.thecochranelibrary.com

Levitan RM, Kinkle WC, Levin WJ, Everett WW. (2006). Laryngeal view during laryngoscopy: A randomized trial comparing cricoid pressure, Backward-Upward-Rightward Pressure and bimanual laryngoscopy. *Ann Emerg Med*, Vol. 47, No. 6, (June 2006), pp. (548–555), ISSN 0196-0644

Lim HC, Goh SH. (2009). Utilization of a glidescope videolaryngoscope for orotracheal intubations in different emergency airway management settings. *Eur J Emerg Med*, Vol. 16, No. 2, (April 2009), pp. (68–73), ISSN 0969-9546

Petrini F et al. (2005). Recommendations for airway control and difficult airway management. *Minerva Anestesiol*, Vol.71, No.11 (Nov 2005), pp.(617-57), ISSN 1827-1596

Pepe PE, Raedler C, Lurie KG & Wigginton JG (2003) Emergency ventilatory management in hemorrhagic states: Elemental or detrimental?. *Journal of Trauma*, Vol. 54, No. 6, (June 2003), pp. (1048–57), ISSN 0022-5282

Rich JM, Mason AM, Ramsay MA (2004). AANA Journal Course: update for nurse anesthetist. The SLAM Emergency Airway Flowchart: a new guide for advanced airway practitioners. AANAJ, Vol 72, (2004), pp (431-439)

Shafi S & Gentilello L. (2005). Pre-hospital endotracheal intubation and positive pressure ventilation is associated with hypotension and decreased survival in hypovolemic trauma patients: An analysis of the National Trauma Data Bank. *Journal of Trauma*, Vol. 59, No. 5, (November 2005), pp. (1140–7), ISSN 0022-5282

Sollid SJM, Heltne JK, Soreide E, Lossius HM. (2008). Pre-hospital advanced airway management by anaesthesiologists: Is there still room for improvement. *Scandinav Journal of Trauma, Resuscitation and Emerg Med*, Vol. 16, No. 2, (July 2008), pp. (2–8), ISSN 1757-7241

Stept & Safar. (1970). Rapid induction-intubation for prevention of gastric-content aspiration. *Anesth Analg*, Vol. 49, No. 4, (July-August 1970), pp. (633–36), ISSN 0003-2999

Thomas S, Judge T, Lowell MJ, MacDonald RD, Madden J, Pickett K, et al. (2010). Airway management and hypoxemia rates in air and round critical care transport: A multicenter study. *Prehosp. Emerg Care*, Vol. 14, No. 3, (July-September 2010), pp. (283-291), ISSN 1545-0066

Timmermann A, Eich C, Russo SG, Natge U, Brauer A, Rosenblatt, et al. (2006) Prehospital airway management: A prospective evaluation of anaesthesia trained emergency physicians. *Resuscitation*, Vol. 70, No. 2, (August 2006), pp.(179-185), ISSN 0300-9572

Timmermann A, Russo SG, Eich C, Rossler M, Braun U, Rosenblatt WH, et al. (2007). The out-of-hospital esophageal and endobronchial intubations performed by emergency physicians. *Anesth Analg*, Vol. 104, No. 3, (March 2007), pp. (619–623), ISSN 0003-2999

Wang HE, Peitzmann AB, Cassidy LD, Adelson PD, Yealy DM. (2004). Out-of-hospital endotracheal intubation and outcome after traumatic brain injury. *Ann Emerg Med*, Vol. 44, No. 5, (November 2004), pp. (439–450), ISSN 0196-0644

Wang HE, Kupas DF, Cooney R, Yealy Dm, Lave JR. (2005). Procedural experience with out-of hospital endotracheal intubation. *Crit Care Med*, Vol. 33, No. 8, (August 2005), pp. (1718-1721), ISSN 0090-3493

Wang HE, Yealy DM. (2006). Out-of-hospital endotracheal intubation: Where are we?. *Ann Emerg Med*, Vol. 47, No. 6, (June 2006), pp. (523–541), ISSN 0196-0644

Wang HE, Abo BN, Lave JR, Yealy DM. (2007). How would minimum experience standards affect distribution of out-of-hospital endotracheal intubations?. *Ann Emerg Med*, Vol. 50, No. 3, (September 2007), pp. (246-252), ISSN 0196-0644

Warner KJ, Carlborn D, Cooke CR, Bulger EM, Copass MK, Sharar SR. (2010). Paramedic training for proficient prehospital endotracheal intubation. *Prehosp Emerg Care*, Vol. 14, No. 1, (January-March 2010), pp. (103-108), ISSN 1545-0066

Wayne MA, McDonnell M. (2010). Comparison of traditional versus video laryngoscopy in out-of-hospital tracheal intubation. *Prehosp Emerg Care*, Vol. 14, No. 2, (April-June 2010, pp. (278–282), ISSN 1545-0066

Wirtz DD, Ortiz C, Newman DH, Zhitomirsky I. (2007). Unrecognized misplacement of endotracheal tubes by ground prehospital providers. *Prehosp Emerg Care*, Vol. 11, No. 2, (April-June 2007), pp. (213–218), ISSN 1545-0066

7

Emergency Medicine in the Czech Republic

Jiri Pokorny
POMAMED, Prague,
Czech Republic

1. Introduction

The history of out-of-hospital emergency medicine begins many centuries ago. Efforts to help patients have been made by mankind for a long time. In principle, two approaches to providing professional medical assistance can be identified; either with medical help called to the affected person, or the person involved being transferred either to a shaman, a physician, or to a medical center. The story of in-hospital emergency medicine begins with the setting up of facilities designed to take care of and treat those affected in hospitals. The traditional model of provision of emergency care includes outpatient departments related to the individual branches of medicine. The 1960s saw the building of the first emergency departments in the United States (2).

Pre-hospital emergency care has a long-standing tradition in this country. The predecessor of Prague's emergency medical service, referred to as the Prague Volunteer Protection Unit, was established as early as 1857 making it, together with the Budapest-based predecessor of emergency service, to the oldest emergency units within Europe. Just as in many other countries, the utmost priority of the emergency service was to transfer the patient to hospital faster and in a more patient-friendly manner than before. While both world wars, and the Korean and Vietnam wars, brought immense suffering to millions of people, they helped mankind make major progress in their knowledge regarding the provision of emergency care and management of trauma-related shock, as well as clearly showing the advantages of early acute surgery. Military experience has necessarily translated into the provision of emergency care outside the battlefield. Additionally, provision of emergency care had to reflect new insights into the pathophysiology and management of various types of shock, intoxication, coronary heart disease, stroke, and so on.

It should be noted here that modern history of emergency medicine in the Czech Republic began to unfold in what was formerly referred to as the Czechoslovak Republic, as a country founded in 1918 and inhabited by the Czech and Slovak nations until its breakup into the Czech Republic and Slovakia in 1992.

2. Milestones of emergency medicine in the Czech Republic

Several milestones can be identified in the evolution of emergency medicine in the Czech Republic including, in particular:

- Building up a service for transferring patients to health care facilities;
- The founding of coronary care units and first departments of anesthesiology/resuscitation;
- The 1968 Soviet-led invasion of Czechoslovakia making hundreds of experienced physicians and nurses flee the country;
- A 1974 decree of the Czechoslovak Ministry of Health dividing health care into several levels to reflect patients' needs and requiring the setting up of emergency medical units across the country (2);
- November 1989, the fall of the Communist regime and the Iron Curtain, liberalization of societal and economic life and, subsequently, the entry of private entities into the health care sector;
- A 1992 decree of the Czech Ministry of Health (No. 434/92 et seq.) governing emergency medical service (EMS);
- The decision by the Health Minister, Ivan David, in 1998 to make emergency medicine a separate branch of medicine requiring each future specialist to pass a board examination (6);
- Widespread floods in 1997 and 2002 (the so called "thousand-year water") and the 9/11 terrorist attacks in the USA in 2001;
- The economic crisis which hit the world in 2008;
- The year 2011 making the Emergency Medical Service a law.

According to a concept developed by the Czech Ministry of Health and published in 1974, patients are provided health care at different levels (1, 2). The top level of differentiated medical care is resuscitation care in patients developing failure of one or several organs. Originally, this type of care should be provided to patients by multidisciplinary teams at units of anesthesiology/resuscitation; also later at newly formed departments of anesthesiology/resuscitation. The next level below is intensive care provided to patients who have not yet developed failure of vital function but are at risk of this. Intensive care is provided at intensive care units (ICUs), set up predominantly at departments related to the respective branch of medicine, thus giving rise to ICUs of internal medicine, neurology, surgery, urology, gynecology, orthopedics, otorhinolaryngology, and psychiatry as well as pediatric ICUs at departments of pediatrics. These units gradually evolved into subspecialty ones, both within internal medicine and other branches of medicine, to become coronary care and metabolic care units, ICUs of neurosurgery, spondylosurgery, spinal, neonatal, and pre-mature baby ICUs, and so on. The historical division of differentiated care into resuscitation units and ICUs is no longer applicable as many ICUs provide resuscitation care in addition to intensive care, while standard care is provided in standard hospital wards. An extension to standard health care is long-term care, and rehabilitation care, as well as care provided at spa facilities. The lowest level of differentiated care is represented by symptomatic care available to those patients who cannot be cured by state-of-the-art medicine.

3. Building of the system of emergency care in the Czech Republic

Up to the 1970s, pre-hospital emergency care was provided by the general practitioner emergency service (called LSPP, in Czech) in most regions of the country. Originally, this state-run type of care was intended to provide pre-hospital emergency care for citizens in the off-hours when general practitioners or outpatient specialists were unavailable. Physicians on duty would visit not only those who could not be transferred to LSPP offices (whatever the reason) but also had to attend to the most serious cases including persons involved in road accidents, those developing spasmodic conditions, unconscious persons, and those requiring resuscitation. Additionally, their duties included inquests into the cause of death. The professional standard of care depended not only on the erudition and skills of the physician on duty but, also, on the availability of equipment to provide emergency care (and its condition). Another important consideration was the driver on duty on that particular day. Ideally, EMS ambulance crews included two members but the driver's only responsibility was to take the physician to the scene of emergency and back, with any other assistance depending solely on the driver's good will and willingness. In cases where the patient's condition required emergency care and the other member was only "a driver", emergency care was provided exclusively in an impromptu manner by the physician with the outcomes necessarily being such. For a long time, LSPP served as a backup to EMS called in cases requiring care for several patients at a time, or when an EMS ambulance was currently unavailable, e.g., because of a mechanical defect, or in cases requiring secondary transfer in a system where only a single EMS ambulance with a physician was operating within the whole region. Upon the setting up of a network of EMS ambulance stations, the list of duties of emergency service became somewhat shorter, soon to be currently trimmed even more and transformed. If serving properly and performing visits to outpatients, then this type of medical care attends to those developing conditions which, while not posing an immediate threat to life, could result in injury to the patient if deferring care, or if making the patient unnecessarily suffer for a prolonged period of time (e.g., intense pain of the spine). Whilst only restricted to shorter working hours in some areas, LSPP has been completely discontinued in other. According to health care managers, health care should be provided by both EMS and emergency departments, as well as by outpatient departments of hospitals instead of LSPP.

In the Czech Republic, out-of hospital emergency care is also provided by:

- General practitioners and outpatient specialists in their offices with, additionally, general practitioners during their visits to patients, particularly where an EMS ambulance is unavailable at the moment or in cases where the patient's condition deteriorates during the visit.
- Specialist emergency (rescue) units in cases where management of the patient's condition requires, in addition to medical knowledge and expertise, additional training and skills not expected from general health care professionals, such as those of fire fighters, mountain rescue service teams, water rescue service, mining rescue service, cavers, and dog trainers.
- The Czech Red Cross, responsible in particular for supervising compliance with safety rules at major cultural and political events as well as during disasters.
- A variety of private entities providing usual or, as an exception, also less demanding emergency, well paid, care to well-off patients, mainly to rich foreigners.

The above decree issued by the Ministry of Health in 1974 became the basis for setting up a network of EMS throughout the Czech Republic. The system selected for emergency care provision is the so-called French-German one whereby the EMS ambulance crew includes a physician. The reasons for this care, for one thing, traditional ones, with the rationale that – if the physician makes decisions in cases involving no risk of a delay in care – then they should logically also establish the diagnosis and treat patients in a much more serious condition. The medical-based reason for the decision was progress in medicine. It is now generally accepted that what actually matters is not to get the patient to hospital "as soon as possible" but to get them there alive. A critical consideration in emergency medicine is often truly a matter of life and death, i.e., timely provision of invasive procedures already when initiating treatment "on the spot", be that resuscitation involving clearing of the airways and early defibrillation, aggressive management of an anaphylactic reaction, or draining of a tense pneumothorax. The building of the emergency service system has been under the supervision of departments of anesthesiology and resuscitation care ever since 1974 (4). Much of the credit for the current EMS in the Czech Republic goes to anesthesiologists. However, those "going out" to attend to patients or the injured at that time included not only anesthesiologists but, also physicians serving at other departments as assigned by the hospital director. The list of enthusiasts laying, under not easy conditions, the foundations of this country's modern emergency service should by no means fail to include Mikeš, Dostál, Hasík, Novotný, Štětina, and Ždichynec, to mention just a few (5). There is little doubt that the concept of building the EMS network, as conceived by the ministry of health, has distinct advantages but, also, a host of drawbacks. It was not a rare occurrence that shifts in emergency service were assigned to junior physicians at the department or even physicians who had not passed board examinations yet, with the rationale being that full-time and senior physicians had "more important commitments" at their departments. Likewise, most hospitals did not then have the lightweight and portable PR-35 handheld transceivers, so physicians listed for EMS on a particular day were told to go to an emergency via regular hospital phone extensions not allocated for that purpose. No wonder then that 5 or 10 minutes were lost before locating and waiting for the physician on duty, and the time lost could not be made up however short the trip to the patient was. Accordingly, the fate of patients often depended not only the seriousness of the emergency but, also, on the department and the physician on duty on that particular day. In the decision-making process about the purchase of medical technology, departments and wards were most often given priority over the emergency service as heads of departments were invariably given priority over physicians in charge of the emergency service in the respective area. Given the need to solve the problems and to coordinate the service of rescue teams, Jiří Pokorný sr, the opinion leader in anesthesiology and resuscitation, established an Advisory Board headed by František Ždichynec, director of Prague's Emergency Medical Service until 1990. The Advisory Board included not only chief physicians of EMS units but, also, a number of accomplished experts in other branches providing emergency care. Thanks to rational argumentation when negotiating with the state bodies, a number of achievements were made. The most important of these was the centralized purchase of a 100 fully-equipped Renault Master ambulances, giving the rescue crew the opportunity to use technology they were aware of only when perusing journals and exhibitions until then. Although this was a major qualitative improvement across much of the territory of what was Czechoslovakia at that time, the number of EMS ambulances was not sufficient for all stations, a fact often resulting in conflicts. In some districts, hospital managers went as far as to dismantle the built-in equipment and rather install it in their hospitals. It was these facts that apparently largely contributed to a situation whereby, in the turbulent years following the so-called Velvet Revolution (1989), proponents seeking complete independence of the EMS eventually had their say. However, not all experts were in favor of such a concept (Hora, Pokorný jr). Upon the resignation of Ždichynec as Head of the Advisory Board, the body was taken over by a group of radical proponents of the concept of independence of the rescue services and their detachment from hospitals as the only possible solution. The legislative basis for complete independence of the rescue services was decree 434/92 Coll. Of Laws on EMS. Thus, after less than 20 years of fruitful cooperation, the year 1993 saw the definitive separation of out-of-hospital emergency care from in-hospital emergency care. On the one hand, the independence of rescue services made it possible to complete the creation of a network of EMS ambulance stations, independent health care dispatch units, markedly improved equipment of ambulance vehicles, and improved organization. As a distinct bonus, the independence of the emergency service also facilitated the creation of an integrated rescue system (EMS, firefighting service, and police). The trauma but, also, whole disaster plans of hospitals and districts were re-defined accordingly. On the other hand, this also resulted in the emergency services moving to facilities outside hospitals (most often shared with firefighting units) as well as in severing the "professional links" of the EMS staff to hospitals with all the negative implications.

The air medical emergency service went into pilot operation in Czechoslovakia in April 1987 in Prague. The medical team consisted most often of a physician and a rescuer. While, in indicated cases, transportation of patients by air is no doubt beneficial for the patient, it is extremely costly and its availability is not infrequently limited by the weather.

From time to time, there have been attempts to provide at least basic emergency care in busy downtown Prague by paramedics riding motorcycles. In the large majority of test operations, the rescuer was a paramedic. However, this type of EMS never gained widespread acceptance to actually go into operation – not even with weather permitting. Currently, tests are underway in central Prague to drive the paramedic to the site of an emergency in a minicar.

4. Hospital-based emergency care

The importance of the quick availability of emergency medical care is clearly highlighted not only by warfare experience. The traditional hospital-based pattern of admitting patients and the injured was simply no longer able to meet the demands of modern medicine. The biggest drawback of this concept has turned out to be what could be referred to as the "admission vacuum", i.e., the period of time from patient arrival at a hospital and the time point at which (the necessary) care begins to be instituted by a fully qualified and experienced staff in facilities adequate to and specifically assigned for this purpose, with continued hospital-based emergency care. The first "resuscitation ward" was founded, thanks to the foresight of Hugo Keszler as early as 1953 in a department of experimental surgery in Prague. The first department of anesthesiology and resuscitation for "field" patients opened in downtown Prague thanks to the enlightenment of Prof.

Špaček, Director of the Institute for Clinical and Experimental Medicine, as early as 15th February 1965 at Prague's Na Františku Hospital, which became the center for the training of physicians and nurses. Facilities for the admission and early management of the most serious cases were also being founded in out-of-Prague hospitals. They were rooms in the vicinity of EMS ambulance arrival points so as not to lose time by transporting the patient along hospital corridors or waiting for lifts (e.g., in Kladno and Mladá Boleslav, districts towns close to the capital). However, these were actually not "emergencies" as we perceive them in the Czech Republic today, or even Anglo-American style "emergencies" but, rather, admission rooms of specialist departments of resuscitation with a "high threshold" of patient admission.

As a legacy from its Communist era, the Czech Republic inherited an absolutely rational division of hospitals from level I to III facilities, which was a source of envy – at that time – of managers organizing health care in so-called developed nations. Type I hospitals of local importance and running just several departments provided health care only in the basic branches of medicine. More important for providing emergency care were type II hospitals serving a district catchment area and having more departments including specialist ones. In addition to attending to patients from their catchment area, these hospitals served as centers offering professional care and experience to type I hospitals. Top level care was available at type III hospitals, that is, regional facilities and university (teaching) hospitals. The extent of care possibly provided by each particular hospital was clearly specified according to its "classification". Interestingly, this division was similar to the pattern of facilities providing traumatology care in the USA. Regrettably, the Velvet Revolution introduced, as a reaction to the countless restrictions by the former regime, the "pendulum" principle whereby any regulation was harmful in the hope that all problems would be eliminated by the "invisible hand of the market". As a result, and quite paradoxically, a brand-new and well-equipped, five-bed department of resuscitation opened in a community (formerly Type I) in Sedlčany (a small town about 70 kms south-west of Prague) in the 1990s whereas one of the country's largest health care facilities – Thomayer University Hospital in Prague – did not have its own resuscitation department until 2001. Until then, patients urgently requiring resuscitation care had to be transferred by EMS ambulances and by air to facilities outside Prague, not infrequently exactly to the hospital at Sedlčany. Some regulation of the spectrum of procedures available was only introduced in recent years, mostly due to the restriction of the list of procedures reimbursed by health care insurance companies.

5. NEZAS and the birth of emergency departments

A most interesting – and to date little appreciated – experiment was the attempt by František Ždichynec, the last pre-Velvet Revolution director of Prague's EMS to ensure hospital-based backup and feedback to their physicians and nurses to maintain their erudition and continuity of pre-hospital and in-hospital emergency care. Ždichynec managed to acquire a Prague-based hospital called NEZAS catering to top Communist party and other top-level officials. The hospital was intended to become the center for the management of acute conditions of all branches of medicine including management of multiple trauma. It should have been the referral facility for a major proportion of patients needing emergency care in Prague. The idea of a hospital specializing in the treatment of acute conditions of all branches was not new, as similar hospitals were already in operation not only in Western nations but, also, in e.g., Sofia, Bulgaria, whereby full-time hospital physicians and those on duty as EMS members serve on a rotation basis. Specifically, after several months in a ward (depending on their specialty) and in the emergency department, they were to replace their colleagues serving as standby EMS members. The most experienced physicians were on duty in the air rescue service. As a result, the hospital set up the most unique unit of centralized admission as one of the first in what was then Czechoslovakia. The central out-of-hospital emergency department included two observation beds. The intention was to create a department, using the Western world pattern as a model, providing smooth and problem-free continuous provision of pre-hospital and in-hospital emergency care without the "admission vacuum". Using current terminology, the centralized admission system served as a high threshold (exclusively for the most critical cases) and, also, as a "shelter" for patients who, while requiring emergency care, could not be referred to other health care facilities. The problem was that a high proportion of these "difficult to refer" patients were also the most critical ones as they necessitated not only a specialist ward with mechanical ventilation and flawless monitoring but, also, an experienced team of physicians and nursing staff. These patients included those in the early stages of serious conditions or critical injury or, possibly, resuscitated patients who were by far not in a stable condition. At that time, Prague was coping with a lack of hospital beds with mechanical ventilation. It was not a rare occurrence that patients admitted to an emergency department were subsequently transferred, by car or by air, to various departments of anesthesiology/resuscitation within the Central Bohemia region and, occasionally, to hospitals even farther away. From 03.30 pm to 07.00 am, the centralized out-of-hospital emergency department worked both as a "low-threshold" one serving as an admission, treatment and observation center normally referred to specialist outpatient departments in the working hours, and patients requiring intensive and resuscitation care. It was just the pattern of work within and without the working hours that made the centralized out-of-hospital emergency department of NEZAS markedly different from Western-type emergency departments. Still, it can be reasonably claimed that it belonged to those most resembling the Anglo-American model of these departments. It turned out to be a good concept to place observation beds and one EMS ambulance station with a physician available direct in the hospital. Regrettably, the original idea actually never came into life. In addition to the "human factor" bursting out after the resignation of Ždichynec, the founding father of the concept, from the post of director, in the spring of 1990, there were objective reasons. NEZAS was a small facility and already in the 1990s with inadequate capacity, small numbers of departments, beds, limited capacity and throughput. The availability of consultations, not to mention super-consultation, was suboptimal. A major drawback of the hospital was its location of a residential, sparsely inhabited area, and a minimal natural catchment area of patients. Arrival times both from downtown Prague and most of the city were fairly long. Its location atop a hill with a fairly steep slope proved an additional disadvantage when there was snowfall. The helipad was by far most inadequate and there was even an accident with the helicopter damaged when landing. It was perhaps these reasons which contributed to the fact that, after the completion and opening of a brand-new section of Motol University Hospital with hundreds of beds and incomparably better location, NEZAS lost its last reason to exist to become a private rehabilitation facility. Perhaps the main lesson drawn from the times of the NEZAS centralized out-of-hospital emergency department is that work in such a department is a major bonus for physicians and nurses involved in emergency care. Still, emergency departments should be set up primarily in large hospitals with well-equipped diagnostic capabilities, a wide range of specialties providing emergency care, and an adequate number of standard and specialist beds including observation ones.

The era after the Velvet Revolution saw, in the 1990s, the setting up of additional emergency departments, unfortunately, in a quite uncoordinated manner, under various names, with differently set thresholds or specialties for admitting patients. With no clear definition of an emergency department, it cannot be reasonably determined how many such facilities – and at what level – currently exist within the country*. In some cases, emergency departments attend exclusively to patients with internal diseases, as is the case of the Department of Medicine III of the Prague-based General University Hospital. Only several departments are of interdisciplinary nature. A most atypical pattern of providing early in-hospital emergency care can be seen in the Prague-based Motol University Hospital, the country's largest. Admitted patients requiring emergency care are divided into several streams. The most serious cases with failing vital functions are transported by EMS direct to two resuscitation units of the Department of Anesthesiology/Resuscitation. A proportion of patients in need of intensive care is referred direct from the field to metabolic or coronary care units. All trauma patients not admitted to the resuscitation units go past the emergency department and are brought to an outpatient trauma unit. Some patients are treated directly at outpatient units of specialties available in the particular hospital. Except for outpatient departments of internal medicine, neurology, and orthopedics, all specialist outpatient departments take care of patients on a 24/7/52 basis. The remaining stream comprises mainly patients presenting with acute internal or neurological conditions, intoxicated individuals, those with acute lung conditions, altered consciousness, and other conditions of unclear etiology. These patients are attended to at the emergency department. Unfortunately, those transferred to the emergency department include drunk individuals and the homeless, who take the beds necessary for true patients. The unit has only seven beds and no observation beds. Moreover, in addition to the in-hospital emergency department, emergency service is available (between 7 pm and 7 am) for those presenting with milder conditions in separate rooms one floor above. This emergency service was set up after several LSPP had been discontinued within the university hospital's catchment area. The emergency admission unit is operated by full-time physicians, out-of-hospital physicians, and EMS physicians. A proportion of these physicians have passed the board examination in emergency medicine, while others are just preparing for the examination. The remaining physicians are board-certified in a basic branch of medicine, most often in internal medicine and anesthesiology/resuscitation. In the section providing care to patients with milder conditions, there are mainly general practitioners and out-of-hospital physicians.

---

* Answer from the Ministry of Health to the author's query

6. Emergency medicine becomes a full-fledged specialty

The separation of the EMS from the specialty of anesthesiology/resuscitation led to the establishing of the Society of Pre-hospital Emergency Care and Disaster Medicine as a member of the Czech Medical Association of J. E. Purkyně. Training has been provided since 1992 by the Chair of Pre-Hospital Emergency Care and Disaster Medicine of the Postgraduate Medical School, later re-named to become Chair of Emergency Care and Disaster Medicine.

In 1998, the then Minister (Ivan David) established emergency medicine as a subspecialty. This made the Czech Republic the 7th European country with emergency medicine acknowledged as a fully-fledged medical specialty. The professional society is currently named the Society of Emergency Medicine and Disaster Medicine of the Czech Medical Association of J. E. Purkyně (5, 6). Quite logically, the specialty of emergency medicine should embrace the same areas as is usual elsewhere in the world. Given its historical development in this country, its theoretical and practical parts focus mainly on emergency pre-hospital care and, partly, also on disaster medicine. The emergency admission section was not founded within the professional society until December 2004 to start working in 2005, that is, 7 years after emergency medicine was recognized as a specialty in the Czech Republic.

Kotlyar et al. (3) classify the standard of emergency medicine in individual nations into three groups by the presence or absence of certain features as follows: undeveloped, developing, and developed. In this classification, the Czech Republic belongs to nations with a developed system, being as it is a mixed one with predominant features of the French-German system. There is a nationwide organization, and emergency medicine is a recognized specialty with its own training program. At the time of its recognition, it was a subspecialty for those who had passed board examinations in the five main branches of medicine: anesthesiology/resuscitation, internal medicine, surgery, pediatrics, and general medicine. Today, emergency medicine is also listed as a basic branch. A journal called *Urgentní medicína* (Emergency medicine, in Czech) is published and distributed on a nationwide basis. The specialty pursues its own special research programs and runs databases as well as training programs in subspecialties. Prague's EMS is among the best in the world. Among other things, it offers training programs and participates in European-wide research projects. However, there are not many emergency departments and the overwhelming majority of Czech hospitals do not operate such units at all. In hospitals with these units, they are run in turns by physicians of several specialties. As it is, it is impossible to speak about quality control by comparing the output of individual units. Perhaps the biggest difference as against the Anglo-American system is that many most critical "cases" actually never enter the emergency department and are transferred directly to emergency units of other specialties. In some hospitals, emergency departments are available only for patients presenting with a condition to be managed by an internist while those suffering an injury receive treatment outside the emergency department.

7. Current status

Early in-hospital emergency care in the majority of Czech hospitals has been and continues to be provided by specialist outpatient departments related to the branches of medicine available in the particular hospital. For a variety of reasons, this traditional system has been in operation, with only minor changes, for dozens of years. Still, the number of emergency departments tends to rise. The first specialists in emergency medicine passed their board examination in 1999, with the number of erudite physicians and paramedics increasing ever since. To date, 18 physicians have qualified as forensic experts in the field of emergency medicine.

The organization of EMS in the Czech Republic resembles the Franco-German system. The most critical "cases" are attended to by a physician arriving by car. In most cases, physicians of EMS do not come in an ambulance, but by car with a driver-paramedic taking them fast to the patient. This system is referred to as a "rendez-vous" one and was introduced, in the Czech Republic, by Prague's EMS Director Ždichynec, in the late 1980s in several points across the capital. Based on the very good experience, the system was quickly adopted by other towns and districts. Since the beginning of the 1990s, emergency medical care has been provided by paramedics, with the extent of their involvement gradually increasing. In Prague itself, ambulance crews without a physician attend to about 80% of cases. As the pattern of emergency care provision is currently being transformed throughout the country, EMS ambulances also transfer to hospitals patients who used to be examined by their general practitioners during their visits and could often stay home once treated. Not infrequently, their transportation does not require the presence of a physician.

In the Czech Republic, EMS is run and controlled by the state through regional authorities and statutory towns. EMS ambulances are very well equipped. Only a small proportion of emergency care facilities is established and run by private entities such as the Samaritan Association CR, the Sovereign Order of Maltese Knights, and Trans-Hospital. Unlike many other European countries, the Czech Red Cross is not involved in the organization and provision of EMS.

In 1997 and 2002, the Czech Republic was hit by immense floods. There has also been a worldwide increase in the number of terrorist attacks, and interventions in larger numbers of affected persons are on the increase. All this has led to increased preparedness and ability to cope with large-scale disasters and accidents.

A phenomenon challenging all emergency departments is what is referred to as "overcrowding", whereby the capacity of a given department is inadequate to treat patients requiring care within a reasonable timeframe. There are many reasons for "overcrowding": reduction of the numbers of emergency departments, understaffing, increasing reluctance on the part of physicians receiving training in other specialties to get involved in the management of acute conditions, and the risk of malpractice with subsequent legal (and professional) consequences, working under stress and pressure, the need to treat also the homeless, addicts, and so on, and all this in a situation where it is uncertain whether – or how late – they will get paid for their job. In the USA, emergency care is provided by out-of-hospital emergency departments to uninsured individuals (and there are many millions of those). Another major problem is where "to place" patients requiring hospitalization as not all out-of-hospital emergency departments occupy part of a hospital. For reasons easy to understand, hospitals are reluctant to keep vacant beds for "potential" admission of acute patients, often without a health insurance policy. These beds may "earn" much more money if used for patients due to undergo, i.e., scheduled for, surgery. In 2004, I was invited to join an international team seeking to address the worldwide problem of overcrowding; admittedly, I was horrified. I was simply unable to believe that the situation in emergency departments could be so upsetting in some hospitals with some patients waiting in corridors for several days for admission to the hospital, and emergency physicians performing classical visits. It had long seemed that overcrowding was not an impending problem for the Czech Republic. However, the repercussions of the worldwide economic crisis, which have resulted in shrinking budgets in the Czech health care system, are beginning to take their toll and overcrowding seems to loom even in this country.

8. Conclusion

There is little doubt that out-of hospital and in-hospital emergency care in the Czech Republic is provided at a very good standard, although there is still much room for improvement. In fact, despite some shortcomings, organization of emergency care in this country is among the best in the world. The nationwide system of EMS came into being by a decision of the ministry of health in 1974. In the 1990s, the number of EMS ambulance stations increased substantially and, based on analyses of arrival times in some areas, it continues to rise, though at a slower pace. At present, emergency out-of-hospital care is provided by a total of 14 regional centers of emergency medical care. Decree 434/92 Coll. of Laws sets arrival times across the country at within 15 minutes from the reception of call unless the case requires special attention. The above interval is complied with in 96% of the territory of the country. Besides, virtually the whole country is covered by air EMS ambulances operating from 10 bases. In terms of EMS ambulance stations, the Czech Republic is among the countries with the most dense network and best accessibility worldwide. These facts actually become most evident when comparing our country with the USA, and are best documented by the experience of a group of American physicians coming as "missionaries" shortly after the Velvet Revolution to visit Prague, the capital of a country they thought of as "Hic sunt leones" uncharted territory; they were left almost speechless when seeing the high-quality system of emergency medical care run in the then Czechoslovakia. Upon departure, the group leader commented "We came here to teach you, now we are leaving educated".

9. References

Drábková et al. Základy anesteziologie (Basics of anesthesiology). 1981 Avicenum, Prague: 8-13.

Drábková et al. Základy resuscitace (Basics of resuscitation). 1982 Avicenum, Prague: 8-10.

Kotlyar S., Arnold J. et al. 2006. Introduction to International Emergency Medicine. Emedicine.com. March 7: 1-11.

Pokorný J., Bohuš O. 1996. Anesteziologie a resuscitace na cestě k oborové samostatnosti v České a Slovenské republice (Anesthesiology and resuscitation on their way to become an independent specialty in the Czech and Slovak Republics.). 1996; Pražská vydavatelská společnost, Prague: 15-62.

Pokorný J. jr. 2 000. Urgentní medicína: historie, současnost, trendy (Emergency medicine: past, present, and trends.). Trendy v medicíně 2: 93-5.

Pokorny J. 2004. Urgentní medicína (Emergency medicine). Galen, Prague: XV-XI.

8

Medical Instructions of the XVIII Century to Resuscitate the Apparently Dead: Rescuing the Drowned to Define the Origins of the Emergency Medicine

Silvia Marinozzi, Giuliano Bertazzoni and Valentina Gazzaniga
"Sapienza" University of Rome
Italy

1. Introduction

The concept of an emergency therapeutic action, defined as an immediate intervention to save dying people, is absent from the ancient medical mind. The Hippocratic physician cures diseases, defined as states of functional alterations of the natural processes: the pathologies are considered to be manifestations of a dyscrasia, or rather an imbalance of the body's components, by excess or by default of quality and moods, which moves the *physis* of the body away from its natural condition. The altered organic processes are explained as a consequence of an inappropriate life style, that is a wrong regime which alters and compromises the functions of the entire organism: the quantity and quality of food and pothos, the relation between waking and sleeping, the hygienic and living conditions, the physical change, sexual activity, in an holistic conception which does not involve a medical intervention in contrast with the process in act. The diseases must follow their course, grow and reach the Krisis, the moment of a definite change, which brings towards death or healing. The physician acts in order to re-establish the original equilibrium of the body, though respecting the natural course of the phenomena and thus avoiding to intervene on those who cannot be saved.

The observation of the signs helps in prognosticating healing or death, thus determining the conduct of the physician who cures and gives therapeutic indications only for those diseases and ailments which are deemed curable. The duration of the medical intervention therefore follows that of pathologic course, without any forced action which would interrupt the natural evolution of the process in course.

Prognosis, or rather the prediction of an illness in course in order to decide whether healing is possible or not, is the highest expression of the clinical reasoning of ancient medicine. It will only be the development of human anatomy as a scientific medical discipline, in the XVI Century, to pave the way to conceive new therapeutic measures and above all to boost surgery, which enables a different approach to the cure so as to contrast the process of death in course, and intervenes promptly in the medications of injuries and wounds, developing new systems of hemorrhagic arrest. But the concept of first aid, that is an immediate medical intervention aimed at saving dying people, finds its specific theoretic connotation only in the XVIII Century, when research and the applications of systems of defense and protection of human life becomes a concrete expression of social medicine and public health policies in the Enlightenment. A specific medical literature of health education is developed in the genres of "instructions" or textbooks addressed to the general public, to inform about the disease's risks the people might be exposed to, to educate on prevention and prophylaxis, and to teach techniques for immediate relief and for the care of victims of frequent accidents. The aim the contribution is to present the most recurrent topics in this medical literature as the first step for the formation of a theoretical basis of emergency medicine, which is reflected in the resuscitation of asphyxiated resuscitation techniques developed by medical authors.

2. Rescuing the drowned: the resuscitation of the apparently dead

The concept of reanimation defined as a group of medical actions coordinated in order to reestablish the basic vital functions of a single being, is historically connected to the matter of sudden deaths and above all of apparent death.

It is in fact the fear of burying live people that represents the crucial point towards the development of a medical doctrine on the causes of sudden deaths and above all on the procedures carried out to assess legal death through a codification of the signs relevant to real death. Following this theory the first guidelines have been developed in order to elaborate systems of reanimation of apparent dead people: the same techniques are used to assess legal death can reactivate those organic functions which expired without actually causing the real death of a person.

In 1707, with De subitaneis mortirbus..., G. M. Lancisi (1654-1720) had explained animal life as the balance among three functions and three fundamental organs: the heart, which coordinates blood circulation; the brain, which elaborates the vital spirit in the animal and sensitivity and infuses it to all the parts of the body through the nervous fluid ; the lungs which purify and invigorates the blood through breathing. Death is therefore caused, according to Lancisi, by the ceasing of one of these three functions as far as the postmortem outcomes have revealed, he had found the cause of sudden deaths in a cardiac hypertrophy, often associated to aneurisms or to the presence of "polyps" in the aorta. If aneurisms, polyps and morphologic alterations of the cardiac apparatus definitely compromise the cardiac-circulatory function as Lancisi had asserted in his work, determining immediate death of a single being, there are also other physio-pathologic conditions as syncope, fainting, apoplexies, that the medical literature of the eighteenth century explained as a simple suspension of the vital functions recoverable through specific stimulus techniques. M. Nurock has well underlined this in the XVIII century the terms reanimation and resuscitation do not mean, like today, the revitalization of a single being but only of specific functions, which in certain conditions are appeased/soothed. (Nurok M, 2003).

Reanimation therefore appears as a therapeutic act aimed at stimulating functions and the apparatus of an apparently not vital body that is not dead yet: the vital force is in fact mixed with the animal essence itself, and its lacking phenomenal reality does not necessarily assume its ceasing. In fact, a medium condition between life and death does exist, where the vital impulses are gradually even more appeased till they become silenced, and only later, in a period of time rarely definable, and eventually cease completely. These are the cases of apparent death. But how is it possible to distinguish between a condition which just appears to be death and certain death? Two are the basic epistemic references which come out: the individuation of the etiological causes which determine a "pathologic" condition of apparent death on one side, and the identification of the signs of legal death on the other. In relation to the latter, in fact, many authors of the eighteenth century refer directly to the evidence of the signs of decomposition of the body for the validation of the certification of death. As for the causes, a precise nosology picture is drawn from a specific pathologic outline and, in particular, from that accidentally induced, which though implying loss of willpower, knowledge and the movement of a single individual, and the lack of a clinical manifestation of vitality.

The basic principle is that the result of random casualties, like tumbling, asphyxia, or those caused by environmental factors or toxic fumes, ingestion of poisonous substances, strangulation or drowning, and some pathological forms which induce a state of apparent death, like syncope or apoplexies, are conditions of suspension of the vital functions and not the complete ceasing of them. Aid mainly consists in recovering those vital functions which have been "suspended" and can be recovered with specific medical-surgical interventions before they cease completely.

John Hunter (1728-1793) distinguished among three types of sudden death: the interruption of the vital action without any damages to the vital components; the result of an injury occurred to a vital part, like excessive bleeding, wounds or the cerebral and/or marrow compression; the immediate loss of vitality in all the parts of the body at the same time, as it happens in the case of fulmination, violent brain affections, or a blow to the stomach.

According to Hunter, the first signs of distinction between a real death condition and a state of suspension of the vital activities, is the presence or absence of spasms and contractions which occur when an individual is about to die, while the state of relaxation of the body can imply that the spastic stimulus preceding death has not aroused yet, and therefore that a drowned person could be possibly reanimated. Rigor mortis is the most evident sign of real death, because it is the consequence of the stimulus induced by the process of death. Vice-versa, in many cases of sudden death, where such phenomena do not occur, blood does not coagulate and rigor mortis does not occur, the muscles stand still and soft. Until the animal preserves its "susceptibility of impression", even in the absence of vitality, can be reanimated, because it is reactive to external stimulus (Hunter J., 1837).

J. Janin too (1731-1811), Surgeon of the Royal Army and member of the Royal College of Surgery, faces the problem of the urgency of a criteria of legal death, which eliminates the risk of burying live people. The systems adopted so far, involving the incision or burning of the feet, or putting the flame of a candle under the nostrils, have in fact proved ineffective to check the effective presence or absence of sensitivity in an animal body. For this reason, it is necessary to find a system of coordinated procedures aimed at reanimating apparently dead people thus avoiding the risk for those who are still alive to be considered dead. According to Janin, sudden deaths are often states of apparent death, except for some specific pathologies, in particular those pertaining to the heart, while the presumed deaths by asphyxiation, indigestion, syncope, hypothermia, drowning, are often just a suspension of vitality which with proper intervention, can be completely restored.

Charles Kite (1768-1811) is in contrast with the conventional methods of legal death by the arrest of the pulsations of the pulse and breathing, diagnosed with the flame of a candle or a tuft of wool or a mirror positioned in front of the mouth and nostrils. Using these methods, many individuals who were still alive, had been declared dead. For this reason it has been later considered the necrotic aspect of the body, like the fixed or flabby opaque state of the eyes, the formation of foam at the mouth and nostrils, the rigidity of the body, of the mouth and of the limbs, as a manifestation of decomposition and therefore as an indicative sign of real death. But it is necessary to distinguish between contraction caused by a spasm and the rigidity which arise by the lack of elasticity of the fibers subsequent to death.

Not even the fluidity of the blood can be an absolute sign itself, therefore death can be determined by a complex group of signs, which is now unanimously proved by the evidence of the beginning of the decomposition process. In apparent death there is the arrest of the circulation, breathing, and of the cerebral functions, though with a subsistence of irritability of the muscular fibers; in certain death (biological death) on the contrary, also the latter is lost. Therefore, according to Kite, the real difference between real death and apparent death consists in the presence or absence of the sensitivity, and the signs of death, which are considered indicative of the decease, are only consequences of the loss of the nervous and cerebral functions, but are not necessarily really certain.

The symptomatic outline of poisoning, drowning, and asphyxia, constitute in fact definite nosological realities, because, even though referring to specific pathologic categories, like apoplexy o paralysis, it is possible to define their causes, in the physio-pathologic processes, and in the therapeutic treatment.

It is this causal difference which creates the epistemological basics of first aid: together with the traditional concept of therapy as a system of healing which involves surgery (bloodletting, cauterization, amputations, extractions) and pharmacology intrinsic to the healing process, which include a proper regime to the specific pathologies, there is a therapeutic model of immediate treatment, where the physician, though remaining the necessary referee, can operate in a later moment, when the person has already been saved from the dangerous situation and has already received first aid, preparatory to the medical intervention itself.

In particular, it is the rescue of drowned people to constitute the basis for the theoretical studies, both on the importance of an immediate medical action and on the definition of the status of apparent death.

A rescue model for drowned people, had already been standardized in the XVII Century, based on the theoretical assumption that the arrest of the vital functions was due to the water flowing into vital organs. For this reason rescue techniques had been developed, aimed at expelling the water entered by hanging the drowned person upside down in order to clear the stomach and the chest, and stimulate those parts of the body by shaking them, slapping feet and palms of the hands, and placing the assisted individuals in a barrel opened on both sides, whirling it in many directions to shake them and stimulate in this way the vital organs and the animal vitality.

In contrast with the seventeenth and early eighteenth century authors, whom have dealt with drowned people, it becomes now relevant the timeliness of first aid in all cases of apparent death. Between the XVII and the XVIII Century, various authors, among which T.

Bartholin, A. Borelli., F. Hoffmann, refer of cases where even after many hours of immersion, some drowned people have showed signs of vitality.

It is now under focus a univocal determination of the time by which the reanimation intervention can result effective and a uniform criteria of the practices of reanimation, so as to produce a corpus of regulations to follow in case of emergency, which could be taught and divulged even to non-medical people.

Through this method the majority of citizens are able to learn quick reanimation techniques, because the duration of transfer to the hospital or awaiting a physician or surgeon can be fatal. So, a specific medical literature on medical education is developed, in forms of "notices", "instructions", or didactic-popular manuals, with the purpose of informing the population on the risks of disease to which they can be exposed, teach them prevention and prophylaxis, systems of first aid and treatments to the victims of the most frequent casualties, in particular for drowned, asphyxiated and poisoned people and the dead born children, whose death is explained, according to the physio-pathologic theories of the time, with the alteration and/or ceasing of breathing induced by the lack of air and the subsequent interruption of the dynamics of blood circulation.

Through the study of these works, it is possible to analyze the effects which contemporary medical scientific studies have on the elaboration of a system of first aid.

2.1 A.S. Tissot's Avis and first aid directions

Recent French historiography has identified in the Avis au peuple sur sa santè... (Lausanne, 1761) by S. A. Tissot (1728-1797) the origin of first aid medicine (Larcan A. et Brullard Ph., 1979), even though such work is generally considered by the historians of medicine as an emblematic example of the process of popularization occurred to the medical culture in the seventeenth century. (Singy P., 2010; Riley J.C., 2001).

Undoubtedly, the wide spread of Tissot's work and other medical popular works, like La Médecine, la Chirurgie et la Pharmacie des Pauvres by P. Hecquet (1661-1737), written in 1740, the Domestic Medicine by W. Buchan (1729-1805) written in 1769, and the medical encyclopedias published in the second half of the eighteenth century, like the Dictionnaire de Santé in 1760 e il Dictionnaire de Médecine in 1772, contribute to the standardization of the treatment "protocols" for the necessity of simplifying therapeutic systems of the medicine of the time, and make them accessible to a public of non-experts.

In Tissot's Avis there are in fact some indications of first aid in specific cases, especially for occasional casualties, like asphyxia induced by environmental circumstances, drowning, asphyxiation caused by ingestion of foreign bodies which remain in the esophagus or obstruct the trachea, but also for blood apoplexy.

According to Tissot, an immediate treatment is necessary for all forms of fainting, defined as the loss of senses and motor faculties. He classifies fainting depending on its causes while the reanimation treatments vary in accordance with the etiology and physiopathology of the fainting state itself. In most cases, the author gives simple remedies, like the administration and inhalation of spirit liquor, specific food and drinks after the patient is reanimated.

But for certain cases of fainting, he also gives more complex first aid indications. In the most serious cases of fainting induced by blood excess, or due to constitution of the body or alcohol or food, it is necessary to immediately put hot water and vinegar on the forehead, temples and wrists; pass the vinegar under the nose; place ligatures to the thighs in order to avoid blood reflux.

If, in spite of this intervention, unconsciousness persists for more than a quarter of an hour, bloodletting from the arm and enema treatments were used; the patient is placed in a bed and every now and then some elderberry tea with vinegar and sugar is administered to him/her. Fainting caused by an excessive organic weakness, induced by hemorrhages, diseases, dysentery, urine flux or hunger, are treated by placing the patient in bed and rubbing the whole body with hot flannels; through the inhalation of spirit substances, like Hungary water, volatile salts or strongly aromatic herbs; some drops of Carmelite water or spirit or other liquor are poured into the mouth; flannel cloths tempered in hot wine or spirit are laid on the abdomen, and if unconsciousness persists the whole body is rubbed.

In case of more serious fainting due to nasal hemorrhages, ligatures of arms and thighs are placed, and to increase the effect, the legs are immersed in warm water up to the knees. Once the hemorrhage has been stopped , it is possible to remove the laces from the limbs, and every half an hour the patient is administered with seven or eight grains of nitre and water and vinegar; tampons made of linen soaked with white vitriol, or some Hoffmann's anodyne mineral liquor are inserted into the nostrils.

Innovative is the section relevant to the systems of first aid in case of asphyxiation due to the presence of foreign bodies in the throat, in the esophagus or in the trachea.

Tissot divides these bodies into those digestible, or rather food, and those indigestible, which can often be lethal, like rocks, pieces of glass or metal, sharpened objects, like nails or needles, which can penetrate the fleshy parts. The first can be pushed towards the stomach, with candlesticks, leeks, wooden sticks, or other tubular objects, possibly soft and very smooth in order not to damage the esophagus.

The indigestible objects instead, especially when sharp, must be extracted in order to avoid damages to the organs of the digestive apparatus. Obviously, the kind of treatment depends on the spot where the foreign body has stopped, on its nature and form: if it remains trapped at the entry of the esophagus, it is possible to extract it with the hands; if on the contrary it has gone deeper, it is possible to grab it with tweezers, and in case they are not available, it is possible to use two crossed wooden sticks. Whether it is not possible to extract it according to this regulation because it has gone too deep, it is possible to use a hook, or create it with a wire curved at one end, to be inserted down to where the body has been blocked and move it so as to hook it up when the instrument is extracted. Thin objects which through the use of the hooks could move away from the esophageal walls and go down into the stomach, must be recovered through the use of a ring, both solid or flexible, in order to hook them up. Tissot also explains how to build this instrument: it is possible to use a wire by bending it in the middle so as to form a circle with a diameter as wide as a finger, and drawing both ends up to use them like a handle and insert the ring into the esophagus in order to grab the object; but it is also possible to use wire rings, one into the other to make the catch even firmer, so that by pulling the ends, rings get tightened up and wrapped around the foreign object. Another system is that of inserting beneath the object a dried sponge that, when properly dampened, could swell up until it is able to un-stick it and lift the element to be extracted, or it is possible to fix a woolen or cotton tuft to a flexible handle or waxed thread, which is slipped below the object to be removed. A chapter of the work is dedicated to rescue drowned people. Tissot explains death by drowning as a consequence of asphyxiation induced by absence of air and presence of water into the respiratory tract, which mixing with the air still present in the lungs, forms a viscose foam that blocks the pulmonary functions; this way the circulatory motor is also arrested, and blood, unable to flow back to the head, remains into the cerebral vessels, where it is congested causing apoplexy. In order to save drowned people, it is therefore necessary to decongest the lungs and the brain and reactivate circulation. He lists in sequential order all of the operations to be carried out to reanimate a drowned person: 1) take off his/her wet clothes, rub him/her immediately with hot cloths and baths, even after having placed him/her in a warm bed; 2) insufflate hot air and tobacco fumes into the lungs, blowing into the patient's mouth through a stem or other tubular instruments aimed for that purpose; in this way the hot air introduced into the respiratory tract relaxes the pulmonary vessel and dissolves the foam, so as to reactivate blood circulation; 3) if there is a surgeon, bloodletting is practiced from the jugular in order to decongest the vessels of the head and neck; 4) tobacco fumes are introduced into the intestine, either with the proper fumigation apparatus or with a pipe, whose stem is inserted into the anus of the assisted person, and whose tobacco bowl is strongly poked, or upon which another pipe is positioned upside down to blow the fumes, or with stems and other tubular instruments; 5) some strong volatile liquors are passed under a patient's nose and powders of strongly aromatic herbs are blown into the nostrils; some drops of stimulating liquor are poured into the patient's mouth, and only after the assisted person shows signs of reanimation other substances can be administered; five or six spoonfuls of oxymel melted in hot water or thistle, sage or chamomile with honey, are recommended; the prescribed treatments are practiced even after the drowned person has been reanimated, till he/she recovers his/her full organic functionality.

Tissot's prescribed interventions show a deep knowledge of the debates of the time and on the physiopathology of drowning and above all on the reanimation systems to adopt in order to save drowned people. This results even clearer from the list of the reanimation operations which are still practiced, but which the author denounces to be useless and even damaging to the patients. He thus insists on avoiding to wrap drowned people with the skin of some sheep, cow or dog just slaughtered to infuse warmness; to roll them in a barrel and hang them up side down by their feet to expel the water. He formulates those remedies which will constitute the foundation of reanimation: the recovery of natural body temperature through baths and rubbing and the reactivation of the respiratory functions are essential interventions for reanimation. Even the paragraph dedicated to suffocation due to mephitic vapors or alcoholic liquors gives indications which are in accordance with the medicine of the time: in closed space, the sulphurous oil coming out from burning coal and the exhalations produced by the alcoholic fermentation saturate , making it so unsuitable for respiration to cause fainting, convulsions and apoplexy. In order to reanimate these asphyxiated persons it is necessary to transfer them immediately to the open air, making them inhale penetrating vapors, like the volatile spirit of sal ammoniac or English salt, and then vinegar vapors; the patient's legs are submerged into tepid water and massaged; in the meantime the patient is administered with some lemonade or water with vinegar and nitre and then receives enemas with acre substances. As soon as the asphyxiated person show signs of life, he/she receive antispasmodic drugs, like the Hoffmann's anodyne mineral liquor or opium.

Many of Tissot's instructions are re-elaborated by W. Buchan (1729-1805) in Domestic Medicine, published for the first time in 1769, which widens the description of the techniques of first aid used to reanimate drowned people.

He illustrates various accidental casualties, describing both the symptoms and the physio-pathologic process induced by them, and the rescue operations to perform. The systems of reanimation indicated by Buchan for the victims of hot or cold asphyxia, as well as for fainting, suffocation caused by toxic vapors and the extraction of foreign bodies from the esophagus, follow the instructions given by Tissot's Avis au peuple. More articulated is the description given on the reanimation of drowned persons, with implicit references to the instructions distributed by Drowning Persons Rescue Company and articles on this topic written by contemporary authors. Like Tissot, he underlines the importance of the time factor: when recuperated in a few minutes (quantified in about fifteen minutes), the reanimation interventions are easier and the result is surely positive; otherwise specific and more complex techniques must be adopted.

Drowned people must be immediately transferred to a proper place, making sure they do not suffer shaking, and once lying in a comfortable place with their head slightly lifted. As for all cases of apparent death, the main operation is the recovery of the natural body heat, basic element of all the vital functions; drowned persons must be therefore stripped of all their wet clothing, rubbed with coarse linen and wrapped in warm clothes or cloths. Hot bricks, wrapped in cloth, or hot water bottles are positioned under the feet and palms of the hands; if there is a fire or other source of heat, the patient is placed near it so as to receive proper warmth; otherwise it is sufficient that one or two people lay with the patients in order to infuse the warmness of their body. Nostrils are stimulated with exhalations of strong volatile spirit liquors, or tobacco or marjoram powder, and the chest and back are rubbed with a cloth soaked in a distilled beverage or spirit of hot wine prepared with volatile spirit of salt ammoniac.

At the same time, air is insufflated into the lungs, blowing exhaled breathe directly into the mouth of the drowned persons, making sure that both nostrils are held till the chest is filled and swelled; then the chest is compressed so as to expel the air introduced, repeating the operation until the patients recover their respiratory function. For artificial respiration, it is possible to use a reed that is inserted into one of the nostrils and closing the other and the mouth. In case the mouth of the patient is closed, it is possible to use a spoon handle to open it by levering the dental arch. Other organs are stimulated by introducing fifteen drops of volatile alkali into the mouth (that is spirit of volatile salt ammoniac) and practicing the insufflation of tobacco fumes into the intestines. If a fumigation apparatus is not available, two pipes may be used, with their bowls covered over, introducing one stem into the anus and blowing into the second pipe's stem to fire the bowl of the first one.

Alternatively, an enema of hot water, salt and vinegar can be practiced, or other stimulating spirit liquor. The drowned person is placed in hot water, or covered with hot ashes or salt or sand or cereals. The throat and the nose are stimulated with a feather, and some tobacco or marjoram powder should be applied to the patient's nostrils, the temples and the stomach area are massaged with brandy or wine spirit, and some drops of these liquors are poured into the mouth of the drowned person. When the patients have been reanimated, they are administered with oxymel melted in warm water, or a thistle, sage or chamomile infusion with honey; above all, it is necessary to keep the patients warm and stimulate them, giving them liquor every now and then. If the patients still cough and show a sense of oppression, bloodletting is practiced. Reanimation instructions for drowned people are true for those apparently dead by strangulation, because the suffocation induced requires the same type of stimulation and recovery of natural heat and of the respiratory function (Buchan W., 1774).

The rescue of asphyxiated and drowned persons described by Tissot and Buchan in their works fully represents the codification of rescue systems elaborated by physicians on behalf of the governmental institutions. In general, in the middle of the eighteenth century, there is a new health organization of local administrations on the rescue of the victims of casualties, especially for the drowned people, which distribute public advises containing instructions on how to save the drowned person and thus codifying a kind of reanimation protocol.

2.2 Assistance to drowned people as a model of first aid

In Paris, already in 1740 there is a planning for a first aid policy, with public advises which indicate the measures to adopt for reanimation.

The avis published in 1740 concerning assistance to drowned people and distributed all over the French provinces, gives many instructions concerning the traditional systems of rescuing people, like the practice of hanging the drowned person by the feet to expel the water ingested and penetrated into the body, which had already been advised against and to which barrel rolling is preferred, consisting in placing the drowned person in a barrel opened on both ends in order to be whirled in different directions, and the tickling of the throat and esophagus with the barb of a feather, rubbing till vomit is induced. It is necessary to strip the drowned person of all his/her wet clothes, wrap him/her in warm blankets, transfer him/her to a warm place and put him/her to bed; in order to restart the solid parts of the body apparatus, the drowned people are shaken repeatedly, spirit liquors are poured into their mouth, among which hot urine and a decoction of pepper and vinagra.

The fibers of the nasal ducts are stimulated with volatile spirits, like those liqueur vapors prescribed for apoplexy, the barb of a feather and insufflations of sneezing powders or tobacco. The insufflations of hot air in the mouth and intestines, through a cannula, a bellows or a syringe and the fumigations of tobacco into the intestines through the use of a broken pipe which blows into the body the amount of fumes which a single pipe would smoke, are largely diffused practices. In the most serious cases, it is recommended to call for a surgeon for bloodletting from the jugular in order to expel thickened blood in the brain, and eventually practice a tracheotomy.

The basic idea is that drowning determines apoplexy, which becomes the ultimate cause of death of a person. The lack of instructions concerning the ways by which interventions can be carried out together with the lack of a reward for those who saved drowned persons, induced the government to draw up a memoir which described all the recognized rescue systems aimed at the reanimation of the drowned persons; but the quantity and complexity of the indications given, involve running the risk that only the easiest and less efficient interventions were practiced. In 1755 Claude-Nicolas Le Cat (1700-1768), Surgeon at the Hôtel-Dieu de Rouen, is designated of examining the memoirs and affirms that air insufflations into the lungs is the operation necessary to reanimate drowned persons. He therefore describes a siphon to be introduced into the trachea, by lifting the epiglottis with a proper instrument; a small bellows is adapted to the siphon in order to blow air directly into the lungs. In the same year other surgeons at La Vile de l'Isle reduce to four the number of basic operations for reanimation: shaking, jugular bloodletting, air insufflations into the lungs and tobacco fumigations into the intestines. Other similar advices are given in that period. The consistent number of persons dead by drowning, induced the Dutch government to adopt safety measures, which eventually brought to the foundation of the Dutch Humane Society of Amsterdam in 1767. Well-defined instructions on the modalities and kinds of interventions to practice for the reanimation of drowned persons, are compiled and distributed thus forming the reference model of future lifesaving societies which would be instituted in other European countries. Rescue operations are officially delegated to city guards and the citizens are instructed through public advices, so as to give immediate assistance and delegate to physicians and surgeons only the specialized operations such as bloodletting and tracheotomy. In order to achieve the charitable aim to save drowned persons, the Dutch government distributed advices and pamphlets concerning the operations necessary to reanimate patients, offering six ducats or a gold medal as a reward to anybody, physician or not, who demonstrated with a certificate to have saved and cured a drowned person by following the proper procedures. Once the patient is recuperated from the water, it is necessary to immediately infuse warmness to the drowned person, even by using the savers' clothes or, when possible, hot woolen blankets; the patient is transferred to a house heated with a moderate fire or to a factory with working boilers, covered with blankets and infused with the heat of the savers' body, who should lie beside him/her; then the body is rubbed, particularly on the back along the spine, with flannel or cloths soaked with brandy, or scattering the patient with salt. At the same time tobacco fumes are insufflated into the intestines, and whenever specific instruments are lacking, a simple pipe, a common bellows or a knife's sheath cut at the tip can be used. A strong volatile salt, like spirit of salt ammoniac, must be applied to temples and nostrils; nostrils and throat must only be tickled, without introducing any liqueur, till the patient has recuperated the respiratory and swallowing faculties. In order to reactivate the lungs, a mouth-to-mouth resuscitation is practiced: the assistant blows into the mouth of the patient, blocking both nostrils with one hands and using the other to exercise pressure on the chest to breath the air out (Cogan T., 1773; Trubuhovich RV., 2006).

In France in 1771, Nicholas Pia, pharmacist and alderman of the Municipal Guards of Paris is in charge of distributing public advices concerning drowned persons life saving techniques, and organizing a police service for the town municipality. It thus constituted the life saving Society for drowned persons. In the instructions in 1771 it is indicated that once the drowned person has been taken out of the water, it is necessary to immediately alert the Guards who must be provided with a box containing the essential instruments for first aid. Pia in fact creates a box with all the instruments needed for the reanimation of the drowned persons to be distributed to the guards all around the cities together with the instructions concerning both the rescue operations to carry out and the way to use the instruments in the box for first aid drowning techniques. The box includes a tobacco container, a bellows to fire it, a flexible cannula. The cannula is inserted in the anus, and the other extremity is connected to the spout of the container of tobacco which is kept lighted through the bellows. In about three quarters of an hour, half an ounce of tobacco is burnt. The box also contains a small shirt and a woolen hat to dress and warm the drowned person, a small bottle of volatile spirit of salt ammoniac to soak some paper to be introduced into the nostrils of the drowned person; two pieces of flannel and a bottle of camphor grapevine water to soak them in order to rub the body with it; two boxes of emetics and an iron spoon. The fumigation instruments are essentially made of a cannula intertwined with a leather tube in order to prevent both the inconveniences of accidental obstructions and the risk of the exhalations coming from the digestive apparatus of the assisted person. Once taken out of the water, the drowned person should be transferred to the nearest Guards' building or other proper place where it is possible to carry out the essential reanimation operations and only later, should he/she be brought to the Hôtel-de-Dieu. A medical guards' regulation is constituted: it is establish that by twenty four hours the Guards' Sergeant is compelled to present a report to the city government on the methods and the outcomes of the saving procedures carried out; the government gives forty-eight lire for each rescue operation to be divided among those that have contributed in the rescue. Municipality Guards provide surveillance and drowning rescue interventions and refers directly to the Health Minister. A proper first-aid manual is codified, with the indications both of the operations and their sequence to be carried out. The drowned person must be undress of his/her clothes, covered with warm cloths and exposed to a source of heat; through the use of a cannula, warm air is insufflated into the mouth, accurately closing both nostrils; the tobacco fumes are inserted into the anus by means of a fumigation instrument which every guards' body should be provided with. When an immediate intervention of reanimation is necessary, due to the late arrival of the Guards, it is necessary to insufflate air through the use of proper tubular objects, like the sheath of a knife cut at the tip, or two common pipes placed with the bowls covered over so that one stem is inserted into the anus and the other is used to insufflate tobacco fumes into the intestines. In the meantime the patient's body must be repeatedly shaken, avoiding to let him/her lie too long on their back. The nostrils and throat are tickled with the barb of a feather and the nostrils are also stimulated with tobacco fumes, sneezing powders and volatile spirit of salt ammoniac. The body is massaged with cloths soaked in camphor distilled water, with the addition of spirit of salt ammoniac. Jugular bloodletting is also useful when practiced by an expert. As soon as the patient shows any sign of vitality and recovers his/her respiratory and swallowing functions, lukewarm water is administered; after that an emetic or camphor distilled water with salt ammoniac can be used. Those who take the drowned person out of the water and give first aid, receive twenty-four lire as a reward, for the same reasons by which eighteen of them are given to the Sergeant and the Guards whom have carried out all the necessary rescue operations.

A summary of such operations is distributed to all the city guards, and constitutes an integral part of Pia's box, with the indications concerning how to use the instruments necessary for the treatment of drowned persons (Pia P.N., 1773; Trépardoux F., 1997).

In England as well, methodic studies on drowning reanimation techniques are developed, above all those concerning pulmonary ventilation.

In 1773 the obstetrician Thomas Cogan (1736-1818) translated into English the *Memoirs of the society instituted at Amsterdam in favour of persons drowned* compiled from 1767 to 1771, which became the basic reference model for the foundation of a similar institution in England. In 1774, together with the pharmacist William Hawes (1736-1808), it is instituted the *Humane Society of London for recovery of persons apparently drowned or dead.*

In the same year, Alexander Johnson compiles a *Short account of a Society of Amsterdam and Hamburg for the recovery of persons drowned*, where it is reported how the Societies of

Amsterdam, Hamburg and Paris dealt with such cases and describes many cases of resuscitation of apparently dead people resuscitated in many European cities, with the aim of founding a similar institution in England (Johnson A., 1773).

Already many publications and reports concerning the rescue experiences of apparently dead people, even written by English authors, have shown how the measures adopted to save drowned persons can be applied with the same success to many different cases where the vital force is only suspended, and it is therefore possible to reactivate all the functions and vital motions (Monthly Review or literary journal, 1776).

The instructions distributed by the Humane Society of London give the basic guidelines, in sequential order, on the treatments to perform in case of drowning resuscitation: first of all, it is recommended not to apply the old systems of barrel rolling, hanging the body upside down, violent shaking and stroking. Once the drowned person is taken out from the water, he/she must be brought to a warm and well-aired location, placed upon a bed with his/her head lifted; he/she must be covered with warm cloths and exposed to a source of heat, though not too close to the fire. In order to warm the body, hot water bottles are applied under the feet, to the knees and armpits, and hot cloths or bricks wrapped in linen and placed on the rest of the body, especially on the back. The best treatment would be that of bringing the patient to a factory where, with the purpose of processing some products, there are working boilers and large and well-aired rooms, and the environmental temperature is lukewarm and not extremely hot. It is necessary to immediately stimulate the vital factors reactivating the lungs and the intestines. Then air is blown directly into the mouth of the patient and tobacco fumes are injected into the anus, at the same time keeping the body warm through rubbing performed with hot cloths or salt, or flannel soaked in brandy or rum or other strong alcoholic or spirituous liqueurs; the sense of smell is stimulated by applying spirit of volatile salt or ammoniac in the nostrils, which must be smeared on the temples to stimulate the head nerves; both throat and nostrils are tickled with a feather to reactivate the functions of the digestive apparatus inducing vomit and sneezing. It is specified that these operations are also efficient for other cases of apparent death, like asphyxia, both caused by strangulation or excess of heat or coldness, fits of convulsions, apoplexy, suffocation caused by air polluted with toxic vapors, as it happens in the mines, shafts, caves or alcohol factories. Even though the reanimation techniques indicated by physicians were certainly more sophisticated, in general the rescue operations concerning apparent deaths, distributed through public advices, satisfy the need to use applicable systems which could be easily performed even by non-expert people, and non specific instruments, in order to guarantee the maximum performance of the first aid operations necessary to resuscitate drowned persons even in the absence of physicians and surgeons.

For tobacco fumes insufflations into the intestines, since the half of the XVII century specific instruments had already been perfected, among which the fumigation instrument created by Th. Bartholin, which constitutes the reference prototype of more complex apparatus developed at the end of the eighteenth century (Portal A., 1810).

But in the popular pamphlets and in the instructions drafted for the drowning lifesaving societies, the physician themselves give alternative indications on how to proceed with anal fumigations and artificial respiration in the absence of a specialized instrument, so that more and more people could operate reanimation.

This is why it is possible to find indications on how to practice intestinal fumigations with two simple pipes, or on the kind of common tubular objects, and on how to use them, for the ventilation of the lungs.

2.3 Drowning physiopathology to explain apparent death

More complex are the disputes about drowning nosology and the reanimation techniques to perform. In particular, we can point out a substantial divergence on the cause of death by drowning, which some identify as the result of apoplexy, others as the arrest of the respiratory function, which determines blood congestion in the venous system, and those who indicate it in the disappearance of sensitivity.

In the first case the authors promote bloodletting, even from the jugular, in order to decongest the blood still present in the cerebral vases; while for the other cases blood evacuation can even be dangerous because it further deprives the body of its warmness and vital principle. In the same way, not everybody agrees on the usefulness and efficacy of electricity, promoted above all by those who find vitality and sensitiveness of the fibers already compromised by the cardio-respiratory arrest. The doctrinal differences on the physio-pathologic interpretation certainly have a relapse on the lifesaving procedures proposed by the authors. In particular, it is possible to identify two different currents concerning the system of insufflations of air into the lungs, and the methods to infuse heat. From a doctrinal point of view, the key element for the ventilation of the lungs is the different quality of the expired air, or the one insufflated directly or through the use of a cannula, or the atmospheric one, introduced with a bellow.

When the drowned persons lifesaving society of Amsterdam is founded, the mouth-to-mouth resuscitation technique is advocated to reanimate respiratory functionality through the insufflations of air into the lungs. But already since the first years of the seventies in the eighteenth century, the Dutch society promotes the use of bellows, one for the injection and the other for the aspiration of air, only by practicing mouth-to-mouth resuscitation in extreme cases, that is in the absence of any instrument that could avoid direct contact with the patient. The fear of tainted vapors coming from the patient induce both the physicians and the lifesaving societies to promote the use of bellows and cannulas which became part of the instruments of lifesaving boxes distributed to the city guards.

In particular, the insufflations of air through a bellow is deemed necessary by those physicians who consider atmospheric air more suitable than burnt air to revitalize nerves and fibers. Especially after the diffusion of the studies concerning the discovery of oxygen (or rather sulfur dioxide) made by Joseph Priestley (1733-1804), and in particular the publication of his "Observations on Respiration and the Use of the Blood" in 1776, many authors do not consider exhaled air suitable for resuscitation, because it is full of tainted phlogiston caused by the combustion occurring in the lungs during respiration. Atmospheric air, or that dephlogisticated through oxygen gas, is the vitalizing principle: by inserting the dephlogisticated air into the lungs of the drowned person, the elaboration of the blood still present in the veins is immediately induced, thus reactivating circulation and respiration. For this reason, many popular works containing the instructions to resuscitate drowned, asphyxiated persons, recommend the use of bellows or inhalation instruments to pump atmospheric air, while mouth-to-mouth resuscitation is only indicated in extreme cases when proper instruments are not available.

J. Fothergill (1712-1780), member of the Royal College of Physicians, fellow of the Royal Society of London and of the Royal College of Physicians, and corresponding member of the Royal Medical society of Paris, in 1745 publishes his "Observations on the recovery of a man dead in appearance ...", where he describes the resuscitation system performed in 1744 by W. Tossach, surgeon of Alloa, in order to save a man, apparently dead by suffocation in a well. Once the body had been taken out of the water, W. Tossach immediately practiced mouth-to-mouth resuscitation, closing both nostrils with one hand and blowing intensely till the chest was full of air; as soon as the heart started beating again, he practiced bloodletting from an arm, stimulating at the same time the body of the patient by rubbing and lightly shaking the body. According to Fothergill, the mouth-to-mouth resuscitation technique performed by Tossach has the merit of being practicable by anyone, even in the absence of specific instruments or specialized personnel. From a theoretic point of view, according to Fothergill, when passing through the lungs, blood undergoes a relevant metamorphosis thanks to the vivifying action of pure air and to the dismissal of the toxic and phlogistic one; during drowning this process is interrupted and blood is immediately filled with phlogiston and noxious principle, thus damaging all the vital parts affected by it. The stagnation of phlogistic air provokes the obliteration of sensitivity, that is the vital factor par excellence together with natural heat, and according to Fothergill, insufflations of a small quantity of pure air (or rather that which is oxygenated) would be sufficient to modify the quality of the phlogistic air still present inside the pulmonary vases; but the complexity of such an operation makes the application difficult, and it is possible to reactivate the respiratory motion mechanically through the injection of atmospheric or expired air. The introduction of air into the lungs communicates the motion to the heart too, and therefore it should be well-balanced and controlled; for this purpose the adoption of bellows, as discussed by the Humane Society of London, can be a disadvantage because it makes it difficult for non-experts to control the quantity of air introduced thus increasing the risks of damaging the lungs, while mouth-to-mouth resuscitation permits one to manage the quantity and modality of ventilation into the lungs (Fothergill J., 1783).

Upon W. Haews' invitation, in 1776 J. Hunter published a research on the experimental studies conducted in 1755, where he gives an account on the outcome of the experiments concerning lung ventilation carried out on a dog. Once the dog's chest was opened, Hunter ascertained that the cardiac impulses and frequency varied according to the activation or the suspension of air insufflations, and that in the absence of it the heart swelled and blood coagulated, becoming thick and black in the left ventricle.

He concluded that resuscitation of drowned persons essentially depends on the reactivation of the respiratory function. For this purpose, he indicates the use of two bellows, one to inject and the other to inspire air, inserting the nozzles either in the mouth or in a nostril, without a connecting tube. According to him, the use of bellows permits one to immediately ventilate the quantity of air necessary to relax the lungs and expel it promptly, reproducing the natural respiratory mechanisms. He underlines the importance of how much time the body is under water to have an efficient reanimation, the faster the rescue operations are of drowned persons' from the water the easier it will be. When there is immediate intervention, it is sufficient to practice artificial respiration to reactivate the vital functions; if, on the contrary, the patient stays on in the water for a long time, a more complex protocol must be carried out, involving many different operations to be performed contemporarily. In these cases, in fact, it is appropriate to insufflate stimulants, like volatile alkali vapors (that is spirit of salt ammoniac), through the mouth or the nostrils in order to stimulate the sense of smell; to apply to the nostrils spirituous acid substances, whose exhalations stimulate the nervous and sensory motions. During air insufflations, it is necessary to press the larynges into the esophagus, both to avoid air penetration into the stomach and into the intestines, and to insert stimulants; in the meantime a warm bed is prepared on which to lie the patient, because only heat can restore the vital principle, but without exposing the drowned person's body to an excessive source of heat, because this could also be lethal. Body temperature must be, in fact, gradually restored, not to create spasms and shocks. For this purpose, volatile alkali can be used, or heating and stimulating balms can be used to soak the blankets to be wrapped around the body, and to be injected into the stomach and the intestines, in order to warm and reactivate internal organs. When all these operations are not efficient, Hunter proposes the use of electricity to stimulate the heart. He considers, in fact, apparent death a condition of permanency of the animal sensitivity, even in the presence of a suspension of the vital functions. The stimulus impressed by the electric shocks on the chest, can reactivate the cardiac fibers and recover their functionality. Disagreeing with the thesis of death by drowning as a result of apoplexy, he discourages bloodletting because bleeding would further deprive the patient of the heat and vital principle. For the same reason he condemns the use of emetics and laxatives, which would weaken even more the animal apparatus (Hunter J., 1837).

William Cullen (1710-1790) draws up a memoir on the resuscitation techniques, on behalf of Lord Cachart, President of the Board Of Police in Scotland and promoter of the drowned persons rescue organizations and the distribution of instructions and public advices on this matter in the Scottish cities.

Contrary to the traditional systems of barrel rolling, hanging people upside down and stroking, Cullen affirms that a light shaking of the body is sufficient to reanimate a person only when promptly taken out of the water, but it is contraindicated in the other cases. According to him life does not cease immediately after the interruption of the pulmonary and cardiac activity, because vitality is also given by the nerves and the fibers, or rather by sensitivity from which heart activity depends on.

An essential assumption to reanimate the persons apparently dead, is the recovery of heat, because it is the necessary element to the vitality of the fibers. It is therefore by acting on this vital principle that it is possible to recover pulmonary and cardiac functions and reactivate blood circulation. The first operation to be carried out is therefore body heating, by undressing the patient of his/her wet clothes, transferring him/her to a warm place where there is a burning fire or a working furnace. When it is possible to have hot water, it would be appropriate to immerge the patient into it, because it is the safest and fastest way to recover the body temperature. If the drowned person is thin, he/she can be warmed with the heat of another person's body, then it would be good to have the patient lying down in bed with one or two people. The drowned person must lie down, preferably on their side, keeping his/her head slightly raised. Disagreeing with rubbing, he recommends to apply spirit of salt ammoniac to wrists and ankles and cover the body with cereals or ashes or hot sand or common salt. In the meantime it is necessary to perform all the intervention required to reactivate the fibers of the organs, starting from the intestines which are the ones that mostly maintain the sensitivity. In order to stimulate the intestinal fibers, he proposes tobacco fumes insufflations. In the absence of a proper fumigation instrument or of two pipes useful for the operation, it is possible to inject hot water with a syringe. Contemporarily lungs ventilation is performed, following the method adopted by Alexander Monro, that is blowing air into the mouth or in the nostrils through a cannula. Against those who consider expired air unsuitable for the reactivation of the vital functions, because it is rich in phlogiston, Cullen believes that hot air exhaled from another animal is the most efficient way to reactivate pulmonary fibers; only when such an operation does not achieve the hoped result, insufflations of air is practiced with two bellows, as proposed by J. Hunter. In order to ease air passage through the trachea, the larynges are kept down so as to alternate air insufflations and pressures on the chest which reproduces the natural motion of the lungs. If it is not possible to introduce air in this way, a cannula is directly inserted into the trachea: the surgeon stands on the right of the patient and introduces the index finger of his left hand into the mouth up to the epiglottis and with his right hand he inserts the catheter below the epiglottis. The external extremity of the cannula is then joined to a syringe full of air. Tracheotomy is practiced only as an extreme measure. As opposed to Hunter, he considers jugular bloodletting as a useful operation to dissipate vein congestion, which he believes being a cause of death by drowning. In order to reanimate the other parts of the body, in the most sensitive areas stimulants are used, such as the lime spirit and salt ammoniac. He rather warns about the risks induced by the usual practice of introducing spirituous fluids into the mouth before the patient recovers the respiratory and swallowing functions, and recommends to inject hot wine directly into the stomach through a catheter inserted into the esophagus. Even though following some of the directions given by W. Cullen, the instructions published and distributed to all of the Guards' Houses by Lord Cathcart faithfully following the advices already provided by the drowned persons lifesaving societies of other countries. To recover the natural temperature of the body, for example, in addition to the application of sand or cereal or hot ashes, it is also recommended to use bricks or bottles of hot water to put on the extremities of the body and the rubbing with alcoholic liqueurs; above all the traditional mouth-to-mouth resuscitation is practiced by closing both the nostrils of the drowned person and exercising alternate pressure on the chest to make him/her exhale the air inside it (Cullen W., 1776).

Other authors, mostly French, editors of popular texts, rather tend to figure drowning to be among the other forms of asphyxia. The different forms of asphyxia are noticeably divided according to the cause which determines them: foul or toxic air, excess of heat or coldness, syncope, strangulation and drowning. It is especially the thickening of viscous humors in the bronchus and in the throat together with blood coagulation, induced by the cold water, to render the reanimation of drowned persons more complex than it could be for those asphyxiated.

According to J. Janin (1731-1799?), with the arrest of respiration and the suspension of blood circulation, the electric fluid is restrained and for this reason natural temperature also fails. Janin compares the nervous fluid to a lantern which enlightens till it can burn air, and when this one expires, the sensitivity of the parts fades away. Consequently, in order to resuscitate drowned persons it is essential to restore the natural temperature of the body necessary to stimulate the nervous fluid which starts again to irritate all the membranous and muscular fibers till they recover the systaltic motion and melt the congested fluids; thanks to the stimulating action of tobacco, the intestines recover their peristaltic motion. Insufflations of air into the lungs is then practiced by blowing directly into the mouth of the patient and closing both nostrils well. Once resuscitated, the patient is administered with some spoonfuls of distilled spirit. As well as his contemporary authors, he considers electricity one of the most efficient instruments to test the existence of the vital fluid which, together with air, are the primary elements of vital motions and animal functions. He also finds a strong analogy between apoplexy and strangulation, because in both cases, there is a complexion of the brain vessels, and it is possible to adopt the same systems of reanimation. In order to save asphyxiated person from mophetic or putrid exhalations, it is necessary above all to remove the patient out of the place where there is foul air, undress him/her and rub him/her with hot water and vinegar to infuse heat; it can also be useful to place under the nose cloths soaked in spirit of vinegar and to tickle the nostrils with a feather (Janin J., 1772).

In a letter published on the Mercure de France in August 1772, Jacquin affirms that, together with the four operations (shaking, bloodletting, insufflations of air into the lungs and fumigation of tobacco fumes into the intestines) indicated in the advices provided by the Prevôt des Merchands et Echevins (Provost of the Merchants and Echevins), it is appropriate to place the drowned person on a bed of hot ashes in order to stimulate with heat the recovery of blood circulation. According to his project, every station of the Guards' House in each city must have a folding bed, a barrel of ashes, an iron heater with its trivet and two stoves to treat the patient as soon as he/she is saved, immediately warming the ashes. All the other operations of resuscitation can be in fact carried out while the patient is lying on the bed under which burning stoves are placed to keep the ashes heated. Thence starts a real debate on whether to use ashes as an essential instrument of intervention for the resuscitation of drowned persons. It appears that the process to obtain and keep them warm is hard and expensive, that the directions provided by the lifesaving society of Amsterdam, on which all the others have been based, does not mention it, and that the same effects can be obtained through other systems of body heating. Besides, those who advocate body aspersion with the ashes are condemned by those who believe that the thin powders coming from it, together with the alkali salt contained in it, can be toxic to the patient, as well as mephitic can be the burning coals used to create and keep the ashes warm (Pia P. N., 1773).

Also Joseph Jacques de Gardane (XVIII cent.) includes drowned persons in the nosology category of asphyxia, or rather apparent death by apoplexy induced by the arrest of the circulatory motion which is due to inhibition of the respiratory function provoked by lack of air.

In the case of asphyxia caused by lack of air, the patient should be taken out of the place where he/she is lying, exposed to open air, placed on his/her side and with his/her head slightly raised, undressed of his/her clothes and rubbed with fresh water, refrigerating and stimulating substances such as vinegar, wine or other spirituous liqueur to stimulate blood circulation. Before administering him/her with any treatment, it is good to wait for the reactivation of the respiratory and swallowing functions.

In the case of asphyxia by mephitism, instead, (that is caused by pathogen exhalations due to decomposition of putrefied organic matter, alcoholic fermentation, coal fumes, or foul air in closed places), the patient must be immediately transferred to open air, undressed and rubbed with cold water and vinegar; insufflations of air into the lungs is practiced, some ice is placed in the armpits, under the feet and on the pit of the stomach; only after resuscitation he/she is exposed to a fire. In asphyxia by coldness, before exposing the patient to any source of heat, he/she is sprinkled with snow or freezing water, because a very violent passage from low to high temperatures could be fatal.

In order to reanimate a person asphyxiated by strangulation, jugular phlebotomy is practiced together with blowing air directly into the mouth; once he/she has recovered, a fan or bellows are used to ventilate with the aim of helping him/her to breath. If the cause is the presence of a foreign body into the throat, it is necessary to push it down or extract it. The persons asphyxiated by drowning, must be transferred to a dry place, covered with cloths soaked either in simple distilled spirit or camphor spirit and exposed to a moderate fire to help recover the natural body temperature. Once the patient has been disposed on his/her side, air is insufflated into his/her lungs through a proper tube or with the stem of a pipe inserted into one of the nostrils while the other is closed, or in the mouth. The fastest way is that of mouth-to-mouth resuscitation to better stimulate the expansion of the bronchus. Then tobacco fumes are introduced into the intestines through an instrument composed of a small cannula. It must be inserted into the anus, whose extremity is successively joined to a flexible tube linked to a pipe which is used to blow air into it. In the absence of such an instrument, it is possible to provide the same treatment with two common pipes, with their stems connected; in the meantime the patient should always be shaken and resuscitated by tickling the nostrils and throat with the barb of a feather, or by insufflating tobacco fumes, stroking his/her feet and the palms of the hands with small sticks. As soon as the drowned person recovers his/her swallowing ability, he/she is administered with some drops of camphor distilled water, volatile salt ammoniac, or other spirituous liqueurs. Recommended are also hot baths and/or aspersion of the ashes, rubbing with salts along the crural arteries, application of bread cooked in distilled water below the mammas and on the pit of the stomach, enemas of decoction of tobacco and common salt, bloodletting(Scelta di opuscoli interessanti tradotti da varie lingue, 1775; Gardanne J. J., 1783).

He holds the thickening of black blood into the heart, discovered in the postmortem examination, responsible for the non-elaboration due to the lack of dephlogisticated atmospheric air. By inserting dephlogisticated air into the lungs of the drowned person, it is possible to induce immediately the elaboration of the blood still present in the vessels thus reactivating circulation and respiration. When water has been accumulated into the small vesicles of the lungs, it is necessary to expel it to insufflate atmospheric air. For such purpose, Gardane creates a special instrument, aiming at both aspiring the water still present in the respiratory tract and introducing in it about a hundred cubic inches of air, to expand them at the maximum level and infuse heat(Biblioteca della più recente letteratura edico-chirurgica 1794).

A key point in the codification of the rescue operations to asphyxiated persons is the work of Antoine Portal (1742-1832), who since 1772 had drawn up a series of reports on resuscitation of asphyxiated persons on behalf of the Science Academy of Paris. In his account in 1772 "Sur les effets des vapeurs méphitiques", he follows some of the directions provided by Tissot concerning the rescue of persons asphyxiated by mephitic vapors, though widening the topic in the light of the new medical doctrines on the resuscitation of the apparently dead people. The patient is to be exposed to fresh air and moistened with cold water to counterbalance heat excess and blood rarefaction. It is then necessary to decrease brain pressure through bloodletting, in particular from the jugular, which would permit the evacuation of foamy blood. The patient is administered with vinegar mixed with cold water and with the same mixture enemas are practiced. Portal instead considers the administration of spirituous liqueurs and emetics dangerous but still largely diffused, because the efforts produced by vomit push blood to the brain. Diverging from his contemporary authors, he denounces the uselessness and dangerousness of tobacco fumigations into the intestines because the organs undergo a violent dilatation which compromises their vital functions and above all because fumes comprise the diaphragm on the lungs, thus obstructing inspiration. Thence he recommends to stimulate the intestines with vinegar or other irritating enemas and to insufflate air into the respiratory tract to reactivate blood circulation and therefore restore its functions.

The insufflations of air into the lungs can be performed by inserting a tube into one of the nostrils closing both the other and the mouth or practicing a tracheotomy and inserting a curved tube. The large diffusion of his work both in France and abroad, definitely asserts lungs ventilation with the rhythmical cardiac massage as the resuscitation technique for those who present a cardio-respiratory arrest. In contrast with other authors, Portal recognizes in water penetration into the lungs the primary cause of death by drowning. The data observed induce him to give value to the etiologic interpretation supplied by A. Borelli: the foamy liqueur is produced by the water entering the lungs and it obstructs respiration so that blood, not being able to flow along the pulmonary vessels, accumulates in the pulmonary artery and the subject dies by suffocation. The interruption of the mechanics of blood circulation, blocked by the accumulation of water into the respiratory organs, causes the death of the persons drowned. Resuscitation procedures of the drowned persons faithfully follow what he proposed for the rescue of asphyxiated by mophectic vapors. First, the drowned person must be undressed, preferably using scissors or other instruments which would permit to remove the clothes off without shaking the patient; it is necessary to transfer him/her to a proper place, with a cot or cart, so that he/she lies down on his/her side in an improvised bed, with his/her head slightly raised to ease foam expulsion thus permitting the blood to penetrate the vessels and reach the brain and the thoracic organs. The physician must check whether on the body there are any injuries or contusions, because the level of seriousness of the lesions can indicate if the patient has already died or, however, he/she has suffered too serious injuries to be saved or if resuscitation operations can be really useful. The rubbing is practiced all over the body with a hot cloth to warm it and eliminate the mucous and glutinous substances which often entirely cover the drowned persons body and obstruct the dynamics of transpiration. In order to decrease the serum thickened in the respiratory tract, it is necessary to blow directly into the trachea and from here into the lungs. To do so, it is necessary to close the nostrils of the patient with one hand to prevent air recovery, while using the other to exercise pressure alternatively on the chest so that the respiration is restored, which is necessary to reactivate the blood circulation. He condemns tobacco fumes fumigations into the intestines which can excessively dilate the organs of the digestive apparatus till they are damaged, or push them towards the top till the diaphragm is compressed thus obstructing further respiration and make artificial respiration useless. As for those asphyxiated by toxic vapors, air insufflation is practiced by blowing in a tube inserted into one of the nostrils or, through tracheotomy, directly into the trachea. In order to infuse heat, blankets are used and hot bricks wrapped in linen cloths are placed under the feet. Jugular bloodletting must be practiced only when the drowned person does not show any signs of life. In order to resuscitate an asphyxiated congealed person, he/she must be wrapped in a blanket, transferred to the closest house and put in a non-heated bed; to reestablish the natural body temperature without causing a shock, the patient must be immersed in room temperature water and every two or three minutes hot water must be poured into the bathtub so that in fifteen minutes a temperature of 20 degrees on the Reaumur thermometer should be reached. As soon as the pulse is felt, more and more hot water is to be added till twenty-five degrees are reached thus restoring the right temperature. In the meantime, compresses of cold water on the face are applied, the nostrils are tickled with the a feather, spirituous substances are passed under the nose and air is insufflated into the lungs through a cannula inserted into one of the nostrils. When the patient is not reanimated or presents congealed limbs, rubbing distilled spirit or camphor vulnerary water is practiced all over the body and he/she is wrapped in blankets and placed in a warm bed. Once reanimated, the asphyxiated person is nourished only with liquids in particular with infusions of vulnerary plants or elderflowers and some drops of volatile alkali (Portal, A. 1810).

To contrast the effects of asphyxia by heat excess, the patient is transferred to a moderately cooler place, so that the body gradually adapts to the temperature change. The intervention of reanimation involves bloodletting (preferably from the jugular even in this case), the application of leeches to the temples and, when the patient can swallow, the administration of cold water with some vinegar, also used for enemas, and a footbath in lukewarm water (Portal, A. 1776).

According to these authors, from a physio-pathological point of view, the differences between the rescue operations aimed at saving drowned persons and those focused on asphyxiated persons by toxic air and heat, depend essentially on their different alteration of blood mass: in the case of drowning, blood thickens and coagulates; in the case of heat strokes and asphyxia caused by foul air, coal smoke and exhalation of alcoholics or putrefied matter, blood becomes foamy and rarefied. In both cases apoplexy is generated and for this reason each person is treated with jugular bloodletting and some treatments and stimulants are used to revitalize the parts of the body; but while the asphyxiated persons are to be exposed to fresh air and moistened with cold water, drowned persons essentially need to recover their natural temperature and reactivate their respiratory function in order to stimulate the recovery of blood circulation and therefore the heart.

3. Conclusions

The rescue methods defined in the 1770s, when drowned persons lifesaving societies were developing, are more or less the same till the beginning of the nineteenth century. In accordance with the medical techniques and Brown's doctrine, the reanimation procedures essentially consist in a stimulation of the vital factors, heat and sensitiveness, and internal motions, which should restore those functions compromised by a violent external event, as it happens in casualties.

The concept of apparent death, defined as an organic state of suspension of the vital functions which does not imply the end of life itself, not only makes it necessary to discover new strategies to certify death, but also interventions aimed at resuscitating those individuals whom, in the absence of a pathological status or injuries to the organs, have preserved the vital force. This is why drowned persons represent an important paradigm, because their condition is induced at least by two different factors of interruption of the natural vital impulses, the coldness of water and lack of air, without even considering the trauma caused by falling in the water. For this reason, reanimation procedures imply both body heating, to restore its natural temperature, and the stimulation of different apparatuses, the respiratory one in particular. The insufflations of air, beyond the doctrinal and technical divergences among various authors, is universally recognized as a good instrument to stimulate pulmonary process and, through the movement inferred to the lungs, the blood still present in the cardiac vessels. The methods used to save drowned persons thus represent the expression of the most complex practical system elaborated to rescue dying people in the seventeenth century and this is why it can be considered as the epistemic model of emergency medicine. This is the presupposition for the creation of effective therapeutic protocols to take care of more specific pathological categories, including resuscitation techniques. In particular, the artificial respiration, obtained by the insufflation of the air in the lungs and the alternating pressure on the chest, forms the basis of the medical resuscitation until the present day. The modern resuscitation developed in the late 50's of the last century, when Peter Safar (1924 - 2003), a specialist in anesthesiology, codified the "mouth to mouth" breathing to revive the patients unable to breathe autonomously. In the early '60, the engineer William Kouwenhoven (1886 - 1975) codified the rules for the external cardiac massage (MCE). Safar continued his studies on this specific medical field, writing the ABC of resuscitation, i.e. A for Airway, B for Breathing and C for Circulation. In the same times, the Laerdal, the Norwegian industry of medical instruments, produced the "Resusci Anne", the first human mannequin for the teaching of the artificial respiration as the first medical step of resuscitation. In the early '70s of the Nineteenth century, the American Heart Association (AHA) codified the guidelines for the teaching of homogenous CPR techniques, still used and taught to the medical practitioners and to the health professionals

4. References

Biblioteca della più recente letteratura medico-chirurgica, Tomo III, parte I (1794), pp. 98-115.

Buchan, W. (1774). Domestic Medicine or the family physician. Philadelphia, USA

Cogan, T. (1773). Memoirs of the society instituted at Amsterdam in favour of drowned persons. London, England

Cullen, W. (1776). *A letter to Lord Cathcart concerning the recovery of persons drowned and seemingly dead*. London, England

Fothergill, J. (1783). The works of John Fothergill, London, England

Gardanne, J. J. de (1783). Catéchisme sur les morts apparentes , dites asphyxies . Dijon, France

Hunter, J. (1837), The works of John Hunter (ed. by J. F. Palmer), London, Vol. IV, pp. 165-175.

Janin, J. (1772). Réflexions sur le triste sort des personnes qui sous une apparence de mort, ont été enterrées vivantes... Paris, France

Johnson, A. (1773). An account of some Societies at Amsterdam and Hamburg... London, England

Kite, C. (1788), An essay on the recovery of the apparently dead, London, England

Larcan, A.; Brullard, Ph. (1979). Remarques concernant la prévention, la notion d'urgence et l'organisation des secours au XVIII siècle. *Histoire des Sciences medicale*, Vol. 13, No. 3, pp. 271-278, ISSN 0440-8888

Monthly Review or literary journal 1776; june 1773-january 1774.

Nurok, M. (2003). Elements of the medical emergency's epistemological alignment: 18-20th perspectives. *Social Studies of Sciences,* Vol. 33, No.4, pp. 563-579, ISSN, 0306-3127

Pia, P. N. (1773). Détail des succès de l'établissement que la vile de Paris a fait en faveur des personnes noyèes..., Paris, France

Portal, A. (1776). Rapporto fatto per ordine dell'Accademia delle Scienze sopra gli effetti dei vapori mofettici, Parigi, France.

Portal, A. (1810). Istruzioni sopra la cura degli annegati, degl' Asfissiaci, delle persone morsicate... Paris, France.

Dalla stamperia di Vincent, ParigiRiley, J. C. (2001), Rising Life Expectancy: A Global History, ISBN 0521802458, Cambridge, England,

Scelta di opuscoli interessanti tradotti da varie lingue (1775). Milano, Lombardia, vol. VII.

Singy, P. (2010). The Popularization of Medicine in the Eighteenth Century: Writing, Reading, and Rewriting Samuel Auguste Tissot's Avis au peuple sur sa santéby. *Journal of Modern History,* Vol.82, pp.769-800, ISSN 00222801.

Tissot, S.A. (1769). Avis au peuple sur sa santè. Lyon, France

Trépardoux, F. (1997). Philippe-Nicolas Pia (1721-1799), échevin de Paris, pionnier du secourisme en faveur des noyés (II partie). *Revue d'Histoire de la Pharmacie,* Vol.85, No.316, pp. 375-384, ISSN 0035-2349.

Trubuhovich, RV. (2006). History of mouth-to-mouth rescue breathing. Part 2: the 18th century. *Critical Care and Resuscitation,* 2006, Vol. 8. No.2, pp. 157-171, ISSN 14412772

9

Considerations in Mass Casualty and Disaster Management

Peter Aitken[1] and Peter Leggat[1,2]
[1]Anton Breinl Centre for Public Health and Tropical Medicine,
James Cook University, Townsville, Queensland
[2]School of Public Health, University of the Witwatersrand, Johannesburg
[1]Australia
[2]South Africa

1. Introduction

Disasters have increased in frequency over the past century. A number of high profile disasters have also dominated news headlines in the past decade raising the media and community awareness, of disasters. This has been across the full spectrum of disasters and as illustrated in Table 1 has included terrorist bombings, hurricanes, earthquakes, tsunamis and floods.

The relevance of mass casualty incidents and disaster management to Emergency Medicine is obvious. Emergency Departments are the 'front door' of the hospital component of the health system. The injured or unwell and also often the worried well, will present for care. Emergency Departments (ED) need to be able to respond effectively, which mandates advance planning and preparedness. Most ED already run beyond capacity so the ability to manage an acute influx of patients in a system with potentially damaged infrastructure is a significant challenge requiring fore-thought and an understanding of disasters. Additionally, the broad skill set of Emergency Physicians may see them working in the pre-hospital arena or as part of international disaster response. This requires additional training to maintain the safety of clinicians in often challenging, and hazardous environments.

The aim of this chapter is to:

- Provide an overview of disaster epidemiology and the definitions and principles of practice;
- Outline common problems associated with mass casualty incidents and disaster management;
- Describe the potential roles of emergency physicians in mass casualty incidents, international response and pandemics and the specific issues associated with these;
- Identify emerging issues in mass casualty incidents and disaster management, future developments and research areas.

Year	Location	Disaster	Dead	Broader Impact
2001	New York	World Trade Centre	> 3,000	Broad societal change
2003	Bam, Iran	Earthquake	>25,000	>30,000 injured
2004	South Asia	Tsunami	>230,000	1.6 million homeless
2004	Russia	Beslan school siege	334	Legislative change
2004	Spain	Madrid train bombing	191	Change of government
2005	London	Subway bombings	52	Societal impact UK
2007	New Orleans	Hurricane Katrina	> 1,800	> $80 billion USD
2008	Myanmar	Cyclone Nargis	>140,000	Politics of aid
2008	China	Earthquake	> 65,000	> $140 billion USD
2009	Haiti	Earthquake	>80,000	1.5 million homeless
2010	Pakistan	Floods	>1000	20 million homeless
2011	New Zealand	Earthquake	181	>$20 billion USD
2011	Japan	Earthquake + Tsunami	> 15,000	> $300 billion USD

Table 1. Examples of Major Disasters in the Past Decade.

2. Definitions

A consistent problem in disaster management is a lack of consistency in definitions. This may lead to research problems and difficulty comparing one database with another or problems comparing outcomes when different definitions of injury or restoration of function are used. Most importantly it can lead to an ineffective response if different systems or organisations use different definitions in the same community.

A number of studies have illustrated the differences in disaster definition (Al-Mahari, 2007; Debacker, 2002). While these tend to focus on the role of the organisation and include finance, transport or health for those organisations, which have these as key roles, there remain a number of common elements. These can be described as:

1. An extraordinary event
2. Damage to existing infrastructure
3. A state of disaster / emergency declared
4. A need for external assistance

Definitions, from the World Association of Disaster and Emergency Medicine (WADEM) (Sundnes & Birnbaum, 2002) and Australian Emergency Management Institute (AEMI, 2011) are shown in Figure 1 and highlight these commonalities.

WADEM has made efforts to standardise the language of disasters. The primary purpose of this was to promote consistency of terms in research through development of their Utstein Template (Sundnes & Birnbaum, 2002). However, use of common language in operational phases is just as important. For example one of the key benefits of the Advanced Trauma Life Support (ATLS) has been the development of a common language in the management of trauma. Confusion also often exists between terns such as 'disaster' and 'mass casualty incident'. Generally speaking, a mass casualty incident, while it may involve large numbers of patients, can be managed within the resources of the affected organisation or health facility. A disaster cannot, and will mean the mobilisation of additional resources using external assistance. This is obviously context dependant with different thresholds for

WADEM Disaster Definition	EMA Disaster Definition
"A serious disruption of the functioning of society, causing widespread human, material and environmental losses which exceed the ability of the affected society to cope using only its own resources; the result of a vast ecological breakdown in the relations between man and his environment, a serious and sudden event (or slow as in drought) on such a scale that the stricken community needs extraordinary efforts to cope with it, often with outside help or international aid."	"A serious disruption to community life which threatens or causes death or injury in that community, and damage to property which is beyond the day-to-day capacity of the prescribed statutory authorities and which requires special mobilisation and organisation of resources other than those normally available to those authorities."

Fig. 1. Examples of Disaster Definitions.

external assistance for different systems (e.g. a small rural hospital versus a large inner city tertiary teaching hospital). This also explains why most definitions of disasters do not use numbers of patients in their definition, while this may be included for specific facilities. Of note is that many definitions of 'disaster' used by databases, also specifically exclude war and complex emergencies (CRED, 2000).

3. Epidemiology of disasters

Disasters have always occurred. Our ability to capture an historical record has improved with development of language and writing skills, just as our awareness of disasters in other countries has improved with the growth of telecommunications and the internet. The great flood in the Bible is likely to have been based on a real event and historically coincides with the description of a major flood event in the Mesopotamian Gilgamesh epic. One of the earliest confirmed descriptions of a disaster was that of Pliny the Elder who witnessed the destruction of Pompeii by the volcano Vesuvius in AD 79.

Table 2 describes selected major disasters from world history. Points to note are that the number of deaths does not always reflect the true impact of the disaster or allow full comparison between disasters. While only 6 official deaths were recorded in the Great Fire of London (the poor and homeless were not included), 80% of the buildings were destroyed. Change the context to the London of today and imagine the impact not just on London, but the whole of the country – socially, psychologically and economically. Similarly while 20-40 million died during the Spanish Flu of 1918-1919, the Black Death killed an estimated 100 million people in the 14th century which was approximately one third to one half of Europe's population at the time.

The frequency of disasters has also increased. Data from the CRED database is reproduced in Figure 2 and clearly shows a rise in disaster numbers each decade from the 1950's to end of the 20th century (CRED, 2000). While improved reporting has no doubt played a role, there are many other reasons for this. The world population has increased significantly, and along with that both population density (Drabek, 1986) and spread of population with large cities located in at risk areas (Dynes, 1998). This means an incident is both more likely to affect larger numbers of people in an inhabited region (e.g. inner city) but also affect people in previously unpopulated zones. The growth in technology has also contributed to not just

Year	Location	Disaster	Dead	Broader Impact
79	Pompeii	Volcano (Vesuvius)	30,000	First recorded description
526	Syria	Antioch Earthquake	250,000	
1300's	Europe	Black Death Plague	1,000,000	1/3 -1/2 population die
1666	London	Great Fire	6 officially	80% of buildings destroyed
1883	Indonesia	Volcano (Krakatoa)	40,000	Global temperature effects
1887	China	Flooding	1-2,000,000	1/2 deaths due disease, famine
1912	North Atlantic	Titanic	1517	Shipping safety (lifeboats)
1918-19	World	Spanish Flu pandemic	20-40,000,000	3% world dead, 27% infected
1931	China	Floods	1-2,000,000	Most dead any natural disaster
1970	Bangladesh	Cyclone Bhola	300,000	Most cyclone deaths
1976	China	Tangshan Earthquake	>300,000	International aid refused
1989	England	Hillsborough	91	Stadium safety

Table 2. Major Disasters in World History (prior to 2000).

industrial disasters but also transport disasters (Quarantelli, 1985), which have evolved from horse and cart to the A380 with potentially 500 passengers aboard, or involve carriage of dangerous goods.

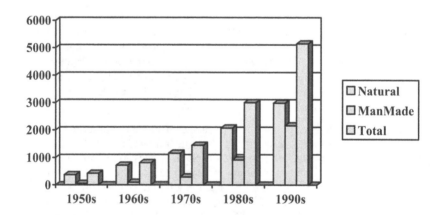

Fig. 2. Frequency of Disasters Each Decade.

There are also many types of disaster evident from this table. The WADEM Utstein Template describes disasters by hazard and separates them into natural disasters, man-made disasters and mixed disasters where both nature and man contribute (Sundnes & Birnbaum, 2002). An abbreviated version is provided in Table 3 describing natural and man-made disasters. Mixed disasters may occur as a result of man's activities influencing desertification processes, flooding due to altered waterways or landslides due to removal of trees.

NATURAL	Seismic	Earthquake
		Volcano
		Tsunami
		Celestial collision
	Climatic	High winds – gales, cyclones, hurricanes, typhoons, tornados
		Precipitation – rain, snow, ice
		Lightening
		Temperature extremes – heat, cold
		Erosion
		Drought
		Desertification
		Floods
		Avalanches
MAN-MADE	Technological	Substance release – chemical, biological, radiological
		Transport
		Structural failure
		Explosions
		Fire
		Environmental interference
	Conflict	Armed conflict – war, civil war, complex emergency, terrorism
		Unarmed conflict – sanctions, embargo

Table 3. Classification of Disasters by Hazard (based on WADEM Utstein template).

Table 4 based on information from the IFRC database shows the frequency of different disaster types by continent (IFRC, 2000). A number of clear messages emerge from this.

- The three most common disaster types are floods, windstorms (including cyclones and hurricanes) and transport disasters. This holds true for all continents except Africa where floods is replaced by drought.
- Disasters are over represented in the developing world, while North America, Europe and Oceania is less affected. This can only partly be explained by population differences. While 90% of disaster related deaths occur in countries with income less than 760 US dollars per year (Haddow & Bullock, 2003), it is not surprising that there are lower levels of disaster preparedness and response capability in those countries. When there is a struggle to put food on the table today, it is difficult to plan for tomorrow. Similarly, some shelter is better than none and some income is better than none. This potentially leads to less developed industrial standards, building codes and response capability of both health and emergency services.

The burden of disasters in developing countries remains one of the major challenges in global emergency medicine and disaster health. There have been efforts to address this through initiatives such as the Decade of Global Disaster Reduction where the focus was on mitigation as the key to addressing natural disasters (Iwan, 1999). Similarly international bodies such as the WHO or Pan American Health Organisation (PAHO) have made efforts to develop cost effective solutions and promote disaster preparedness. The real solution lies in improving local capacity with linkages between development and preparedness, all of which has financial implications.

Disaster Type	Asia	Americas	Africa	Europe	Oceania	Total
Transport	668	233	437	186	11	1535
Floods	362	216	207	153	25	963
Windstorms	322	283	49	71	58	783
Industrial	225	55	37	67	2	386
Misc. accidents	178	45	57	53	5	338
Droughts / Famines	77	39	113	13	11	253
Earthquakes	112	48	10	37	8	215
Avalanche / Landslide	101	40	12	25	5	183
Forest fires	18	55	11	39	9	132
Extreme temperatures	35	30	6	51	4	126
Volcanic eruptions	16	23	3	2	6	50

Table 4. Frequency of Disaster Types by Continent (Based on data from IFRC).

It is also important for Emergency Physicians to remember that health and medical issues are just one component of the damage caused by a disaster. Mortality is a poor indicator of the severity of a disaster. Communities can be affected in many ways, including disruption of transport, education, security, water and sanitation, to name just a few. These have been described as "Basic Societal Functions' by WADEM and are described in Table 6 (Sundnes & Birnbaum, 2002). Health workers need to appreciate that they are simply one part of the disaster effort and that their needs may not be considered the main priority at that particular stage by those responsible for overall coordination of the response. This broad extent of damage may also impact on the health effort. It may affect the ability of staff to report to work, while power and water failures may lead to secondary health hazards that need to be pro-actively planned for and addressed. An example of this broad impact is seen in the effects of Hurricane Mitch on Honduras in 1997. While approximately 9000 people were killed, more than 3 million were displaced with 75% of the Honduran population affected. The damage bill of 8.5 billion US dollars was more than the GDP of Honduras and was estimated to set development back by more than 20 years (Lichtenstein, 2001).

(1) Medical
(2) Public Health
(3) Sanitation / H2O
(4) Shelter / Clothing
(5) Food
(6) Energy Supplies
(7) Search & Rescue
(8) Public Works & Engineering
(9) Environment
(10) Logistics / Transport
(11) Security
(12) Communication
(13) Economy
(14) Education

Table 5. Basic Societal Functions as Defined by WADEM.

4. Major principles of care

Disaster Management is "the aggregate of all measures taken to reduce the likelihood of damage that will occur related to a hazard(s), and to minimise the damage once an event is occurring or has occurred and to direct recovery from the damage" (Sundnes & Birnbaum, 2002). Disaster management, like any profession or health sub-specialty has its own language to describe the components of this. It is important to fully understand these major models, principles of care and key concepts, which are described below.

4.1 Disaster models

A number of models have emerged in recent years. The disaster cycle (Hogan, 2002) describes a series of phases from warning, impact, rescue, recovery and the quiescent phase. While this describes the life cycle of a disaster it should not be interpreted as when activities occur. For example, recovery should begin as early as possible in the response phase and is not simply a transition. A Venn diagram style model developed by Bradt et al (2003), describes the interface between public health, clinical medicine and emergency management as the core focus of disaster medicine. This has since been expanded by WADEM in a model that illustrates the complexity and multi-disciplinary nature of disaster medicine (Archer & Synaeve, 2007).

4.2 Comprehensive approach

The Comprehensive Approach consists of Prevention / Mitigation; Preparation, Response and Recovery (AEMI, 2011). It is important to recognise that these are NOT sequential phases, but simply different areas of emphasis. Recovery, for example, should start early in the response phase rather than after this has finished. Recovery for maximum effect should also address mitigation issues.

4.2.1 Prevention and mitigation

Prevention refers to activities undertaken to stop a disaster happening. This is obviously impossible for many disasters - despite scientific advances we cannot stop an earthquake or a cyclone from occurring. While it may conceivably be easier to stop manmade disasters, there are often hidden costs associated with this that stop it happening. For example we could stop aircraft disasters by banning air flight but the effect on the global economy and world culture would be prohibitive. Mitigation is the usual alternative and refers to activities undertaken to lessen the effects of a disaster. Examples include building codes and town planning with inclusion of flood zones. A definition is the "regulatory and physical measures to ensure that emergencies are prevented, or their effects mitigated" (AEMI, 2011).

4.2.2 Preparedness

Preparedness refers to those activities undertaken beforehand to lessen the impact of the disaster. This consists primarily of planning but examples also include the education, training and exercising of staff and the development of warning systems fro communities. A definition is the "arrangements to ensure that, should a disaster occur, all those resources and services which may be needed to cope with the effects can be rapidly mobilised and deployed" (AEMI, 2011).

4.2.3 Response

Response refers to the actions taken directly following a disaster. Examples include deployment of teams and emergency services, rescue services and acute health care. A definition is the "actions taken in anticipation of, during and immediately after impact to ensure that its effects are minimised and that people are given immediate relief and support" (AEMI, 2011).

4.2.4 Recovery

Recovery refers to the process of restoring the affected community to normal. This includes psychosocial issues, the economy and reconstruction. A definition is "the coordinated process of supporting disaster affected communities in reconstructing their physical infrastructure and restoration of emotional, social, economic and physical well being" (AEMI, 2011).

4.3 All agencies

The All Agencies approach emphasises the multiple agencies that come together in disaster management. Nobody responds alone and preparations should ensure the ability to work together and 'play happily together in the sandpit'. For this to occur, organisations need to come together in advance as part of preparedness. It is not just a common language and interoperability of systems that is important. A common finding in post incident reviews is that the pre-incident development of networks, relationships and trust between individuals is an important determinant of successful outcomes.

4.4 All hazards

The All Hazards principle promotes the concept of planning for a consistent response across disaster types. There can be issues in having a separate plan for every type of disaster, as this can lead to a shelf of plans, which are unlikely to be used. Many elements of a plan are common to each disaster type. These might include for example the activation arrangements, recall of staff, triage, surge arrangements and documentation (AEMI, 2011).

4.5 Prepared community

The prepared community recognises that the initial response will be from those in the affected community. External assistance will take time to arrive and in the meantime local people will have rescued people from the rubble, commenced first aid and initiated treatment as best able. People by nature will turn to local agencies and organisations for assistance. They will present to local facilities, whether they be health or government. Increasing the ability of the local community to respond increases the ability of the community to manage the disaster. This can be defined as "a prepared community is one which has developed effective emergency and disaster management arrangements at the local level, resulting in:

- Alert, informed and active community, which supports its voluntary organisations.
- Active and involved local government.
- Agreed and coordinated arrangement for PPRR" (AEMI, 2011).

4.6 Risk management

The principles of risk management can be described as identification of the risk, analysis of the risk and management of the risk. Risk can be defined as 'the systematic application of management policies, procedures and practices to the tasks of identifying, analysing, evaluating, treating and monitoring risk' (AEMI, 2011)

A key issue in the identification and prioritisation of risks is consideration of the likelihood of an event and the likely impact if it occurs. This can be done as formal risk assessment scoring systems, classic 2 x 2 risk tables (likelihood and impact), knowledge of local disaster history and answering the question "what if?". An example of a 2 x 2 table is shown in Figure 3 with Cell B (high impact and high likelihood) the obvious focus of initial planning. Increasingly organisations are required to perform a formal risk analysis. This should still be supplemented by local knowledge and review of what might happen as a result. Once recognised, risks should be modified - this can either be by prevention or mitigation strategies. Strategies should also be reviewed.

A High Impact Low Likelihood	B High Impact High Likelihood
C Low Impact Low Likelihood	D Low Impact High Likelihood

Fig. 3. Risk Management using Risk Tables.

4.7 Resilience

There has been a major focus in recent years on recognising the importance of resilience (Castleden, 2011). There are many definitions of resilience in use, but simply put it is "the ability of a community to 'bounce back' following a disaster". Factors contributing to community resilience include past experiences, preparedness, and degrees of dependence or independence. Many rural or regional communities are thought to be more resilient than their urban counterparts, although this varies between communities, disaster type and even disaster frequency.

5. Common problems

The analysis of different disasters illustrates a number of common issues. It is important to note that in many reports these are described as 'lessons learned'. This is not true – they have usually only been observed. Lessons have only been learned once strategies have been devised and implemented to successfully address these issues.

A selection of these problems is described below, with examples of research work trying to address these included as potential solutions.

5.1 Communication

Communication is THE most common problem identified in most disaster reviews (Arnold, 2004; Braham, 2001; Chan, 2004; Gerace, 1979; McEntire, 1998). This may occur as a result of problems with the medium, the message and the messenger, all of which may vary depending on the intended target audience. It is also essential to remember that communication is not simply disseminating information but is a two way street and as much care needs to be taken ensuring the ability to receive messages and information as disseminating them. While it may be impossible to avoid all communication problems, these can be minimised with advance preparation and ensuring redundancy of methods.

There may be a failure of the communication medium and having a pre-identified fall back solution is a mandatory part of preparedness. Hospital switchboards may be overwhelmed, phone systems (including mobile or cell networks) may collapse, and email may fail. Reach of the message is also important. Not everyone is able to receive the message using the same medium. This applies just as much to hospitals as communities. The elderly may be less likely to access email than younger groups, some pockets of the population may be geographically isolated, have poor phone or television reception, speak a different language, or not have a fixed abode. Similarly, clinical or operational staff are unlikely to access email regularly, while administrative staff will be able to. Staff work different shifts or in different buildings, on or off campus.

Reliance on one communication method alone is a recipe for disaster, as this may fail, be overloaded or not have sufficient reach. Planning should consider the use of alternatives such as use of runners, Public Address (PA) systems, SMS messaging, and social networks including personal communication and tools such as Facebook and Twitter. When using multiple modes of communication, it is essential that the message is consistent, to avoid confusion. A standard structure, with use of a pre-developed template, helps achieve this. Radios are a commonly used alternative but staff must be trained in proper radio use and a system put in place to ensure radios are charged and accessible when needed.

Community information should remember potentially isolated groups and distribute information in multiple languages (selection of which to be guided by knowledge of local community) as well as use of sign language for television broadcasts. The message structure should be clear and concise while at the same time not causing undue alarm or panic.

Communication planning should also recognise that there is a need to also receive information. Clear contact points and lines of communication should be established with logging of calls and communication. While it is important to be able to be aware of large scale or strategic developments through monitoring of news channels and regular updates from higher-level committees, it is also important to be able to receive information from 'the coalface'. A member of the Incident Management Team walking through operational areas may provide this opportunity in an informal way. Use of electronic media also provides an opportunity if developed properly. An open email account for staff feedback can assist this process. A more formal solution is the use of tools such as 'survey monkey', which allow analysis of feedback patterns, potential prioritisation of issues and recognition of gaps in message coverage. This approach also allows real time improvement, during the life cycle of the disaster, rather than waiting for feedback in the operational debrief and initiating changes in practice for 'next time' (Seidl et al., 2010). It is also possible to learn from other industries by analysis of their management of communication (Seidl et al., 2011).

5.2 Command, control, coordination

Command, control and coordination arrangements became a point of emphasis after the California wildfires in the 1970's. This recognised that there are limited spans of control and a need for clear lines of command within organisations and communication across organisations. Failure to do this may lead to difficulties with an integrated response and either task omission or task duplication. Figure 4 illustrates some of the key elements of Command, Control and Co-ordination.

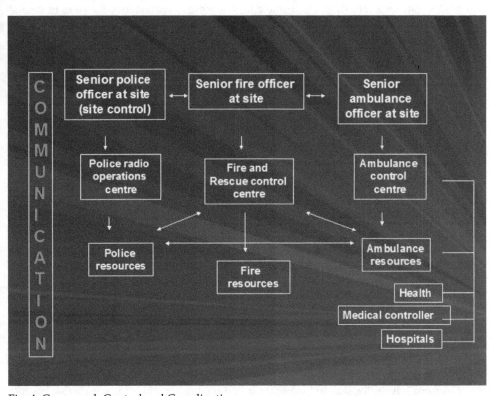

Fig. 4. Command, Control and Coordination.

Command is the direction of members of an organisation in the performance of roles and tasks.

• It operates vertically within an organisation.

Control is the overall direction of emergency management activities in an emergency situation.

• It operates horizontally across organisations.

Coordination bringing together of organisations and elements to ensure an effective response, mainly concerned with systematic acquisition and application of resources in accordance with threat or impact.

- It operates both vertically and horizontally as functions of authority to command and control.

Incident Command Systems or Incident Management Systems have many guises but are all essentially similar (see Figure 5). They have a person in charge and then people supporting them by adopting functions such as "planning" (what might happen?); "operations" (what do we need to do?); "logistics" (how do we make this happen?); "admin / finance" (keeping track of costs) and "media". It is important staff are trained to work in these roles, or they will tend to fall back into their usual role and that there is redundancy for roles in case of either illness or a prolonged response and the need for shifts.

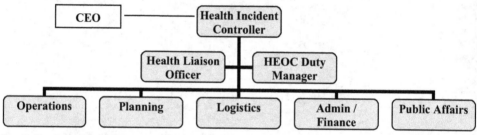

Fig. 5. Typical ICS Structure.

5.3 Activation procedures

Activation procedures need to be clearly defined and able to occur 24 hours a day, seven days a week. Common causes of delays are the failure of staff receiving the information to recognise the need for activation, inability to locate a senior staff member with the authority to activate the plan and difficulties with dissemination of the activation message. Solutions to this include:

- A pre-determined point of contact for notification of disasters, which applies equally to Health Districts, Health Facilities and Clinical Departments.
- Delegation of authority to activate to individuals on site after hours,
- A dedicated phone for calls from other organisations such as ambulance services and / or airport flight control.
- Clear procedures for staff to follow, including notification of senior staff, if they receive a call,
- Visibility of action cards close to phones.
- Cascading activation procedures to expedite spread of the message
- Use of group message systems such as SMS or pagers
- Avoidance of switchboards to avoid congestion and failure of message dissemination

5.4 Surge management

Health systems need to be able to expand their capability as part of disaster response. This can be thought of in terms of "space", "staff", "stuff" and the "system" (Kaji et al., 2006). Table 6 summarises a number of suggested approaches to surge management across this spectrum. Each facility is different however and strategies need to be developed that recognise local issues including barriers and potential solutions. Staff action cards should include some of these tasks as key prompts. Expert working groups have also developed 'surge cards' that summarise key emergency department actions to facilitate surge management both before and during an incident (Bradt et al., 2009).

	Space	Staff	Stuff	System / Flow
ED	Decant patients Divert patients Expand ED Absorb into existing ED space	Reception area "Buddy" non ED staff with regular ED staff Call in lists Group page	Preparation of essential equipment Preparation of functional kits (e.g. crush or burns)	Triage Control entry Cohort areas One way flow
OT	Cancellation Extra theatres	Staggered recall	Preparation of essential equipment	Case selection for early OT Prioritise life saving surgery Delay minor orthopaedic work until after this Damage control surgery
ICU	Discharge as possible Expand bed space	Staggered recall Staff expansion programs	Additional ventilators, monitors, fluid pumps	Case selection re futility and early care
Wards	Discharge Absorb extra patients as 'over-census' Cohort patient group	Staggered recall Prior identification of double skilled staff (e.g. ICU, OT)	Preparation of discharge medications	Cohort area Ward staff coming to get patients from ED or OT
Across Organisation	Alternative care areas for acute patients (expansion) Use of community facilities, outreach or fever clinics Liaison with private facilities Liaison across state borders	Support services Use of students Volunteer system Runners plan Fatigue policy Indemnity	Early identification of resource gaps Resupply routes protected Pre-event stock piles for seasonal risks	Incident Management Team and Emergency Operations Centre established with rapid activation protocols and redundancy

Table 6. Surge Management Strategies.

5.5 Vulnerable groups

While we traditionally think of women, children, the elderly and the disabled the concept of vulnerability is much broader than this. All of us can be vulnerable to disasters. Travel in a different city, particularly overseas, loss of prescription lenses or medications and even minor injuries such as a sprained ankle can increase our personal vulnerability regardless of other factors. Emergency Departments should consider vulnerability from three perspectives.

5.5.1 General community

Women, children, the elderly and the disabled are vulnerable. This list should also include tourists, migrants, the homeless and those in communities easily isolated or in at risk zones. Buildings may be vulnerable also because of their location and / or their occupants. Buildings with at risk occupants include nursing homes, schools, prisons, mental health institutions and hospitals themselves. These facilities should be encouraged to link with local government to ensure adequate arrangements are in place to support occupants during a disaster or be able to evacuate. Evacuation to a hospital is generally only recommended as a last resort to preserve surge capacity and capability to care for the rest of the community.

5.5.2 Vulnerable groups likely to impact on directly on the ED

These are people who are more likely to present to ED for care as a result of a disaster. Common groups include:

5.5.2.1 Those who are dependent on power supplies

Those dependent on power supplies may have the following facilities interrupted:

- Home oxygen (especially use of power dependant oxygen generators)
- Home ventilators
- Other power dependant medical services e.g. suction; electric wheelchairs
- Refrigeration dependant medicines such as insulin

5.5.2.2 Those dependant on home support

Many elderly or disabled in particular are dependant on community organisations to supply meals, assist with showers and bathing dress chronic wounds or deliver medications. The interruption of these due to staff injury or illness, disrupted transport infrastructure (e.g. damage to roads or cars, petrol availability) or destroyed pharmacies may see these patients brought to the ED for care. Alternatively these people may have previously coped with support from family but lose this support when the family home or business is damaged.

5.5.2.3 Those with chronic disease

Many chronic diseases may be exacerbated by the stress of involvement in a disaster. This may include increased presentation rates of patients with ischaemic heart disease or unstable diabetes for example. The other 'chronic disease' worth noting is drug use. In the early stages of large disasters there may be increased presentation of patients with acute drug withdrawal as supply lines are interrupted. The logistic supply chains of drug supply are remarkably effective and ingenious however and this phase is usually short lived. It may in fact be replaced by presentations with overdose due to either overly enthusiastic use patterns or the introduction of stronger substances from different suppliers filling the market gap.

5.5.3 Vulnerable staff

Staff vulnerability has the ability to impact on staffing levels and service capability. Staff may not be able to present for work because of disruption to transport (e.g. public transport not working, roads closed), school closure and need to care for children or the effects of the disaster on their own family (illness, injury, damage to dwelling). Staff, also need to be considered during pandemics or work in altered conditions. This may include the ability, or inability, of pregnant staff or those with chronic disease, to work in flu clinics. Arrangements that can be made in advance include the ability to offer a shuttle service for staff transport, accredited child-care arrangements on campus, pre-planning for redundancy of the workforce so that 'essential' positions can be covered.

5.6 Recovery

Emergency Physicians also need to remember the 'long tail' of recovery. The response phase is relatively short lived in comparison to the recovery phase. Recovery can be thought of in terms of reconstruction, emotional or psychosocial, economic and the community. Planning for recovery should start with the early phases of the response. This is important for a number of reasons. Firstly any fund raising is much easier to achieve in the early stages of a disaster with heightened media attention. Part of monies raised or donated should be kept aside for the recovery process. Secondly it is also important for the affected community to see their future recovery needs being planned for and addressed. Recovery planning should ensure that the affected community has a voice and that there is consistent, and on going, communication with community members. Often insurance is one of the major issues. In developing countries, recovery is even harder. The opportunity cost of the disaster means that development may be set back many years.

5.7 Post incident review and debrief

A post incident review and debrief should be conducted after any disaster. This should consist of both a hot and cold debrief as well as a formal report and longer term follow up arrangements of staff.

The 'hot debrief' is important to conduct soon after the disaster. It should focus on operational issues and is best conducted within work units. It is not a time to criticise performance as emotions can run high. The 'cold debrief' occurs later and should allow time for functional, or work, areas to review their own performance before a whole of organisation meeting between department representatives. The focus, again, should be on system improvement rather than blame. A formal report needs to be developed from this to help guide system improvements and satisfy reporting and governance arrangements. The formal report should also provide an objective evaluation of performance against standards and indicators. This is important if we are to improve the delivery of care.

Staff need to be cared for, as well as the community. Forced psychological debriefing, is now thought to be associated with worse outcomes. Instead staff should be made aware of follow up arrangements and provided with contact numbers if needed.

5.8 Planning

Planning is the most important element of preparedness. In many ways it is the planning process that is as important as the plan itself. The planning process should bring a representative group of people and organisations together to develop the plan. This allows relationships to be developed that will support the ability to operationalise the plan later and ensure planning arrangements are valid across agencies. All of this helps prevent the concept of a plan sitting on a shelf because it is not meaningful to the users - the 'paper plan' concept. Other key concepts in planning are to base planning on normal arrangements and build on these rather than starting afresh and plan for both what is likely to happen and what people are likely to do. The diagram below (See Figure 6) describes the sequence of activities for disaster planning based on the Emergency Management Australia guidelines (AEMI, 2011). It is also important to recognise that following review of the plan that the planning objectives are revisited as part of a continuous improvement process.

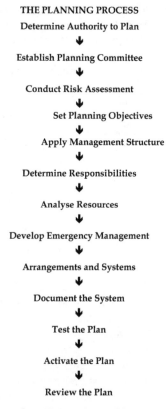

THE PLANNING PROCESS
Determine Authority to Plan
↓
Establish Planning Committee
↓
Conduct Risk Assessment
↓
Set Planning Objectives
↓
Apply Management Structure
↓
Determine Responsibilities
↓
Analyse Resources
↓
Develop Emergency Management
↓
Arrangements and Systems
↓
Document the System
↓
Test the Plan
↓
Activate the Plan
↓
Review the Plan

Fig. 6. Approach to Planning (based on EMA approach).

5.9 Education, training and exercises

There is widespread agreement on the need for improved education and training in disaster medicine. (Birch, 2005; Birnbaum, 2005; Gaudette, 2002; Marmor, 2005; PAHO, 1999; Russbach, 1990; Sharp, 2001; VanRooyen, 2005.) As Birnbaum has noted, we need to move from the era of the well-intentioned amateur, to that of the well-trained professional (Birnbaum, 2005).

Current training for health staff, with its need to focus on hospital and community care, does not adequately prepare personnel for work in a disaster. Disaster medicine is not just more patients but more patients in a system with damaged infrastructure. In the words of Quarantelli (1988) – 'there are both quantitative and qualitative differences' to normal care.

There are often significant intervals between training and exposure and there may be difficulties in application due to different conditions (Ford, 2000). Also many of those who are involved in disaster response do not experience this again. This means they do not have a chance to pass on the lessons of experience and each responding group consists of novice disaster practitioners (Birnbaum, 2005). The growing need for disaster relief, and time sensitive demands, has led to inexperienced or inadequately trained personnel in the field who may be of limited and decreasing usefulness (Campbell, 2005; Moresky et al., 2001). Key areas are decision making (Frisch, 2005), with trained staff able to make better decisions (Moresky, 2001; VanRooyen, 2001). Teamwork skills also need to be specifically addressed (Ford 2000) to improve team efficiency during a crisis (DeVita, 2004).

A number of developments have occurred to improve disaster health education.

- An education framework has been developed by WADEM, which consists of seven levels (Archer & Synaeve, 2007). This has also been adapted so that it is consistent with national qualification frameworks (FitzGerald et al., 2010).
- A model curriculum has been developed by the International Society for Disaster Medicine (ISDM 1993).
- Curricula and frameworks have been inked for national context.
- Competencies have been developed, particularly in public health.
- A number of education programs have been developed, ranging from short courses to post graduate university programs.
- While standard educational approaches are used mainly a number of novel instructional methodologies have been developed and include on line formats, aide memoires and use of case studies to provide vicarious experience with use of video as a substitute for the real environment. If possible immersive learning with use of simulation is ideal but costly and more difficult to organise than for traditional one on one patient care.

Exercises are essential to test the plan, or elements of it, as well as provide the opportunity to both practice and test individual skills. While many different exercise classifications exist, a simple approach is to consider the following:

- Discussion Exercises – These are theoretical 'talk throughs' of the response to a particular scenario and useful as a preliminary activity.
- Tabletop Exercises (with or without props): These have additional information and inputs but are still usually a hypothetical activity.

- Functional Exercises: These test specific elements of a plan such as the activation or call-in procedures.
- Full Field Exercises: These involve mock patients but use real resources including staff, vehicles and other equipment including communications channels.

The first step in development of an exercise is identification of the objectives. This allows selection of the appropriate exercise type (budget issues and time line of need with standing). The design and development of full field exercises in particular needs significant resources

5.10 Research, evidence and standards

There has been a remarkable growth in published disaster medicine literature over the past few decades. Research in disaster health is still an emerging area however, with disaster literature traditionally anecdotal in nature and dominated by case reports. Research during disasters is difficult. It is hard to conduct formal trials and there are ethical concerns with use of personnel to collect data rather than assist with the response. Solutions include use of standard definitions (Sundnes & Birnbaum, 2002), standardised reporting of case studies to allow contextual comparison (Bradt & Aitken, 2010), and improved reporting to allow collation of data, recognition of the value of qualitative and mixed methods research and use of novel methods.

The development of standards allows objective assessment of performance while also guiding evidence based response that assists effective use of resources. The SPHERE guidelines have been one of the first systematic efforts to improve accountability. They provide key indicators across 5 sectors: water supply and sanitation, nutrition, food aid, shelter and site management and health services (Sondorp et al., 2001). They provide clearly defined guidelines and minimum standards (Brennan et al., 2001) and are used by both NGOs and military and may be a common link between them (Dufour et al., 2004).

5.11 Media management

Media will be present in a disaster. There is no point in ignoring them and instead efforts should be made to ensure the media are pro-actively managed. To do this there is a need to understand what the media want, what health needs from the media and how to achieve this. The media will initially focus on the scope of the disaster. Questions will want to determine the numbers killed, numbers injured, types of injuries and special groups involved such as children. The next phase will want human-interest stories with a focus on heroes or tales of sacrifice or despair. International media will be interested in whether any of those affected were from their home country. The next phase will focus on blame and who was or is responsible. The timeline of media interest has also been compressed with the development of 24 hour news channels and the transition may occur much more rapidly.

The media can also assist health facilities by passing on health warnings to the community or advice about what health services are available and how to access them. Staff can also be advised about the need to return to work. To achieve this compromise means managing the media. Ideally this should be done in conjunction with a professional public relations or media advisor. Even if not available a number of basic rules can be used as a guideline. These include:

- Have a designated venue for media statements
- Have a designated media spokesperson so there is a familiar 'talking head'
- Have a scheduled time for media conferences, and keep to it.
- Develop a small number of key messages that you want to convey
- Anticipate problem questions and how to respond to these
- Provide media training for those likely to be used as media spokespeople

Other issues to consider are the use of media images. Having multiple film crews or photographers may be disruptive to operational staff and potentially compromise the privacy of those affected. Most media will be happy to cooperate if it means access to vision. Allowing one cameraman access and asking media to 'pool' images is one option to consider. It is also inevitable that with large disasters there may also be political pressures to manage the media at a high level. While this is helpful in promotion of a consistent message it may lead to delays in ability to use the media to pass information to affected local communities.

6. Mass casualty management

Emergency physicians have an important role in mass casualty management. This extends from the pre-hospital response at the site, to care during transport and once in the Emergency Department. All of this requires planning and it is important that pre-hospital care and hospital based care form part of a continuum so that both the therapeutic vacuum is minimised and the disaster is simply not moved from one site to another.

6.1 Site management

While this does differ in some countries, in most environments the police service has overall responsibility for the disaster site. They will normally establish an outer cordon and restrict access to the area. Health responders need to not only have appropriate personal protective equipment, but should have identification and be clearly identified as health staff. Fire may have responsibility for any central hazardous zone. An example of site structure based is shown in Figure 7.

It is important that structure is established early in the response. While the cordon assists this process, care should be taken in identifying access and egress routes for emergency vehicles, location of a casualty clearing post (if needed) and areas to both hold ambulances and areas to load them. One of the issues can be that failure to establish this early leads to a congested site with difficulties in loading ambulances and transporting patients. Another essential early task is the establishment of a command post so that all agencies responding to the scene can report in, and provide updates and input across their respective areas of expertise.

For health teams deployed to a site a number of helpful mnemonics exist. The MIMMS course (Major Incident Medical Management System) uses the CSCATT mnemonic for tasks at a scene and the (M)ETHANE for the initial report from the site (Advanced Life Support Group, 2005). These are described in Figure 8 and 9.

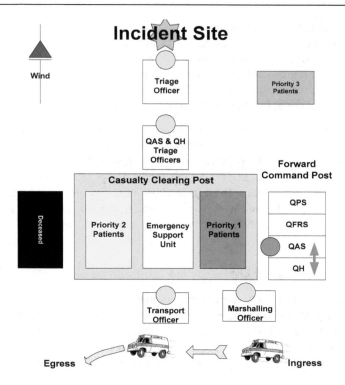

Fig. 7. Site Structure. Legend: QAS = Ambulance; QFRS = Fire and Rescue; QH = Health; QPS = Police (Source: Queensland Health, 2011).

C	Command
S	Safety
C	Communication
A	Assessment
T	Triage
T	Treatment
T	Transport

Fig. 8. CSCATT mnemonic for scene tasks (from MIMMS).

M	Mass casualty incident or not?
E	Exact location
T	Type of incident
H	Hazards present at site
A	Access to site
N	Numbers of casualties (and specific types of injury)
E	Emergency services present and required

Fig. 9. METHANE mnemonic for reports for scenes (from MIMMS).

6.2 Triage

Triage in disasters is based on a priority-based system and colour coded. Most systems use red as the most urgent category, followed by yellow with green as minor injuries or 'walking wounded' and black as dead (see Figure 10). The expectant category, those not expected to survive, is controversial, with some systems using blue tags for this, while others include this in the red group or do not recognise at all. Triage accuracy is also important. Under triage may mean patients with high acuity injuries do not receive timely care while over triage may consume resources which may also delay access of some patients to care. The two main systems in use are "Sieve and Sort" and "Start and Save". Both of these use simple algorithms in the initial component (Sieve or Start) as a screening mechanism, with more complex anatomical and injury score based approaches on subsequent arrival at the Casualty Clearing Post (Sort or Save).

Priority	Treatment	Colour	Comment
Immediate	1	Red	Need immediate care and transport
Urgent	2	Yellow	Need urgent care and transport – usually 6 hours
Delayed	3	Green	Initial separation by ability to walk in sieve / start
Deceased		Black	

Fig. 10. Summary of Triage Systems.

There is no perfect triage tag and many varieties exist. These include single coloured cards, folding cards, cruciform tags, flags and wristbands. Some problems with use of tags include visibility, the ability to record information, waterproofing of cards and ability to change triage category (either inability to change or ability to change by patient).

6.3 Care on site and casualty clearing post

The principles of care on site are aimed at 'doing the most for the most'. This includes simple measures to assist immediate preservation of life, life saving interventions and those that ensure the ability to safely transport to hospital. This is a simplistic view however and needs to be reconciled with degree of resources on scene that are able to provide care (may be surplus or overwhelmed), the availability of transport platforms able to move patients (and provide care en route) and the distances to hospital. Figure 11 summarises the key elements of care on site.

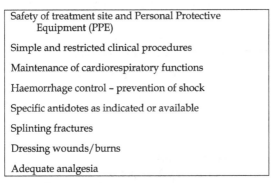

Safety of treatment site and Personal Protective Equipment (PPE)

Simple and restricted clinical procedures

Maintenance of cardiorespiratory functions

Haemorrhage control – prevention of shock

Specific antidotes as indicated or available

Splinting fractures

Dressing wounds/burns

Adequate analgesia

Fig. 11. Elements of care on site.

6.4 Transport

The best transport platform to use is one that is normally used to carry patients. This means staff are familiar with the transport environment and vehicles are configured appropriately with stretchers, equipment, drugs and communications. Care also needs to be provided en route and this provision of care is equally as important as the transport platform.

There may be a need to improvise when there are large numbers of patients and ideally this will have been considered prior to any event. Large numbers of 'walking wounded' may need to be transported by bus or train, with health care worker escort rather than relying on use of ambulances. This not only moves these people away from the scene so they can access health care as required but preserves specialised ambulance resources for those most severely injured.

6.5 Disposition

The disposition of patients from the scene should consider a number of principles. These are principles only though and it may not be possible to keep to them.

- The most severely injured should be transferred first (Triage Category Red)
- Where possible normal policies, such as trauma bypass, should be maintained with major trauma sent to those facilities capable of managing this and smaller facilities receiving those with lesser injuries.
- Those with special injuries should be transferred to specialist units initially (if possible) to avoid secondary transfer and increase passage of these patients in cohorts (e.g. burns, spinal or paediatrics)
- Patients should be distributed between centres so that the disaster is not simply moved from the site to the hospital. This 'carousel' style model should also recognise facility expertise and patient requirements as well as patient volumes.
- Ideally families should be kept together if possible (and if known or recognised)

This needs close liaison between the site and a central control point. This allows: information on bed availability to be conveyed to the site commander (and stops them from either having to make multiple phone calls to ascertain this information or simply sending patients without knowledge of bed availability). It also allows the central control point to have increased knowledge of incoming patients, which assist distribution of information flow, as well as on going planning.

6.6 Care in the emergency department and the hospital

The ED has a key role as the 'front door' to the hospital. Many of the issues described previously, such as communication, surge capacity, planning, education and training apply equally to ED. A number of key messages and myths are presented below. Key activities include the following examples:

- Having a plan!!
- Having defined activation procedures
- Having maintained, and current, staff recall lists
- Having an over flow area for surge capacity (ideally for less injured)

- Having tabards so that key staff roles in ED can be identified
- Having surgical and ICU liaison in ED which helps to prioritise OT cases and also establish futility early in a consensus manner
- Having an ultrasonographer in ED
- Limiting radiological investigations in the initial stages
- Recognising the 'dual wave' phenomenon where minor injuries arrive first, and may fill operating theatres, before pre-hospital personnel evacuate the more seriously injured.

Whole of hospital activities include:

- Having a plan that is linked to site and ED response as well as jurisdiction and national arrangements
- Having defined activation procedures that operate 24 hours a day, 7 days a week
- Being able to empty the ED rapidly to supply immediate surge capacity
- Being able to discharge patients from wards and ICU to create bed capacity
- Being able to create OT capacity
- Ensuring consistent information flow across the facility
- Planning for communications failure so that redundancy measures, such as radio, runners and PA system announcements, are in place
- Establishing a specific centre for family re-union
- Establishing a media centre and providing regular media updates
- Capturing all information flows including tracking and data management systems
- Capturing all costs for possible reimbursement if jurisdiction or national disaster declarations

Myths to be aware of include the following examples:

- The ED will always receive prior notice of incoming patients from a disaster. Patients will self evacuate and will present to hospital either on foot or using any means of transport available. Plan to have no notice.
- Patients will only present to designated hospitals. Patients who self evacuate from a site will present to the closest health facility. This may be a hospital designated for obstetric or cancer services, however regardless of this some patients will present.
- The ED will always receive regular, and accurate, updates from the scene. Communications channels may be interrupted or accurate information may not be available. Plan to
- All patients arriving at ED will have been already triaged. Patients may self present and plan for this to occur with triage tags available on arrival.
- All patients arriving at ED will have been decontaminated following CBR disasters. Again, patients will self-present and may bypass decontamination services. Plan to have to deal with non-decontaminated patients.

6.7 Volunteers

Volunteers may be a useful resource or a minefield of regret if not managed properly. Consideration should be given in advance to how best to manage these arrangements. This can include pre-event credentialing of local medical and nursing practitioners as well as standing arrangements to grant emergency credentialing powers to individuals under and approved process. The reasons for ensuring this occurs includes:

- Avoiding volunteers who may really be media or simply those with a morbid curiosity
- Ability to 'buddy' volunteers with regular staff to (a) maximise their efficiency by providing a system chaperone (b) ensure their safety by being able to log their presence
- Avoid issues with liability for the department, hospital and organisation
- Indemnity of volunteers

It is also important to provide volunteers with identification so they can move around the allocated area without being challenged or not used appropriately. Ideally this should consist of both an ID card and a tabard to aid recognition.

6.8 Predictors of numbers

Having an idea of numbers is important. While communication from the site may provide this information, it does not always hold. The Centers for Disease Control and Prevention (CDC) has developed a 'calculator' based on analysis of a number of disasters (CDC, 2005). For sudden onset urban disasters (this distinction is important) an ED can expect in total, twice the number of patients that present in the hour following the arrival of the first patient. Two axioms should also be remembered - in widespread natural disasters (e.g. tsunamis) the initial estimates are likely to be under while in localised man-made disasters (e.g. transport / industrial) the initial estimates are usually over the actual figure.

6.9 Chemical, Biological or Radiological (CBR) incidents and decontamination

A special consideration is the potential for patients to be involved in chemical, biological or radiological

Incidents (CBR). This may occur as a discrete incident in its own right (e.g. chemical spill, nuclear reactor incident) where the causative agent is easily identified or as part of a more complex scenario involving a 'dirty bomb'. In this scenario biological or radiological material is mixed in with a standard explosive device.

A CBR scenario poses a series of new, and different, concerns. These include:

- The ability to ensure decontamination prior to entry to ED
- Who provides decontamination – is this hospital staff or fire services?
- What happens to any residual run off? Is simple dilution sufficient for all substances?
- The provision of PPE to ED staff – and ensuring they are trained in use of equipment
- The ability to offer antidotes to staff and patients if exposure has occurred

The level of preparedness of most ED, for a CBR event has been questioned (Caldicott et al., 2008).

7. International humanitarian response

Emergency physicians may play a role in international response. Key considerations include:

7.1 International diplomacy and politics

The affected country must, first invite international teams that deploy overseas. Failure to wait for this, despite good intentions, may result in diplomatic incidents and can even considered being invasion. The process for securing diplomatic approval may take days, and while clinical staff may feel frustrated by this delay, failure to do this prior to arrival, may result in teams being refused entry, spend hours or days at airports or ports or even returned home. Similarly, their equipment may not be allowed entry with significant effects on the team's effectiveness.

It is also likely there will be increased calls for disaster medical assistance from developing countries. (McEntire, 1998; Lennquist 2004; Burkle 2001). This is underpinned by the precept that health and security are a basic human right (Judd, 1992; WHO, 2005). There have also been changes in how disasters are viewed by the world community with disaster relief being seen not as a magnanimous gesture but as a humanitarian obligation and claimed as a right by affected countries (Gunn, 2005).

While cost effective mitigation is seen as the key to natural disasters (Iwan, 1999), most governments provide little assistance for mitigation in comparison to response. While disaster aid should be seen as part of long-term development (Gunn, 2005), "silent", long term investments in mitigation are rarely viewed with favour by politicians (Stephenson et al., 2005).

7.2 Epidemiology of aid

The timeline of injury must be understood when planning to deploy teams and the selection of the team should reflect the injuries or illnesses likely to be present. Different disasters produce different injury patterns, which helps estimate needs and timelines (Milsten, 2000; Noji, 2000; Van Rooyen, 2001). There is also at tri-modal distribution of medical issues post sudden onset disasters (Maegele et al., 2005, Taylor et al., 1998). Phase 1 occurs in seconds to minutes and has a high mortality, phase 2 occurs in minutes to hours and consists of medical care with a focus on trauma management, and phase 3 occurs days to weeks afterwards and consist of complications such as sepsis, multi-organ failure and mental health issues; the care of displaced persons and a lack resources and trauma from the clean up and recovery.

Three phases of care have been described for deployment of foreign field hospitals, in a guideline document developed by WHO and PAHO (2003). These are outlined in Table 7 and are based on an appreciation of the following key issues:

- The timeline of survival
- Types of injury can be predicted for different types of disasters
- Chronic disease is often exacerbated by the disaster due to stress, loss of access to usual care (e.g. dialysis or home oxygen) or loss of usual medications
- Women and children still have babies
- Disruption of water and sewage may have significant impact on infectious disease, as may power loss and refrigeration failure
- Vector control may be problematic with disasters caused by flooding or rainfall

Unfortunately international medical assistance teams are rarely on site soon enough to deal with the acutely injured (Judd, 1992; Hsu, 2002; Asari, 2000; Noji, 2000; Redmond, 2005;

Wallace, 2002). Following the Gujarat earthquake, outside help arrived only after local health services had provided emergency assistance and immediate care with specialised field hospitals arriving too late to reduce mortality and morbidity (Bremer, 2003, Roy, 2002). Similarly following the Chi Chi earthquake of the 104 teams that responded, 80% needed more than 24 hours to be able to provide care (Hsu, 2002).

7.3 Type of aid

International assistance is often best supplied by means other than through deployment of an international health team, in fact this should be a provider of last resort. Cash rather than goods, is often more appropriate (Campbell 2005; de Ville de Goyet 2000; Martone 2005; Redmond 2005b). Money is often the most useful resource as it allows:

- Increased local control of resource allocation and how the money is spent.
- Purchase of goods, and personnel locally, which helps stimulate the local disaster affected economy (Martone 2005, Redmond 2005b).
- Purchase of local goods, and use of local personnel, often at a significantly lower cost
- Use of local staff, familiar with local health care standards as well as language and culture

Phase	PHASE 1 EARLY EMERGENCY CARE	PHASE 2 FOLLOW UP TRAUMA AND MEDICAL CARE	PHASE 3 TEMPORARY HEALTH FACILITY
Primary Role	Provide early emergency medical care, including ATLS.	Temporarily fill the gaps in emergency medical assistance during the period when health services are progressively overwhelmed by the need for ongoing secondary care of trauma victims and routine medical care.	To substitute for damaged installations pending repair or reconstruction.
Timeline	Initial 48 hours following the onset of an event.	From day 3 to day 15, and should not exceed 15 days.	From second month to two or more years.
Essential Requirements	Be operational on site within 24 hours of event Be entirely self sufficient Offer similar or higher standards of medical care than were available in the affected country prior to the precipitating event.	Be fully operational within 3-5 days of event Minimal need for support from local communities Basic knowledge of health situation, language and respect for culture Availability of selected specialties. e.g. general surgery, anaesthetics, internal medicine, obstetrics / gynaecology, paediatrics with appropriate paramedic and support staff. Equipment should allow treatment of all patients regardless of age / gender. Sustainability Evaluation of the cost effectiveness and cost benefit associated with use of foreign field hospital	Lack of other cost effective alternatives Appropriate standards for patients and staff Designed for use by final reconstruction Installation and maintenance support provided at no cost to affected country

Table 7. WHO / PAHO Guidelines.

Donated goods may create a problem in their own right. Common problems include:

- Being unusable (Rubin et al 2000) due to expiry dates, (particularly for medications and food) and the language that instructions are written in (particularly for medications or technical equipment)
- The appropriateness of donated goods, such as revealing swim wear to cold climates or Muslim countries
- Consume personnel and space for storage, cataloguing and transport or destruction (Frisch 2005; Noji 2000; Rubin et al 2000).
- Undermining local practice rather than supporting it (Redmond 2005b).
- Technical support, and consumables, for medical equipment. Power sources and plug configuration should also be considered.
- Ability to actually enter the country through posts and customs

The 1988 Armenia Earthquake is an example of this. More than 5000 tons of drugs were donated, which occupied more than 30 warehouses and took 50 people 6 months to sort through. Of these only 30% were relevant and useful with 8% expired. There are also concerns about how donations are used and the risk of corruption with donations of money. This should not prevent donations. Donations should instead be based on assessed needs and the requests of the affected community

7.4 Based on needs

Any assistance offered should be based on the needs of the affected community. As Redmond notes "if aid is to do the most good for the most people it must be targeted" (Redmond, 2005b). Rapid needs assessments have thus become the norm for gathering information about the status of an affected population (Keim et al., 2001; Malilay, 2000; Redmond, 2005 Asari et al., 2000; Chen et al, 2003).

The United Nations use Disaster Assessment and Coordination teams (UNDAC), which are a 2-6 person team drawn from member countries that travels quickly to a disaster scene to report the immediate needs to the international community (Redmond, 2005). Needs assessment is a specialised area of expertise, and without use of personnel with appropriate experience and training multiple problems may occur. These include:

- May be inaccurate (Asari et al, 2000; Birnbaum, 2005; Braham et al., 2001; Malilay, 2000; Maury et al., 2004; McEntire, 1998; 1999; Rubin, 2000).
- May be incomplete (Asari et al., 2000; Mallilay, 2000; Maury et al., 2004).
- May be delayed (Asari et al., 2000; Braham, 2001; Malilay, 2000; Maury, 2004; McEntire, 1998; 1999).
- May be repeated multiple times by different agencies leading to assessment fatigue (Malilay, 2000; Nabarro, 2005; PAHO, 1999; Redmond, 2005).
- Need for a validated tool (Malilay, 2000)
- Need for standardisation of the content (Bradt, 2003; Malilay, 2000).
- Need for timeline to determine what information is needed from assessments at various times post disaster (Malilay, 2000).
- Level of experience of those performing the needs assessment (Redmond, 2005b).
- Assessment may not involve local population (Redmond, 2005b).

7.5 Integration with existing services

Deployed teams need to integrate with local services. It is the local services who will have provided the initial care and it is the local services who will continue to provide care after the deployed team has left. The local population should ideally be involved in all phases of relief operations as it enhances capacity building, empowers local communities and helps regain control over their lives (Brennan et al., 2001; Leus et al., 2001). Failure to do so can lead to mistrust, resentment, lack of cooperation (Brennan et al., 2001) and undermine the capacity of local people to solve their own problems (Judd, 1992). It may also lead to undermining of the local health system or problems with on going care for those treated by deployed teams.

Common problems are:

- Different standards used by deployed team to local health services
  - This may undermine local health services by raising expectations of care to a level that is unable to be continued locally due to resource or funding issues
  - This may leave patients with no adequate follow up post procedure, with risk of complications
- Free care and impact on economic recovery and livelihood of health workers

7.6 Self sufficiency

Deployed teams must be self sufficient (Nabarro, 2005; Redmond, 2005; Roschin, 2002) to ensure they do not pose an additional burden on affected communities. This applies not just to medical equipment but also to their ability to support themselves. All teams should have a basic self-sufficiency capability, which should include shelter, sleep gear, food and water at a minimum. Ideally teams should be self-sufficient for the duration of their stay but this will depend on the context of the disaster and the ability to provide re-supply. It may actually provide assistance to the affected community to contribute to the local economy by purchasing local products, including accommodation, if these are not in short supply.

7.7 Language and culture

Communication is a cornerstone of health care unfortunately language barriers are common with international deployment. This may occur between the team and the affected population or between responding teams. Solutions include bilingual staff, language training and interpreters. Use of bilingual staff is the optimal arrangement but difficult to achieve, while few deployments have time to arrange language lessons in time to be more effective than the basics of 'please' and 'thank you'. Interpreters are the most common option for most NGOs (Moresky, 2001). The use of interpreters from the local community may also assist integration with local services, provide local knowledge and local cultural advice and, if paid, stimulate the local economy (Redmond, 1991; McCurdy, 1999). While the most efficient solution is use of interpreters, this needs to be approached with caution. Payment well above local rates may result in loss of staff from local essential functions, including health services. Care also needs to be taken with selection of interpreters that isolation of cultural groups does not inadvertently occur. This may result in other groups not wishing to seek care or perceived favouritism.

Culture is unfortunately often over looked as a potential issue (Moresky, 2001). Cultural factors must be addressed in order to appreciate the context of disasters for a population (Keim et al., 2001). Common problems include dress codes of international responders, especially for women, the ability of men to examine or treat women (Roshchin et al., 2002) and the cultural appropriateness of donated goods. All team members should be aware of cultural issues before deploying as failure to do this may compromise the personal safety of team members and effectiveness of the mission.

7.8 Safety and security

Safety and security is becoming an increasing problem (Brennan, 2001; Burkle, 1995; Holland, 2004; Schull, 2001; VanRooyen, 2001). The major cause of death and injury in the 1970s was MVA (Birch. 2005; Brennan, 2001), while the major cause of death in the 1990s was violent trauma (Brennan, 2001). Sheik (2000) looked at the deaths of 382 aid workers and found 67% were from intentional violence, with the number of deaths from hostile acts increasing. Unfortunately combatants in complex humanitarian emergencies (CHE) increasingly regard medical workers as targets (Bricknell, 2005). Deployed teams need to be cognisant of their own safety and security. All deployed teams should have safety and security training and have considered the elements in Table 8 as a minimum.

Grouping	Details
Vehicle safety and travel	Vehicle inspection Vehicle safety Convoy planning and driving Driver training Basic mechanics Trip planning (routes, access points, petrol, what to carry)
Basic Navigation Skills	Map reading Use of GPS Use of compass
Basic Communications Skills	Use of radios including radio protocols Use of specific team communications equipment
Camp Safety	Perimeters Guards Lighting Curfews Equipment security
Personal Safety	Grab bags Avoiding being out alone (especially after dark) Identification
Team Safety	Buddy strategies and monitor systems Rendezvous points Team musters and regular team meetings
Critical Incident Safety	Actions on Evacuation plans Hostage negotiation Weapons awareness

Table 8. Essential Safety and Security Training.

7.9 Health and welfare of deployed team

The health and welfare of deployed teams is important. Team members becoming ill or injured may compromise the mission by altering the level of care able to be provided. It may also increase the workload for other members as yet one more patient is added to the load, and the morale of team members may be adversely affected. The sponsoring organisation may also be adversely affected either by reputation, or through costs of evacuation, care and rehabilitation of the unwell team member(s), which may be prolonged and even possibly litigation.

The health and welfare of deployed teams involves a systematic approach that recognises the need for pre and post health support; health support during deployment and appropriate team selection, education and training and logistic support (Aitken et al., 2009a; 2009b; 2011).

Processes should be in place to ensure that all team members who deploy:

- Are in good physical health and have had a recent medical and dental check up
- Have access to regular personal medications (if appropriate to deploy with these) and have a spare set of eyeglasses if needed
- Have received appropriate vaccinations prior to deployment and access to any chemoprophylaxis necessary
- Have an appropriate degree of physical fitness
- Ideally have acclimatisation schedules considered, especially for any deployment from temperate to hot environments
- Have access to medical care while deployed, including a team medical kit
- Have access to clean water and safe food supply while deployed
- Have access to uniforms appropriate to both climate and work environment
- Have task appropriate personal protective equipment
- Are protected from vector borne diseases by an appropriate combination of vector control, prophylactic measures and access to treatment
- Have access to post deployment follow up health care, with both physical and mental health issues addressed

7.10 Coordination

Deployed teams should not only integrate with local health services but also coordinate their activities with other deployed teams. This is to ensure that all needs are addressed and that there is appropriate coverage of aid needs to all geographical areas. Otherwise, both task omission and task duplication can easily occur. This is especially important in large-scale disasters where coordination and logistics issues can be immense. As an example consider the problems faced in Haiti. At one stage there were over 1000 NGO on ground, in a country with virtually all infrastructures (including government) destroyed and the native language was different to nearly all deployed teams.

Efforts to improve global coordination of disasters have led to the development of the Cluster approach, which is now an essential component of international humanitarian work. The clusters are open to all contributing agencies with each of the nine clusters (Protection, Camp Coordination and Management, Water Sanitation and Hygiene, Health, Emergency Shelter, Nutrition, Emergency Telecommunications, Logistics, and Early Recovery) led by a designated agency. Two additional clusters, Education and Agriculture, were later added. For the Health Cluster the lead agency is the World Health Organisation. There are also efforts currently to ensure only appropriately trained and prepared teams deploy internationally with development of an international register of accredited teams.

8. Pandemics

The recent experience with Pandemic (H1N1) 2009, while not the severe disease initially expected, has highlighted a number of issues confronting emergency medicine.

8.1 ED design

Emergency Departments, as a rule, are not designed to manage large numbers of patients with infectious disease. Open plan design, which meets the need to maintain the visibility of patients with acute presentations, sacrifices not only privacy but also offers little ability to isolate patients. As FitzGerald et al (2010) note, "curtains make poor barriers to the spread of disease". Few ED have designs well suited to management of infectious patients with ability to isolate from time of presentation to triage and through their ED 'journey'.

8.2 Identification of index cases

This can only happen as a result of raised awareness and heightened suspicion. EDs need to recognise that they are part of the broader health system as well as the front door of the hospital. There should be strong links with local public health and communicable disease networks. This allows ED staff to be aware of communicable disease alerts and have a clear reporting structure if cases are identified.

8.3 Alternative care sites

The use of "flu clinics" is intended to divert patients from Emergency Departments and preserve ED capacity. The establishment of 'flu clinics' needs careful planning for it to be successful:

- It is important to avoid using ED staff for this role or ED capacity may be actually reduced;
- There must be an ability to provide immediate care for those with more severe illness at flu clinics as well as the ability to transfer to higher levels of care
- There must be clear case definitions and protocols in place to ensure standardised and consistent care across the community
- The community must be informed of where to attend to seek care.

8.4 Controlling entry to ED

Patients with flu, or any infectious disease, should not enter EDs and mingle freely with other patients and staff. Pathways should be established so that patients with suspected infectious diseases are diverted to alternative care sites (flu clinics) or if unwell have a clear route to areas capable of isolation or ideally negative pressure rooms.

8.5 Integrated care

It is imperative that EDs have established links with the public health system, primary health care and the full hospital system. Planning needs to ensure that this is a 'whole of health' response. This enables early notice of emerging infectious diseases, clear reporting lines, support for alternative care sites and consistent care pathways with in the hospital for admitted patients to both the ward and Intensive Care. It is also essential that microbiology and laboratory services as well as hospital administration are included in this.

8.6 The workforce

Staff welfare is an essential element of pandemic management. This not only protects the health and safety of health personnel but also ensures the on going ability of the ED to provide care. This needs to include access to PPE, vaccination and antiviral medications. Staff in high-risk groups may also need to be re-deployed from their primary place of employment. While this may differ for specific disease processes, for H1N1 this included pregnancy, immunosuppression and chronic disease. There is a need for clear processes to be in place for sick leave and staff absence as carers during the pandemic (Considine et al., 2011). The latter is particularly important when schools are closed, or staff quarantined as the primary carers of those with confirmed illness.

The willingness of staff to present for work also needs to be considered. Conflicting opinions have been presented, however the severity of the disease and levels of personal risk are probably the best guide. Health workers are altruistic by nature, however personal and family risk may limit this. The personal risk for health workers when caring for patients in an environment similar to the 1918 pandemic (see Figure 12) should not be under estimated.

9. Emerging issues

Disaster health does not stand still. As the world changes and new technology is developed, different threats emerge. Risk assessment is a continuous process and needs to recognise new hazards as they emerge. Some of these are discussed briefly below.

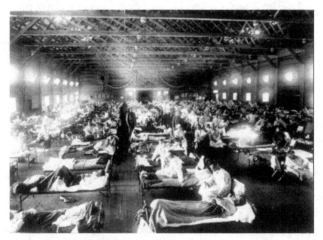

Fig. 12. Patient care during the 1918 Flu Pandemic.

9.1 Climate change

It has been proposed that climate change will bring with it an increased number of severe storms, cyclones and hurricanes. Additionally global warming may cause the endemic regions for vector borne disease to expand. The most serious concern is the spread of malaria while other diseases such as dengue fever are also of concern. The exposure of disease naive populations increases the potential to cause significant morbidity and mortality.

9.2 Heatwave

Heatwaves are generally an under recognised disaster and have caused significant mortality. Most of this occurs in populations in which buildings have been adapted for the cold and keep heat in. Buildings reliant on air conditioning to keep cool, including hospitals, are particularly at risk with power failures. Recent work has identified standard definitions, the influence of biometeorological influences (Vaneckova et al 2011) and population susceptibility (Wang et al 2011). Local temperature, and the variation from this, is one of the most important factors with the elderly and those with chronic disease particularly ischaemic heart disease and diabetes, at risk.

9.3 Pandemics and emerging infectious disease

The advent of cheap global travel and expansion of international trade has its own risks, with the spread of disease able to occur much more readily as a result of this. Emerging infectious diseases have the potential to be spread quickly with transcontinental flight and may not be noticed initially if diseases have a longer incubation period allowing disembarkation before onset of symptoms and negating the effectiveness of pre-flight screening. This is particularly relevant given that the majority of travellers would not postpone their travel, even if they exhibited flu-like symptoms (Leggat et al., 2010). Pandemics occur regularly and while Pandemic (H1N1) 2009 was not the disease initially feared, diseases with higher case fatality rates such as SARS and 'Bird Flu' and emergence of novel viruses associated with animal reservoirs continues to pose concerns. Fortunately, almost everyone reported that they would comply with physician's advice to stay at home for seven days if they were diagnosed with Pandemic (H1N1) 2009 (Brown et al., 2010). Interestingly, most of these people also indicated that they would have sufficient food supplies to cope with isolation for a period of three days, although they would cope less well if there was a disruption in utilities (Aitken et al., 2010).

9.4 Conflict and war

War is not included as a disaster in many databases. However both war and complex health emergencies have accounted for millions of deaths in the past century. This is not just as a result of direct violence but occurs due to disruption of the health system, loss of access to basic food and water, loss of immunisation programs and general loss of infrastructure including transport systems. The crisis in the Democratic Republic of the Congo (DCR) resulted in the deaths of ten million people over a two year period with more than 50% dying as a result of infectious disease. Of the 15% who died from battlefield injuries many of these occurred in inaccessible places away from help (Brennan & Nandy, 2001).

9.5 Information technology

The development of information technology has enhanced our ability to respond and manage disasters (Arnold et al., 2004). However many of our systems, including health systems, are so reliant on computers that a major disruption of the information technology infrastructure may result in complete system failures. This may range from patient data systems, refrigeration and cooling of medical and blood-stocks to digital radiology systems. Indirect effects include the impact on public transport, economic breakdown and other components of critical infrastructure.

9.6 Standards of care

An emerging, and necessary, discussion is the concept of standards of care during a disaster. The modern community has an expectation that care will continue, at the same standard, during a disaster. Depending on both the imbalance between supply and demand and the level of infrastructure damage this may not be possible.

10. The future

The ability to predict the future is in the realm of crystal balls and Nostradamus. Novel disasters will occur, or 'traditional' disasters in less likely locations. However it is likely that future developments will include work on the emerging issues described above with a focus on:

- standards of care (and altered standards of care),
- accountability and credentialing of disaster health care providers and managers,
- the integration of health care into the disaster 'system',
- improved communication with improved visibility of communication and sharing of information,
- the impact of ED overcrowding on surge capacity
- the implications of an aging population on disaster response in the developed world.

11. Conclusion

Disasters are of special significance to Emergency Physicians and all those who work in Emergency Departments. As the front door of the hospital, ED staff need to be aware of local risk profiles, prepare their department and ensure they become involved in a 'whole of hospital' and 'whole of community' approach to disaster planning. Emergency Physicians and ED nurses are well suited to acute humanitarian roles with their broad skill mix and familiarity with uncertainty. These personnel do however; need additional training across public health, safety and security to be most effective as aid workers.

Increasingly, disaster medicine is moving from good intentions to good practice, with growth as a professional discipline in its own right. There has been a recent growth in research, development of standards and indicators of effectiveness and moves to not just improved education and training of responders, but credentialing as well. One of the challenges for the future, with the high likelihood of future disasters, is to build on this so that lessons identified are put into practice to become lessons learned and that these innovations are formally assessed to determine effectiveness and whether outcomes are improved.

12. Acknowledgment

The authors would like to acknowledge the assistance and contributions of all authors, co-authors and researchers involved in the papers presented in this chapter. More importantly, this chapter is dedicated to all those who have been victims of disasters.

13. References

Aitken, P., Leggat, P.A., Robertson, A.G., Harley, H., Leclerq, M.G. & Speare, R. (2009a). Pre and post deployment health support provided to Australian Disaster Medical Assistance Team members: Results of a national survey. *Travel Medicine and Infectious Disease*, 7: 305-11.

Aitken, P., Leggat, P.A, Robertson, A.G., Harley, H., Leclerq, M.G. & Speare, R. (2009b). Health and safety aspects of deployment of Australian Disaster Medical Assistance Team members: Results of a national survey. *Travel Medicine and Infectious Disease*, 7: 284-90.

Aitken, P., Brown, L.H., Leggat, P.A. & Speare, R. (2010). Preparedness for Short Term Isolation among Queensland Residents: Implications for Pandemic and Disaster Planning". *Emergency Medicine Australasia*, 22: 435-41.

Aitken, P., Leggat, P.A., Robertson, A.G., Harley, H., Speare R. & Leclerq, M.G. (2011). Education and Training Requirements for Australian Disaster Medical Assistance Team members: Results of a national survey. *Prehospital and Disaster Medicine*, 26(1): 41-8.

Al-Mahari, A.F. & Keller, A.Z. (2007). A review of disaster definitions. *Prehospital and Disaster Medicine*, 12(1): 17-21.

Advanced Life Support Group. (2005). *Major Incident Medical Management and Support: The Practical Approach at the Scene* (MIMMS), 2nd edition. London: John Wiley & Sons (Wiley-Blackwell). ISBN:978-0-7279-1868-0.

Archer, F. & Seynaeve, G. (2007). International guidelines and standards for education and training to reduce the consequences of events that may threaten the health status of a community. *Prehospital and Disaster Medicine*, 22: 120–30.

Arnold, J.L., Levine, B.N., Manmatha, R., Lee, F., Shenoy, P., Tsai ,M.C., Ibrahim, T.K., O'Brien, D.J. & Walsh, D.A. (2004). Information sharing in out-of-hospital disaster response: The future role of information technology. *Prehospital and Disaster Medicine*, 19(2): 201-7.

Asari, Y., Koido, Y., Nakamura, K., Yamamoto, Y. & Ohta, M. (2000). Analysis of medical needs on day 7 after the tsunami disaster in Papua New Guinea. *Prehospital and Disaster Medicine*, 15(2): 81-5.

Australian Emergency Management Institute. (2011). Australian Emergency Management Handbook Series Series. Handbook 1. Disaster Health. 1st edition. Canberra: Commonwealth Attorney-General's Department.

Birch, M. & Miller, S. (2005). Humanitarian assistance: Standards, skills, training and experience. *British Medical Journal*, 330: 1199-201.

Birnbaum, M.L. (2005) Professionalisation and credentialing. *Prehospital and Disaster Medicine*, 20(4): 210-1.

Bradt, D.A., Abraham, K. & Franks, R. (2003). A strategic plan for disaster medicine in Australasia. *Emergency Medicine*, 15: 271-82.

Bradt, D.A. & Drummond, C.M. (2002). Rapid epidemiological assessment of health status in displaced populations – an evolution towards standardized minimum, essential data sets. *Prehospital and Disaster Medicine*, 17(4): 178-85.

Bradt, D.A. & Drummond, C.M. (2003). From complex emergencies to terrorism – new tools for health sector coordination in conflict associated disasters. *Prehospital and Disaster Medicine*, 18(3): 263-71.

Bradt, D.A., Aitken, P., Fitzgerald, G., Swift, R., O'Reilly, G. & Bartley. B. (2009). *Emergency department surge capacity: Recommendations of the Australasian Surge Strategy Working Group. Academic Emergency Medicine* 16: 1350-8.

Braham, M., Aghababian, R., Andrews, R.A., Austin, C., Brown, R., Yao-Zhong, C., Engindeniz, Z., Girouard, R., Leaman, P., Masellis, M., Nakayama, S., Polentsov, Y.O. & Suserud, B.O. (2001). 5th Asia-Pacific conference on disaster medicine. Theme 7. Sharing international experiences in disasters: Summary and action plan. *Prehospital and Disaster Medicine*, 16(1): 42-5.

Bremer, R. (2003). Policy development in disaster preparedness and management: Lessons learned from the January 2001 earthquake in Gujarat, India. *Prehospital and Disaster Medicine*, 18(4): 370-82.

Brennan, R.J. & Nandy, R. (2001a). Complex humanitarian emergencies: A major global health challenge. *Emergency Medicine*, 13: 147-56.

Brennan, R.J., Valderrama, C., MacKenzie, W.R., Raj, K. & Nandy, R. (2001b). Rehabilitating public health infrastructure in the post conflict setting: Epidemic prevention and preparedness in Kosovo. *Prehospital and Disaster Medicine*, 16(4): 244-51.

Bricknell, M.C.M. & MacCormack, T. (2005). Military approach to medical planning in humanitarian operations, *British Medical Journal*, 330: 1437-9.

Brown, L.H., Aitken, P., Leggat, P.A. & Speare, R. (2010). Self-reported anticipated compliance with physician advice to stay home during pandemic (H1N1) 2009: Results from the 2009 Queensland Social Survey. *BMC Public Health*, 10: 138.

Burkle, F.M., Isaac-Renton, J., Beck, A., Belgica, C.P., Blatherwick, J., Brunet, L.A., Hardy, N.E., Kendall, P., Kunii, O., Lokey, W., Sansom, G. & Stewart, R. (2001). 5th Asia-Pacific conference on disaster medicine. Theme 5. Application of international standards to disasters: Summary and action plan. *Prehospital and Disaster Medicine*, 16(1): 36-8.

Caldicott, D., Edwards, N., Aitken, P., Lee, C. & Eliseo, T. (2008). Terror Australis 2004: preparedness of Australian hospitals for disasters and incidents involving chemical, biological and radiological agents. *Critical Care and Resuscitation*, 10(2): 125-36.

Campbell, S. (2005). Responding to international disasters. *Nursing Standard*, 19(21): 33-6.

Castleden, M., McKeel, M., Murray, V. & Leonardi, G. (2011). Resilience thinking in health protection. *Journal of Public Health*, 33(3): 369–77.

Centers for Disease Control and Prevention. (2005). *Mass casualties predictor*. Accessed 4 April 2006. Available from: http://www.bt.cdc.gov/masstrauma/predictor.asp

Chan, T.C., Killeen, J., Griswold, W., Lenert, L. (2004). Information technology and emergency medical care during disasters. *Academic Emergency Medicine*, 11(11): 1229-36.

Chen, K.T., Chen, W.J., Mallilay, J. & Twu, S.J. (2003). The public health response to the Chi-Chi earthquake in Taiwan, 1999. *Public Health Reports*, 118: 493-9.

Considine, J., Shaban, R., Patrick, J., Holzhauser, K., Aitken, P., Clark, M., Fielding, E. & FitzGerald, G. (2011). Pandemic (H1N1) 2009 influenza in Australia: absenteeism and redeployment of emergency medicine and nursing staff. *Emergency Medicine Australasia*. (in Press)

Centre for Research on the Epidemiology of Disasters (CRED). (2011) Homepage. Accessed 5 December 2011. Available from: http://www.cred.be/emdat

Debacker, M. (2002). *Definition of disaster and disaster medicine*. CEMEC: European Masters in Disaster Medicine. Course Notes 2002.

de Ville de Goyet, C. (2000). Stop propagating disaster myths. *Lancet*, 356(9231): 762-4.

DeVita, M.A., Schaefer, J., Lutz, J., Dongilli, T. & Wang, H. (2004). Improving medical crisis team performance', *Critical Care Medicine*, 33(2): 61-5s.

Drabek, T. (1986). *The human system responses to disaster: an inventory of sociological findings*. Springer-Verlag, New York, 1986.

Dufour, C., Geoffrey, V., Maury, H. & Grunewald, F. (2004). Rights, standards and quality in a complex humanitarian space: is SPHERE the right tool? *Disasters*, 28(2): 124-41.

Dynes, R.R. (1998) *Dealing with disasters in the 21st century*. University of Delaware - Disaster Research Centre.

FitzGerald, G.J., Patrick, J.R., Fielding, E., Shaban, R., Arbon, P., Aitken, P., Considine, J., Clark, M., Finucane, J., McCarthy, S., Cloughessy, L. & Holzhauser, K. (2010). H1N1 Influenza 2009 outbreak in Australia: Impact on Emergency Departments. (ISBN: 978-1-74107-322-5) Brisbane: Queensland University of Technology.

Fitzgerald, G., Aitken, P., Arbon, P., Archer, F., Cooper, D., Leggat, P., Myers, C., Robertson, A., Tarrant, M. & Davis, E. (2010). A National Framework for Disaster Health Education in Australia. *Prehospital and Disaster Medicine*, 25(1): 70-7.

Ford, J.K. & Schmidt, A.M. (2000). Emergency response training: Strategies for enhancing real-world performance. *Journal of Hazardous Materials*, 75: 195-215.

Frisch, T. (2005). The international aid perspective. *Crisis Response Journal*, 1(2): 22-3.

Gaudette, R., Schnitzer, J., George, E. & Briggs, S.M. (2002). Lessons learned from the September 11th World Trade Centre Disaster: pharmacy preparedness and participation in an international medical and surgical response team. *Pharmacotherapy*, 22(3): 271-81.

Gerace, R.V. (1979). Role of medical teams in a community disaster plan. *Canadian Medical Association Journal*, 120: 923-8.

Gunn, S.W.A. (2005). The humanitarian imperative in disaster management – A memorial tribute to Professor Peter Safar. *Prehospital and Disaster Medicine*, 20(2): 89-92.

Haddow, G.D. & Bullock, J.A. (2003). International disaster management. In Haddow GD, Bullock JA (eds), *Introduction to Emergency Management*, Butterworth Heinemann, USA.

Hogan, D.E. (2002). Education and Training in Disaster Medicine. Chapter 37 In. Hogan DE *Disaster Medicine*. Lippincott, Williams and Wilkins.

Holland, J. & Wooster, P. (2004). International rescue team: selection and training. *Crisis Response J*, 1(1): 51-4.

Hsu, E.B., Ma, M., Lin, F.Y., VanRooyen, M.J. & Burkle, F.M. (2002). Emergency medical assistance team response following Taiwan Chi-Chi earthquake. *Prehospital and Disaster Medicine*, 17(1): 17-22.

International Society for Disaster Medicine, Scientific Committee. (1993). *Curriculum: Education and Training in Disaster Medicine*. Geneva, Switzerland 1993: Available from the Secretariat of the International Society for Disaster Medicine.

International Federation of Red Cross and Red Crescent Societies (IFRC). (2001). *World Disasters Report 2000*, International Federation of Red Cross and Red Crescent Societies, Geneva.

Iwan, W.D., Cluff, L.S., Kimpel, J.F., Kunreuther, N.H., Masaki-Schatz, S.H., Nigg, J.M., Roth, R.S., Ryland, H., Stanley, E. & Thomas, F.H. (1999). Mitigation emerges as major strategy for reducing losses caused by natural disasters. *Science*, 284(5422): 1943-7.

Judd, Lord. (1992). Disaster relief or relief disaster?   A challenge to the international community. *Disasters*, 16(1): 1-8.

Kaji, A., Koenig, K.L. & Bey, T. (2006). Surge capacity for health- care systems: a conceptual framework. *Academic Emergency Medicine*, 13: 1157-9.

Keim, M.E. & Rhyne, G.J. (2001). The CDC Pacific emergency health initiative: A pilot study of emergency preparedness in Oceania. *Emergency Medicine*, 13: 157-64.

Leggat, P.A., Brown, L.H., Aitken, P. &, Speare, R. (2010). Level of concern and precaution taking amongst Australians regarding travel during Pandemic (H1N1) 2009: Results from the 2009 Queensland Social Survey. *Journal of Travel Medicine*, 17(5): 291-5.

Lennquist, S. (2004). The tsunami disaster – new lessons learned and old lessons to be learned better. *International Journal of Disaster Medicine*, 2: 71-3.

Leonard, R.B., Spangler, H.M. & Stringer, L.W. (1997). Medical outreach after Hurricane Marilyn. *Prehospital and Disaster Medicine*, 12: 189-94.

Leus, X.R. (2000). The road ahead. *Prehospital and Disaster Medicine*, 15(4): 136-43.

Lichtenstein, J. (2001). After Hurricane Mitch: United States Agency for International Development, Reconstruction, and the Stockholm Principles. Report prepared for Oxfam-America. Washington, DC: Oxfam.

Maegele, M., Gregor, S., Steinhausen, E., Bouillon, B., Heiss, M.M., Perbix, W., Wappler, F., Rixen, D., Geisen, J., Berger-Schreck, B. & Schwarz, R. (2005). The long distance tertiary air transfer and care of tsunami victims: Injury patterns and microbiological and psychological aspects. *Critical Care Medicine*, 33(5): 1136-40.

Malilay, J. (2000). Public health assessments in disaster settings: Recommendations for a multidisciplinary approach. *Prehospital and Disaster Medicine*, 15(4): 167-72.

Marmor, M., Goldstein, L., Levi, Y., Onn, E., Blumenfield, A., Kosashvili, Y., Levy, G., Hirschorn, G., Heldenberg, E., Or, J., Setton, E., Goldberg, A. & Bar-Dayan, Y. (2005). Mass medical repatriation of injured civilians after terrorist attack in Mombassa, Kenya: Medical needs, resources utilized, and lessons learned. *Prehospital and Disaster Medicine*, 20(2): 98-102.

Martone, G. (2005). Tsunami aftermath: Community regeneration is the focus of relief efforts in Indonesia. *American Journal of Nursing*, 105(7): 70-2.

Maury, H. & Russbach, R. (2004). The Quality Compass – A new tool to manage and evaluate humanitarian assistance. *International Journal of Disaster Medicine*, 2: 106-10.

McCurdy, I. (1999). DART: disaster assistance response team. *IAEM Bulletin*, 16(10): 19-20.

McEntire, D.A. (1998). Balancing international approaches to disaster: rethinking prevention instead of relief. *Australian Journal of Emergency Management*, 13(2): 50-55.

McEntire, D.A. (1999). Issues in disaster relief: progress, perpetual problems and prospective solutions. *Disaster Prevention and Management*, 8 (5): 351-61.

Milsten, A. (2000). Hospital responses to acute onset disasters: A review. *Prehospital and Disaster Medicine*, 15(1): 32-45.

Moresky, R.T., Eliades, M.J., Bhimani, M.A., Bunney, E.B. & VanRooyen, M.J. (2001). Preparing international relief workers for health care in the field: An evaluation of organisational practices. *Prehospital and Disaster Medicine*, 16(4): 257-62.

Nabarro D. (2005). Putting it together: stronger public health capacity within disaster management systems. *Prehospital and Disaster Medicine*, 20(6): 483-5.

Noji, E.K. (2000). The public health consequences of disasters. *Prehospital and Disaster Medicine*, 15(4): 147-57.

Pan American Health Organization/World Health Organization. (1999). *Evaluation of preparedness and response to hurricanes Georges and Mitch: Conclusions and recommendations*. Accessed 4 April 2006. Available from: http://www.paho.org/english/dd/ped/concleng.htm

Quarantelli, E.L. (1985). Disaster planning : small and large – past, present and future. *University of Delaware - Disaster Research Centre Report*, 84: 8.

Quarantelli, E.L. (1988). Assessing disaster preparedness planning. *Regional Development Dialogue*, 9: 48-69.

Queensland Health. (2011). Mass Casualty Sub-Plan to the Queensland Health Disaster Plan. Version September 2011. Accessed 4 March 2012. Available from: http://qheps.health.qld.gov.au/emu/docs/mascas-subplan-2011.pdf

Redmond, A.D. (2005a). Natural disasters. *British Medical Journal*, 330: 1259-61.

Redmond, A.D. (2005b). Needs assessment of humanitarian crises. *British Medical Journal*, 330: 1320-2.

Roshchin, G.G. & Mazurenko, O.V. (2002). Ukraine's disaster medicine team mission to India following the earthquake of 2001. *Prehospital and Disaster Medicine*, 17(3): 163-6.

Roy, N., Shah, H., Patel, V. & Coughlin, R.R. (2002). The Gujurat earthquake (2001), experience in a seismically unprepared area: Community hospital medical response. *Prehospital and Disaster Medicine*, 17(4): 186-95.

Rubin, M., Heuvelmans, J.H.A., Tomic-Cica, A. & Birnbaum, M.L. (2000). Health related relief in the former Yogoslavia: Needs, demands and supplies. *Prehospital and Disaster Medicine*, 15(1): 1-11.

Russbach, R. (1990). International assistance operations in disaster situations. *Prehospital and Disaster Medicine*, 5(3): 247-9.

Schull, M.J. & Shanks, L. (2001). Complex emergencies: Expected and unexpected consequences. *Prehospital and Disaster Medicine*, 16(4): 192-6.

Seidl, I., Daly, M., Johnson, A. & Aitken, P. (2011). A tale of two cities: airline responses to the Eyjafjallajökull eruption and lessons for health disaster management. *Australian Health Review*, 35: 294–6.

Seidl, I., Johnson, A., Mantel, P. & Aitken, P. (2010). A strategy for real time improvement (RTI) in communication during the H1N1 emergency response. *Australian Health Review*, 34: 493–8.

Sharp, T.W., Wightman, J.M., Davis, M.J., Sherman, S.S. & Burkle, F.M. (2001). Military assistance in complex emergencies : What have we learned since the Kurdish relief effort?, *Prehospital and Disaster Medicine*, 16(4): 197-208.

Sheik, M., Gutierrez, M.I., Bolton, P., Spiegel, P., Thieren, M. & Burnham, G. (2000) Deaths among humanitarian workers. *British Medical Journal*, 321: 166-8.

Sondorp, E., Kaiser, T. & Zwi, A. (2001) Editorial: Beyond emergency care: Challenges to health planning in complex emergencies. *Tropical Medicine and International Health*, 6(12): 965-70.

Stephenson, R.S. & DuFrane, C. (2005). Disasters and development: Part 2: Understanding and exploiting disaster-development linkages' and 'Disasters and development: Part 3: Assessing tradeoffs in investing in vulnerability reduction. *Prehospital and Disaster Medicine*, 20(1): 61-9.

Sundnes, K.O. & Birnbaum, M.L. (2002). *Health disaster management: guidelines for evaluation and research in the utstein style. Prehospital and Disaster Medicine*, 17 (Supp 3):

Taylor, P.R., Emonson, D.L. & Schlimmer, J.E. (1998). Operation Shaddock – the Australian Defence Force response to the tsunami disaster in Papua New Guinea. *Medical Journal of Australia*, 169(11-12): 602-6.

Vaneckova, P., Neville, G., Tippett, V., Aitken, P., FitzGerald, G. & Tong, S. (2011) Do biometeorological indices improve modeling outcomes of heat-related mortality? *Journal of Applied Meteorology and Climatology*, 50: 1165-76.

VanRooyen, M. & Leaning, J. (2005).After the tsunami – Facing the public health challenges. *New England Journal of Medicine*, 352(5): 435-8.

VanRooyen, M.J., Hansch, S., Curtis, D. & Burnham, G. (2001). Emerging issues and future needs in humanitarian assistance. *Prehospital and Disaster Medicine*, 16(4): 216-22.

Wallace, A.G. (2002). National disaster medical system: Disaster medical assistance teams. In. Hogan DE & Burstein JL (eds), *Disaster Medicine*. Lippincott Williams and Wilkins, Philadelphia.

Wang, X.Y., Barnett, A.G., Vaneckova, P., Yu, W., Fitzgerald, G., Wolff, R., Tippett, V., Aitken, P., Neville, G., McRae, M., Verall, K. & Tong, S. (2011). The impact of heatwaves on mortality and emergency hospital admissions in Brisbane, Australia. *Occupational and Environmental Medicine*. (in Press)

World Health Organization. (2005). *Health and human rights*. Geneva: WHO. Accessed 4 April 2006. Available from: http://www.who.int/hhr/en

World Health Organization/Pan-American Health Organisation. (2003). Guidelines for the use of foreign field hospitals in the aftermath of sudden impact disasters. *Prehospital and Disaster Medicine*, 18(4): 278-90.

10

Traumatic Brain Injury

Zahra Gardezi
University of Toledo
Toledo, Ohio,
USA

1. Introduction

Almost 1.7 million Americans sustain traumatic brain injury (TBI) annually according to the center for disease control,275,000 get hospitalized while 52,000 die of traumatic brain injury. 1.365 million are treated and released from the Emergency Department . About 80 to 90,000 sustain long term disability. The rate of death from TBI remains low, 6/100,000, but the cost to society remains high. Survivors suffer from long term sequelae such as seizures, loss of memory and cognitive impairment. According to one estimate, half of the hospitalized patients end up requiring neuro-rehabilitation. Falls are the leading cause of TBI in children and adults over the age of 65. TBI in patients under the age of 19 have increased in the United States over the last decade (Morbidity and Mortality Weekly Report (MMWR) Nonfatal Traumatic Brain Injuries Related to Sports and Recreation Activities Among Persons Aged ≤19 Years --- United States, 2001--2009 October 7, 2011 / 60(39);1337-1342). MVA s are the major cause of TBI and TBI related death in young adults.

Types of Injury:

- Scalp laceration
- Skull fractures
- Epidural hematoma
- Subdural hematoma
- Intra-cranial hemorrhage

2. Scalp Injuries and skull fractures

Scalp lacerations tend to bleed profusely and while bleeding can easily be controlled with surgical staples, they may be associated with penetrating injury to the brain parenchyma. Motor vehicle crashes (MVCs) and blast injuries are also associated with fractures of the skull. The parietal bone is mostly commonly fractured and is associated with epidural hematomas due to tearing of the middle meningeal artery. Linear skull fractures are associated with delayed epidural hematomas and may be cause of sudden neurological worsening. Depressed skull fractures are associated with high kinetic energy resulting in CSF leaks presenting as otorrhoea or rhinorrhea (shattered cribriform plate.). Immunofixation with beta-2 transferrin can help differentiate CSF from other body fluids. Depressed skull fractures and fractures involving the sinuses have a high incidence of infection. It is therefore prudent to start the patient on antibiotic prophylaxis. Both, Clindamycin 600 mg IV Q6hr and Vancomycin 1G Q12 is also acceptable. Radiographs have no role in the diagnosis of skull fractures due to their low sensitivity and specifity in defining underlying brain damage. Head CT with bone windows should be done in the emergency department. The Brain Trauma Foundation recommends all fractures depressed greater than the thickness of the cranium be surgically elevated.

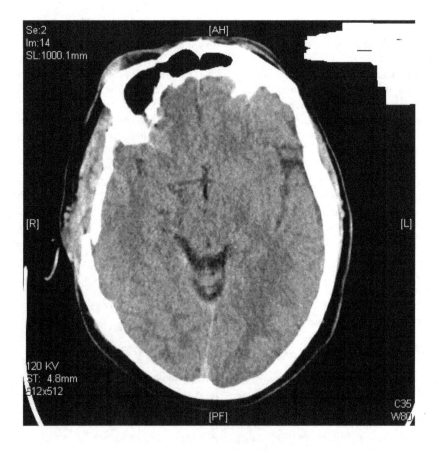

Fig. 1. Depressed Right temporal Bone Fracture requiring surgical elevation. Image coutesy: Dr. Azedine Medhkour, MD, Neurosurgery, University of Toledo Medical Center.

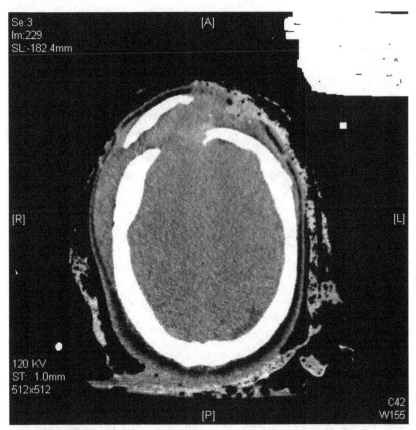

Fig. 2. Anterior displacement of comminuted frontal bone fracture. Image coutesy:
Dr. Azedine Medhkour, MD, Neurosurgery, University of Toledo Medical Center.

3. Intra-cranial hemorrage

3.1 Epidural hematoma

Epidural hematoma forms secondary to trauma to the skull and underlying vessels e.g. torn
meningeal artery. 9 to 10% present as a delayed hematoma. Anisocoria (papillary difference
or >2 mm) is present in 67% of the patients.

3.2 Subdural hematoma

Subdural hematoma is seen in 0.5 to 5% of head injuries and is usually associated with
traffic trauma and falls in the elderly especially those on anticoagulants. All patients
reporting LoC should be evaluated for a syncopal episode prior to fall or MVA. The
evaluation should include 2D trans-thoracic echo for undiagnosed aortic and mitral valve
stenosis, EKG and cardiac enzymes to rule out myocardial infarction as well as a carotid
ultrasound to detect plaques and/or critical narrowing. 24 hr. Holter monitoring and tilt
table may also be necessary as arrhythmias and postural hypotention could be possible

causes of loss of consciousness. Patients over the age of 65 are frequently on anti-hypertensive medications and diuretics.

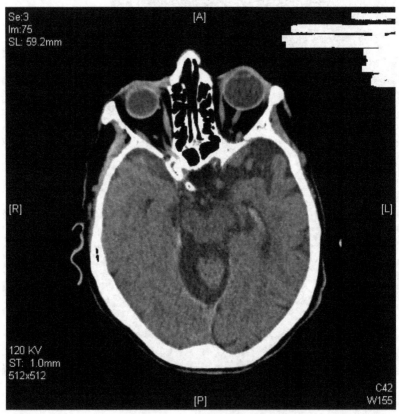

Fig. 3. Subarachanoid hemorrhage in anterior brainstem. Image coutesy: Dr. Azedine Medhkour, MD, Neurosurgery, University of Toledo Medical Center.

4. Intra-parenchymal hemorrhage

In 4 to 23% of TBI the brain is injured as it accelerates along the irregularities of the inner table of the skull.

- *50% pts are unconscious at presentation
- *2/3 rd require Surgery in the 1st 48 hrs.
- *70% of delayed ICH occurs in the 1st 48 hrs.

4.1 Contusion

Contusions are the most commonly identified injuries on CT and are due to sudden deceleration injury with brain impacting on the inner table of the frontal or middle fossa . Contusions may also appear distant from the area of impact (counter-coup). The resulting multi-polar areas of injury, ischemia and edema lead to rapid rise of ICP and chances of herniation. Patients usually have focal neurologic deficits with contusions but sudden deterioration may be a sign of hemorrhage into the contusion. A repeat CT may be indicated under the circumstances.

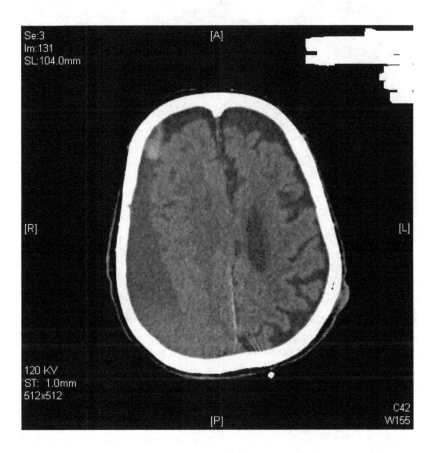

Fig. 4. Acute on chronic, mutipolar subdural hemorrhage with midline shift. Image coutesy: Dr. Azedine Medhkour, MD, Neurosurgery, University of Toledo Medical Center.

4.2 Concussion / diffuse axonal injury

Concussion is the temporary loss of consciousness and is on the same continuum as diffuse axonal injury (DAI) . DAI refers to disruption of intra-cerebral axons at the grey/ white matter junction due to angular forces. DAI carries the worst prognosis of all TBIs. The extent of damage may not be visible on the first CT scan. Unconsciousness lasting over 6 hours without sedation should raise suspicion for DAI and may warrant a gradient echo MRI for definitive diagnosis.

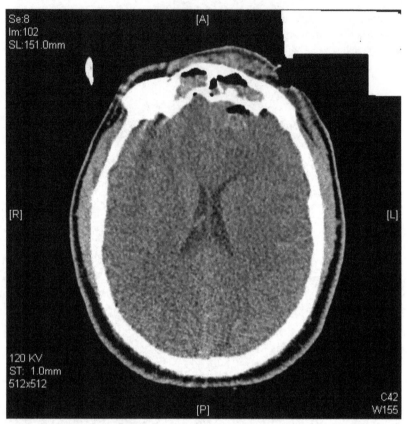

Fig. 5. Severe DAI with loss of grey and white matter differentiation. Image coutesy: Dr. Azedine Medhkour, MD, Neurosurgery, University of Toledo Medical Center.

5. Early evaluation and treatment

The Glasgow Coma Scale (GCS) remains the cornerstone of early assessment by clinicians in the ED . But in the pre-hospital setting simple observations such as combativeness, alcohol intoxication, high speed MVA, loss of short term memory ,vomiting, age over 60 and trauma above the clavicles are signs that underlying brain injury is likely and early interventions such as airway protection may be necessary. All patients with suspected head injury should be immobilized due to high incidence of co-existing spine injuries. Evaluation of ABCs i.e. Airway , breathing and circulation should be the first priority Tracheal intubation for GCS less than 6 should be performed, when possible prior to transport. All patients should be resuscitated with isotonic saline. (0.9% NaCl) Hypotonic and dextrose containing fluids should be avoided as they can worsen brain edema. Small volume resuscitation with hypertonic saline in patients with poly-trauma involving the head is also acceptable. 3% saline (8ml/kg) was associated with similar hemodynamic benefits when compared with high volume isotonic resuscitation i.e. Lactated ringer at 33 ml/kg. in experimental models of head injury. Contrary to popular belief LR infusion is not associated with Calcium influx or progression of neuronal injury. However recipients of HS had higher serum Na and lower ICPs.

6. Principles of management

6.1 Prevent secondary injury

The initial insult to the brain at the time of primary impact is only a portion of the damage sustained in TBI. Secondary insults compound the initial injury. Secondary injury is caused by hypotension and hypoxia. Early hypotension, especially in the field, strongly correlates with poor outcome and mortality. The prognosis of TBI is primarily dependant on the ability to escape secondary injury. Threshold values for intervention are:

- S_aO_2 <90,
- ICP >20,
- CPP <60,
- SBP <90.
- Hypo and Hypercarbia i.e. <28 or>45.

Hypoxia occurs in 22.4 % of severe TBI patients and 55% of patients are hypoxic on tracheal intubation. Hypoxia for 10 to 20 min i.e. S_aO_2 less than 90% is an independent predictor of poor outcome.

Goals of Management	
O2 sat	>97%
SBP	>90mmHg
CPP	>60mmHg
Blood Glucose	100-150mg/dl
ICP	<20
Temp.	<37.5

Table 1.

6.2 Sedation

Light sedation may be indicated for anxious patients. Sedation decreases $CMRO_2$ while agitation and combativeness can raise ICP considerably. Midazolam, lorazepam and propofol can be used for this purpose.

7. Elevated ICP

7.1 Head position

Keeping the head of bed elevated to 30 degrees and in a midline position may prevent kinking of internal jugular veins and obstruction of venous outflow. Patients with spine injuries and log roll precautions should be kept in reverse Trendelenberg to aid venous drainage.

7.2 Mannitol therapy

Mannitol is an osmotic diuretic used to reduce intracranial pressure and brain edema. It expands plasma volume by creating an osmotic gradient and improves cerebral blood flow. However, it should only be used with caution patients with congestive heart disease (CHF) or renal disease. Mannitol is typically given as a bolus 0.25grams to 1.5 grams per kilogram IV in hemo-dynamically stable with no active source of intracranial bleeding. It has consistently been shown in studies to reduce ICP and can help temporize the patient's condition while definitive therapy is determined. At present there is no evidence to support its use as a continuous infusion. An ICP monitor may be placed before a second bolus is administered to determine the effect on ICP. Serum osmolality should be maintained between 300 to 320 Osm/L. Higher values are associated with acute kidney injury.

7.3 Hypertonic saline

3 % saline can be used to decrease cerebral edema and decrease ICP. HS can be started at 20 to 50 cc/hr. with serial monitoring of serum sodium every 4 hours. Rate of rise of serum sodium should not be greater 0.5meq/l /hr or 2 meq/l/ 2 hrs. The maximum allowable rise is 10 meq/24 hrs. Central pontine myelinolyis (locked-in-syndrome) can occur in patients with pre-existing hyponatremia. HS can also be given as a 250 cc bolus. Effects of HS are mediated not only by its ability to expand plasma blood volume but also by its ability to attenuate the immunolgic response by preventing neutrophil activation and improving cerebral blood flow.

7.4 ICP Monitoring

ICP monitoring is indicated in all salvageable patients with: severe TBI i.e. GCS 3-8 after resuscitation; patients with CT scans showing hematoma, contusion, swelling or herniation; and in all patients with normal CT but 2 or more of the following features: age>40,unitaleral or bilateral posturing or SBP< 90. All these are at significant risk for intra-cranial hypertension. CT scans cannot reliably predict ICH. The incidence of intracranial hypertension can be greater than 60 % in comatose patients with GCS<9. ICP monitors are usually intra-parenchymal with a fiber-optic transducer at the tip. Epidural and sub-arachanoid bolts are also inserted and offer a high degree of accuracy.Intra-ventricular devices offer the additional advantage of draining CSF with rapid reduction of ICP in patients who cannot tolerate mannitol due to hemodynamic instability. ICP monitoring also allows the clinician to identify patients with intra-cranial hypertension that is refractory to medical management who require decompressive craniotomy.

8. Seizure prophylaxis

Reduced CBF (<20cc/ml/100g/min) or loss of consciousness stimulates in a threshold pattern the release of excitatory neuro-transmitters. The CSF concentrations of glutamate, glycine and aspartate increase up to 8 fold. These levels remain elevated up to a week after the initial inciting factor. These increased levels have been described as the mechanism for post-traumatic seizures. Seizures dramatically increase $CMRO_2$ and are associated with a worse prognosis. Current practice is to use levectiectetam 500 mg q12 hours for a week. Phenytoin, phosphenytoin and valproic acid can also be used. Unlike levectiectetam, phenytoin requires frequent lab checks to monitor therapeutic levels and is associated with adverse effects such as enzyme induction, myocardial depression, and fever. In one study almost half of the patients with post-injury seizures had therapeutic blood levels of phenytoin. Valproic acid has been associated with a higher incidence of death than the other antiepileptic medications.

8.1 Reversal of anti-coagulation

Elderly patients are frequently on anti-thrombotics for a variety of conditions such as DVT, chronic atrial fibrillation, ischemic stroke, coronary artery disease, or stent placements. Urgent reversal of anti-coagulation is necessary in this patient population. Rapid enlargement of an intracranial hematoma can lead to midline shift, mass effect, herniation and deterioration of neurological status. The incidence of re-bleeding is also very high . 10-15ml/kg of FFP should be given for urgent reversal of warfarin. Vitamin K should be added unless the reversal is meant to be transient. Administration of prothrombin complex concentrate (Profilnine) contains factors II,VII, IX and X and leads to normalization of INR within 10 min and has a half life of 6 to 8 hours. PCC has the advantage of a predictable response, rapid correction of INR and low volume which makes it ideal in patients with CHF. A dose of 25 U/Kg should be given for INR <4.0 and 50U/Kg for INR >4.0. Platelet transfusions may be required for patients on aspirin or clopidogrel. Recombinant activated factor VII was originally developed for hemophiliacs but its use had recently been extended to coagulopathic trauma patients. Factor VII at a dose of 90 mcg/kg leads to a more rapid reversal of coagulopathy and reduces the time to neurosurgical intervention. But, its use is limited by cost and thrombo-embolic complications especially in patients with coronary stents.

Apixaban and Dabigatran, are two of the new drugs being prescribed both for DVT and stroke prophylaxis to patients with history of pulmonary embolism, mechanical valve and chronic Atrial fibrillation. The former is a Factor Xa inhibitor and the reversal would be the same as heparin and lovenox i.e. FFP and RBC transfusions. However, the latter is a direct thrombin inhibitor, no specific antidotes exist at this time. This drug was approved by FDA in Oct. 2011. We don't have enough experience with it yet. We do know that prothrombin complex does not reverse it well. And that Factor II inhibition is one of its mechanisms of action which makes Factor VII a potential reversal agent. But no definitive recommendations can be made at this time.

8.2 Normothermia

Mild hypothermia is beneficial. Fever increases $CMRO_2$ so the patient's temperature should always be maintained at less than 37.5°C. While blood in the subarachanoid space and infection are the two leading causes of fever, diencephalic seizures can manifest themselves as a paroxysmal increase in temperature, heart rate , respiratory rate, and rigors . They can occur in the absence of any blood in the brain. Paroxysmal autonomic instability with dystonia or PAID is another term coined to describe the episodic nature of this syndrome.

8.3 Vasospasm prophylaxis

Vasospasm occurs in 20 to 35% of severe TBI and is especially common in blast injuries and are a cause of neurologic decline. Transcranial Doppler studies can be performed at the bedside where there is a high index of suspicion. Peak velocities greater than 200 cm/sec or less than 120 cm/sec are reasonably accurate in including or excluding vasospasm. However computed tomography angiography (CTA) should be used to confirm the diagnosis for values lying in the intermediate range. Nicardipine infusions can be used in patients with an established diagnosis of vasospasm. Magnesium infusions can be used to keep serum Mg above 3.5 for patients at high risk for vasospasm to reduce the incidence.

8.4 Steroids

Steroids have no role in the management of traumatic brain injury. They are not associated with decreased ICP or improved outcome. Methylpredisolone was found to be associated with worsened outcome in the CRASH(Corticosteroid randomization After Significant Head Injury) Trial in 2004.

8.5 Beta-blockade

Survivors of traumatic brain injury are subjected to catecholamine surge manifested by hyperthermia, tachycardia, tachypnea, arrhythmias and eventually cardiac necrosis. All of which may contribute to secondary insults. There is some evidence to suggest immunosuppression as a cause of catecholamine excess. Beta blockers offer survival benefit by suppressing the systemic effects of catecholamines.

9. Neurologic recovery

Amantidine is increasingly being used in TBI patients who develop diffuse axonal injury. It has shown to improve neurologic status by increasing dopamine levels in the brain. It can also be used in patients with frontal lobe lesions who are difficult to arouse. Atypical anti-psychotics like Aripiprazole (Abilify) is increasingly being used for improve cognitive function in TBI patients. Incidentally, Patients whoever were on Statins pre-injury were found to have better outcomes in a retrospective study.

9.1 Intravenous estrogens

Recent interest in IV estrogen use for TBI stems from the clinical observation that women in the reproductive age group generally do better than male cohorts after TBI. Also, levels of CSF estradiol were considerably higher in the male survivors compared to non-survivors. Estrogens are believed to induce the synthesis of heat shock proteins, reduce levels of cytokines and are anti-apoptotic. Animal studies have shown up to a 60 % reduction in the area of ischemic injury when IV estrogens were administered within 30 min. post-injury. Similar benefits were observed in spinal cord injury. The dose currently recommended for resuscitative purposes is a one time dose of 0.5mg/kg. The National Institute of Health Resuscitation Consortium is now considering implementation of a multi-centered trial after positive results from their pilot study.

10. Conclusion

Traumatic brain injury is one of the leading causes of death and disability in adults. Care of the TBI patients in the emergency department should be protocolized based on ATLS guidelines i.e. Airway, Breathing and Circulation. Definitive airway in the form of endotracheal intubation should be performed in moderate to severe TBI. Hypotension and hypoxia must be avoided. Early CT imaging and neurosurgical consultation/intervention should be sought.

11. References

[1] Selassie A W, Zaloshnja E, Langlois, JA,Miller T, Jones P, Steiner C. Incidence of Long-term Disability Following Traumatic Brain Injury Hospitalization, United States, 2003. *Journal of Head Trauma Rehabilitation. Focus on Clinical Research and Practice.* 23(2):123-131, March/April 2008.

[2] Centers for Disease Control and Prevention. Report to Congress on Mild Traumatic Brain Injury in the United States: Steps to Prevent a Serious Public Health Problem. Atlanta (GA): Department of Health and Human Services (US), CDC, National Center for Injury Prevention and Control; 2003.

[3] Bartlett J, Kett-White R, Mendelow AD, Miller JD, Pickard J, Teasdale G. Guidelines for the initial management of head injuries. Recommendations from the Society of British Neurological Surgeons. British Journal of Neurosurgery. 1998;12(4):349–52. [PubMed] (Role of CT scan)

[4] Livingston DH, Lavery RF, Passannante MR, Skurnick JH, Baker S, Fabian TC, et al. Emergency department discharge of patients with a negative cranial computed tomography scan after minimal head injury. Annals of Surgery. 2000;232(1):126–32. [PubMed]

[5] Surgical management of depressed cranial fractures. Bullock MR, Chesnut R, Ghajar J, Gordon D, Hartl R, Newell DW, Servadei F, Walters BC, Wilberger J, Surgical Management of Traumatic Brain Injury Author Group. Neurosurgery. 2006;58(3 Suppl):S56

[6] Woiciechowsky C, Asadullah K, Nestler D, et al. Sympathetic activation triggers systemic interleukin-10 release in immunodepression induced by brain injury. Nat Med. 1998;4:808–813.

[7] Jones PA, et al, Measuring the burden of secondary insults in head injured patients during intensive care, J of Neurosurg, Anesthesiol 1994: 6: 4-14

[8] Effects of cortisosteroids on death within 14 days in clinically significant head injury.:Roberts I, Yates D, Sandercock P, Farrell B, Wasserberg J, Lomas G, Cottingham R, Svoboda P, Brayley N, Mazairac G, Laloë V, Muñoz-Sánchez A, Arango M, Hartzenberg B, Khamis H, Yutthakasemsunt S, Komolafe E, Olldashi F, Yadav Y, Murillo-Cabezas F, Shakur H, Edwards P; CRASH trial collaborators. Lancet. 2004 Oct 9-15;364(9442):1321-8.

[9] Estradiol facilitates the release of neuropeptide Y to suppress hippocampus-dependent seizures:Ledoux VA, Smejkalova T, May RM, Cooke BM, Woolley CS;J Neurosci. 2009 Feb 4;29(5):1457-68.

[10] Surgical management of acute epidural hematomas. Bullock MR, Chesnut R, Ghajar J, Gordon D, Hartl R, Newell DW, Servadei F, Walters BC, Wilberger JE, Surgical Management of Traumatic Brain Injury Author Group. Neurosurgery. 2006;58(3 Suppl):S7.

[11] Holland L, Warkentin TE, Refaai M, et al, "Suboptimal Effect of a Three-Factor Prothrombin Complex Concentrate (Profilnine-SD) in Correcting Supratherapeutic

International Normalized Ratio Due to Warfarin Overdose," *Transfusion*, 2009, 49(6):1171-7. [PubMed 19210325]

[12] Impact of early pharmacological treatment on cognitive and behavioral outcome after traumatic brain injury in adults: a meta-analysis. Wheaton P, Mathias JL, Vink R.J Clin Psychopharmacol. 2009 Oct;29(5):468-77.

[13] The Use of Atypical Antipsychotics After Traumatic Brain Injury. Elovic, Elie Paul MD; Jasey, Neil N. Jr MD; Eisenberg, Michal E. MD. Section Editor(s): Glenn, Mel B. MD

[14] Hypertonic Saline Resuscitation: Efficacy May Require Early Treatment in Severely Injured Patients. Hashiguchi, Naoyuki MD; Lum, Linda RN; Romeril, Elizabeth RN; Chen, Yu MD; Yip, Linda PhD; Hoyt, David B. MD; Junger, Wolfgang G. PhD. The Journal of Trauma: Injury, Infection, and Critical Care Issue: Volume 62(2), February 2007, pp 299-306

[15] Piloto C: University of Texas Southwestern, Parkland test hormone; study examines use of single dose of estrogen after severe traumatic brain injury. *Center Times*, publication of University of Texas Southwestern Medical Center, Dallas, TX, September 2009; p 3

[16] The impact of hyperglycemia on patients with severe brain injuryJ. Trauma. 2005 Jan;58(1):47-50.Jeremitsky E, Omert LA, Dunham CM, Wilberger J, Rodriguez A.

[17] Effect of Secondary Prehospital Risk Factors on Outcome in Severe Traumatic Brain Injury in the Context of Fast Access to Trauma CareThe Journal of Trauma: Injury, Infection, and Critical Care. Issue: Volume 71(4), October 2011, pp 826-832

[18] Zumstein, Matthias A. MD; Moser, Mario MD; Mottini, Matthias MD; Ott, Sebastian R. MD; Sadowski-Cron, Charlotte MD; Radanov, Bogdan P. MD; Zimmermann, Heinz MD; Exadaktylos, Aristomenis MD. Long-Term Outcome in Patients With Mild Traumatic Brain Injury: A Prospective Observational StudyThe Journal of Trauma: Injury, Infection, and Critical Care. Issue: Volume 71(1), July 2011, pp 120-127

[19] Hoge CW, McGurk D, Thomas JL, Cox AL, Engel CC, Castro CA. Mild traumatic brain injury in U.S. Soldiers returning from Iraq. *N Engl J Med*. 2008;358:453–463.

[20] Anglois J, Rutland-Brown W, Wald M. The epidemiology and impact of traumatic brain injury: a brief overview. J Head Trauma Rehabil. 2006;21:375–378.

[21] Thurman D, Guerro J. Trends in hospitalization associated with traumatic brain injury. JAMA. 1999;282:954–957

[22] Beta-Adrenergic Blockade and Traumatic Brain Injury: Protective? The Journal of Trauma: Injury, Infection, and Critical Care. Issue: Volume 69(4), October 2010, pp 776-782. [

[23] Balbino, Marcos MD; Capone Neto, Antonio MD; Prist, Ricardo BS; Ferreira, Alice Teixeira MD; Poli-de-Figueiredo, Luiz F. MD. Fluid Resuscitation With Isotonic or Hypertonic Saline Solution Avoids Intraneural Calcium Influx After Traumatic Brain Injury Associated with Hemorrhagic Shock: The Journal of Trauma: Injury, Infection, and Critical Care. Issue: Volume 68(4), April 2010, pp 859-864

[24] Brain Trauma Foundation and AANS/CNS Joint Section on Neurotrauma and Critical Care. Guidelines for the management of severe traumatic brain injury. *J Neurotrauma (Suppl)*. 2007;24:S1–S106. [Context Link]

[24] Reversal of Coagulopathy in Critically Ill Patients With Traumatic Brain Injury: Recombinant Factor VIIa is More Cost-Effective Than Plasma.he Journal of Trauma: Injury, Infection, and Critical Care. Issue: Volume 66(1), January 2009, pp 63-75 Copyright: © 2009 Lippincott Williams & Wilkins, Inc.

11

Procedural Sedation and Analgesia in Emergency Department

Balwinder Singh[1], Akhilesh Kumar Tiwari[3], Sanjay Kumar Verma[2],
Pedro Whatts[4], Dipti Agarwal[5] and Subhash Chandra[6]

[1]*Division of Pulmonary & Critical Care Medicine, Mayo Clinic, Rochester, Minnesota;*
[2]*Department of Anesthesia, All India Instituteof Medical Sciences (A.I.I.M.S.), New Delhi,*
[3]*Department of Anesthesia, St. Stephen's Hospital New Delhi,*
[4]*Department of Anesthesia, Saint Luke's Episcopal Hospital, Ponce,*
[5]*Department of Emergency Medicine, Mayo Clinic, Rochester, MN*
[6]*Department of Medicine, Greater Baltimore Medical Center, Towson, MD*
[1,5,6]*USA*
[2,3]*India*
[4]*Puerto Rico*

1. Introduction

Emergency department (ED) is one place in the hospital where variety of patients encounter happen on a routine basis, of varied nature and severity, many of which are associated with varying degree of pain and anxiety. Hence, sedation and analgesia is an important component of acute care provided in the ED. Use of appropriate analgesia and sedation is about striking balance between patient comfort and needs and avoidance of hindering clinical findings to deliver a safe, appropriate and effective care but in comfortable and humane in nature.

2. Definitions

Conscious sedation, being used loosely in the ED for all form of sedations, was first described in 1985 as "light level of sedation where patient retains the ability to independently maintain an airway and respond appropriately to verbal commands" (1). In reality, the level of sedation used in ED is deeper than what was described as conscious sedation. In 2001, Joint Commission on Accreditation of Healthcare Organizations replaced term conscious sedation with moderate sedation/analgesia; a drug-induced depression of consciousness during which patients respond purposefully to verbal commands, either alone or accompanied by light tactile stimulation and maintain adequate spontaneous ventilation and cardiovascular function. Reflex withdrawal from a painful stimulus is not considered a purposeful response. (2) Definitions of recently launched terminology "procedural sedation" vary widely.

Procedural sedation and analgesia (PSA) is a more accurate and appropriate description. The term procedural sedation has emerged from the American College of Emergency Physician (ACEP) (3).

The concept behind PSA is to produce a state of sedation and analgesia with a minimal depression of consciousness where patient can tolerate unpleasant procedures but can maintain spontaneous respiration and airway-protective reflexes. Airway assistance ideally should not be required and the patient should be capable of responding to physical and verbal stimulus. PSA is also helpful for managing uncooperative patients in almost all the allied disciplines of healthcare including dentistry.

3. Who can perform PSA

The person performing the procedure should have sound understanding of medications used and able to monitor response and intervene to manage all potential complications. Expertise in airway management is mandatory, and the provider must be able to identify signs of airway complications both early and late in the course of procedure. Provider should be capable of maintaining airway during spontaneous ventilation and intermittent positive pressure ventilation with a mask and self-inflating resuscitation bag.

PSA is a core competency in emergency medicine residency training and existing evidence supports the PSA administration by ED physician is as safe as by anesthesiologist. Hence, graduates of emergency medicine residency are qualified to for PSA in all age group. For other ED practitioner such as physician assistants, nurse practitioners and physician's from other specialties such as family medicine working in ED; the chief of ED grants privileges for use of PSA.(3, 4)

4. Patient selection

Various patients requiring PSA in ED would be better served if the objectives of PSA are clear. Main objectives include patient safety, minimizing pain, anxiety and physical discomfort, negative psychological impact to treatment by providing analgesia and anxiolysis along with maximal potential for amnesia, patient movements during the procedure and maximizing the chances of success of procedure and returning the patient to pre-sedated state where safe discharge is possible.

Physical Status Classification

I: A normal healthy patient
II: A patient with mild systemic disease
III: A patient with severe systemic disease
IV: A patient with severe systemic disease that is a constant threat to life
V: A moribund patient who is not expected to survive without the operation
VI: A declared brain-dead patient whose organs are being removed for donor purposes

---

Patients undergoing PSA should be assessed for physical status. It could be done using Physical Status Classification issued by American Society of Anesthesiologists. Procedural sedation is appropriate for patients in Classes I, II and III. Procedures for class IV and higher are done in operating room.

There are no absolute contraindications, but things to consider are patients' co-morbid illness or injuries, problems with prior PSA, the ability of provider and facilities to manage the patient's airway. Patients with significant co-morbidity, minimal cardiopulmonary reserve and anticipated difficult airway should be cautiously approached. Another relative contraindication is ingestion of large food or fluid volumes shortly before procedure, less than 2 hours, for risk of aspiration. Role of fasting in emergency PSA is not very clear and risk of aspiration should be weighted over risk from delay in procedure.(5)

5. Preparation

Preparation for PSA includes pre-sedation patient assessment, arranging equipments and choosing right pharmacological agent. Equipments necessary consists equipments to perform the procedure, monitoring and to manage potential complications. Performing time-out prior to the procedure is vital in performing right procedure in right patient. The most common reported complication of moderate sedation is respiratory depression. In PSA, multiple studies have concluded that respiratory depression can be detected early measuring end-tidal CO_2 when compared to oxygen saturation. A change of 10% in end-tidal CO_2 and loss of wave pattern in capnography are indicators of respiratory depression. Use of supplemental oxygen has not been promoted much. American society of Anesthesiologists recommends using supplemental oxygen in deep sedation but does not have similar recommendation for moderate sedation. In many EDs, PSA is performed with 3 litres of supplemental but other ED physician raise concern on use of supplemental oxygen concealing respiratory depression. Current evidence on routine use of supplemental oxygen to avoid hypoxia from respiratory depression is controversial. Low dose oxygen supplemental oxygen doesn't decrease the risk of hypoxia but high dose does. Fortunately, hypoxemia induced by respiratory depression is either self-limiting or reversible with oxygen supplementation. Hence, routine use is not recommended.

Equipments for PSA
1. Intravenous access, peripheral is adequate
2. Monitoring equipments; cardiac monitor, pulse oximetry, blood pressure cuff, capnography
3. Pharmacological agent
4. Reversal agents
5. Equipments for procedure
6. Airway equipments; oxygen supply, face mask/nasal cannula, bag-valve-mask, suction
7. Rescue airway equipments; endotracheal tube, direct laryngoscope, laryngeal mask airway
8. Normal saline

6. Pharmacological agents

A perfect agent for PSA should have rapid onset of action, short duration, rapid, smooth and complete recovery, devoid of adverse effects and able to produce adequate sedation, analgesia and amnesia. Till date, there is no perfect agent available which has all the above-mentioned properties.

7. Deep sedative agents

7.1 Propofol

Propofol is an ultrashort-acting sedative-hypnotic agent that produces dose-dependent, progressive suppression of awareness. Clinical sedation usually begins within 30 seconds from the time of injection and resolves within 6 minutes. Serum concentration drops from rapid distribution and metabolic clearance. It was first used in 1996 for PSA in ED and gained popularity after year 2000 because of its short duration of action, early and complete recovery and cost-effectiveness. Currently, it is most popular deep sedative being used in ED with over 90% satisfaction in both patients and physicians. (6) Based on current evidences, propofol is safe and efficacious in ED procedures requiring deeper level of sedation such as fracture and dislocation reduction, cardioversion, incision and drainage of abscess. It is not an optimal agent to induce minimal to moderate level of sedation. Another disadvantage is not having analgesic properties. Synergistic use of opiate analgesics is associated with higher respiratory depression and achieving near-complete analgesia using opiates prior to propofol infusion is advisable.

Cautions: There are no absolute contraindications apart from allergy to propofol, egg or soy products. Propofol is known for dose dependent hypotension that is reversible with level of sedation. Hypotension is more pronounced in volume-depleted patients and should be replete prior to procedure. Advance age is found to have higher incidence of hypotension and respiratory depression. (7) This effect is most likely related with high serum peak concentration but exact pathophysiology is not yet clear.

Monitoring: Overall, propofol is safe property but due to highly potent sedative agent and little alteration in serum concentration can make swings in level of consciousness and also produce cumulative sedation. Hence, sound understanding of pharmacological properties of propofol, abilities to monitor, intervene and resuscitate if needed for complications from deeper sedation are must for ED physician performing PSA. A dedicated nurse should be available during the procedure. At this point it is not very clear if another ED physician is needed to perform PSA in addition to physician performing procedure.

Recovery: Patients should be monitored until they return to their baseline mental status. Once they reach to baseline mental status, it is unlikely to have suppression of consciousness from redistribution but caution is advised in cases with use of protocol for longer duration with multiple doses. Emesis during recovery is infrequent, in less than 3% and no adverse events is reported post-discharge.

7.2 Etomidate

Etomidate is an ultra-short acting non-barbiturate imidazole derivative, which is well known inducing agent for rapid sequence intubation in the ED. It produces deep sedation similar to propofol. Onset of action is usually within one minute when administered intravenously and patient recovers from sedation with-in 6 to 16 minutes. It has minimal, if any, analgesic property but gained popularity for minimal effect on hemodynamic stability. The liver metabolizes etomidate rapidly, and the duration of effect may be longer in patients with liver failure. Indication profile for etomidate is similar to propofol but gets priority when hemodynamic stability is matter of concern. Additionally, etomidate provides excellent amnesia of the procedure; over 70% of patients have no recall of procedure.

Etomidate Administration

0.1mg/kg body weight IV as initial dose followed by half dose every 3-5 minutes titrating for clinical sedation.

Cautions: The only contraindication to etomidate is hypersensitivity to the medication, but caution should be taken during pregnancy (etomidate is a pregnancy category C drug), and the general precautions regarding procedural sedation and patient selection also should be considered. Side effects are usually rare, and there is no histamine release and hence minimal hemodynamic usability. Myoclonus is commonly reported side effect, up to 20% of cases, but not evident in rapid sequence intubation secondary to concomitant use of paralytic agent. In most cases, it is transient and does not cause respiratory distress and does not need intervention. The ED physician using etomidate should be competent in managing severe myoclonus which happens very rarely and in that scenario, opening airway is difficult. Use of benzodiazepines can decrease the probability of myoclonus. Another commonly reported side effect is emesis, up to 4% of cases, which is self-limiting. Adrenocortical suppression has been reported after the use of a single bolus of etomidate, but one time use of etomidate in otherwise healthy patient is believed to be inconsequential.

Monitoring: Monitoring in use of etomidate is similar to any deep sedative, using pulse oximetry, capnography and hemodynamic monitoring. Respiratory depression and hypoxia are possible as part of deep sedation for which supplemental oxygen is enough but rarely might require bag-and-mask ventilation.

Recovery and discharge: Recovery with use of etomidate is rapid and complete and once patient is back to baseline level of awareness, could be discharged and no adverse effect reported post discharge.

Overall, both deep sedative agents provide similar level of sedation, respiratory suppression but propofol is devoid of myoclonus and emesis and have better success rate of procedure.

8. Dissociative anesthetic agent

8.1 Ketamine

Ketamine is a dissociative agent that dissociates central nervous system from outside stimuli and produces a state of analgesia, amnesia and sedation but maintains spontaneous respiration, protective airway reflexes and hemodynamic stability. Dissociation is produced at a dosing threshold below which patient has analgesia and disorientation and higher dose does not deepen the level of sedation. It is commonly used in short painful and emotionally disturbing procedures such as laceration repair, incision and drainage, reduction of orthopedic fractures and dislocation in children and in mentally disabled patients who are often uncooperative. It is not very popular for procedures where motionless sedation is required as occasional random movements are common in dissociative sedation.

Ketamine Administration

IV route: 1.5mg/kg in children and 1mg/kg in adults as initial dose and repeat half doses for prolonged sedation
IM route: used if no IV access, 4 to 5mg/kg as initial dose to induce sedation and repeated as half dose

---

Cautions: Ketamine is absolutely contraindicated in infants younger than 3-month for laryngospasm and apnea and in schizophrenia as it exacerbates the condition. To prevent the risk of laryngospasm – avoid vigorous stimulation of posterior pharyngeal wall, use in anatomical defect of airway such as stenosis or recent surgery etc, upper respiratory tract infection and in asthma. Ketamine decreases re-uptake of catecholamines, which leads to increased sympathomimetic activity. For this reason ketamine should be avoided in children and adult with known or possible coronary artery disease, congestive heart failure and hypertension. Sympathomimetic action is exacerbated in patients with porphyria and thyroid disease, hence should be used with caution. Ketamine increases intracranial and intraocular pressure and should be avoided in hydrocephalus, intracranial masses/abnormalities, acute globe injury and glaucoma but no more contraindicated in head injury as cerebral vasodilatation caused by ketamine is potentially beneficial.

Monitoring: Pulse oximetry, cardiac monitoring and capnography are recommended. Capnography is increasingly recommended for early detection of respiratory compromise. Co-administration of anti-cholinergic agents to decrease oral secretions, benzodiazepines to decrease recovery reaction, antiemetic agents for emesis that is common with intramuscular administration of ketamine is being practiced. Based on current evidences, prophylactic use of these agents is no superior than as needed basis use. Respiratory depression is uncommon with ketamine but can happen with IV dosing, 1-2 minutes after dose.

Recovery and discharge: Ketamine is known for hallucinations, agitation and emesis during recovery. Recovery reactions are more common in late adolescents and can be rapidly taken care of with use of short acting benzodiazepines. Emesis could occur hours after the procedure. Ataxia has been reported post-discharge and close observation by family member is recommended. At this point, there are no standard guidelines for discharge. Once patient returns to pre-treatment level of awareness, vocalization and activity is achieved, could be discharged.

8.2 Benzodiazepines and opioids

Benzodiazepines act by binding to benzodiazepine-specific receptors on the gamma-aminobutyric acid (GABA)-benzodiazepine receptor complex and potentiate GABA inhibitory action in the CNS and produce sedation, amnesia, anxiolysis, anticonvulsant effects and respiratory depression.

Midazolam is the most commonly used benzodiazepines for PSA, as it has early onset of action producing more complete amnesia, less pain on injection and improved awakening when compared with diazepam. Midazolam possesses a relatively high volume of distribution (Vd) compared with other benzodiazepines because of its lipophilicity. The Vd is greatly amplified in obese patients, resulting in an increased half-life from 2.7 hours to 8.4 hours. On usual dose, sedation is induced within 1-2 minutes and lasts up-to 30 minutes. Midazolam is frequently combined with a short acting opioid; this combination is titrated easily and widely available.

Midazolam Administration

0.02 mg/kg body weight IV in adults and 0.1 mg/kg IV in children less than 5 years of age as initial dose followed by 1mg IV every 3 minutes during prolonged sedation

---

Fentanyl is a favored opioid as it has prompt onset and short duration of action, and it also has minimal cardiovascular depressive effects and hypotension unlike morphine. Fentanyl binds with stereospecific receptors at many sites within the CNS and increases pain threshold, alters pain reception, and inhibits ascending pain pathways. In addition to analgesia, opioid agonists suppress the cough reflex and cause respiratory depression, drowsiness, and sedation. Onset of analgesia begins within 1-2 minutes and lasts up-to 30 to 60 minutes.

Fentanyl Administration

1 to 1.5mcg/kg body weight IV in adults as initial dose followed by 1mcg/kg every three minutes for prolonged analgesia

---

8.3 Barbiturates

This group of drug is one of the oldest classes of drug and their role is mostly restricted to operating room and occasionally ICU, occasionally they may be used for providing sedation outside operating rooms setting. They have been traditionally classified on the basis of their duration of action. Methohexital, thiopental and thiamylal are short acting; pentobarbital is intermediate and phenobarbital fall under long acting group. Their have been few studies on their role in providing sedation to pediatric population in radiological suite during early and late 90s, however due to availability of better and safe alternative they are not the preferred drugs to provide sedation among anesthesiologists and emergency care physician anymore.

8.4 Remifentanyl

Remifentanyl is a recent addition in the list of pharmacological agents that has gained popularity amongst anesthetist and emergency physician, it's a short acting μ-receptor opioid agonist and achieves peak analgesic effect in less than a minute and has an elimination half life of about ten minutes. Due to this short action of the drug, sustained analgesia may require an additional dose or an intravenous infusion. Different dose regimens are in use but the most often used ones were an intravenous bolus dose of 1 μg/kg over 1 minute. Alternatively it can also be titrated to individual needs with an infusion rates ranging from 0.025 - 0.1 μg/kg/min for conscious sedation (8). Recent studies have proved safety and efficacy of remifentanil for PSA when used along with propofol (9 - 11).

Caution: Combination of propofol and remifentanyl has good safety profile as compared to the combination of remifentanyl and midazolam and is being increasingly used due to its safety profile as compared to other agents.

Monitoring: Standard monitoring of PSA is recommended, using pulse oximetry, capnography, and cardiac monitoring

8.5 Dexmedetomidine

Dexmedetomidine is a selective α-2 adrenoceptor agonist was approved by FDA in the year 1999 for sedation in intensive care (13). It causes hyperpolarization of noradrenergic neurons, thereby suppressing the neuronal firing in locus ceruleus along with inhibition of norepinephrine release and activity in descending medullospinal nor-adrenergic pathways. This drug has recently being in focus due to its sedative, analgesic, perioperative sympatholytic properties. Along with all these properties, it is also hemodynamically stable with minimal effect on respiratory drive making it an ideal sedative agent and useful in various clinical scenarios. This drug has now become a safe alternative to benzodiazepine/opioid combination for monitored anesthesia care (14). The recommended dose range for dexmedetomidine is 0.2 – 0.7 μg / kg/hr. Although it preserves respiratory drive at higher doses it may lead to hypotension and bradycardia.

8.6 Reversal of sedation

Reversal of sedation is rarely required if pharmacological agents are carefully chosen based on nature of procedure. The commonly used agents are:

Naloxone: It is administered to antagonize opioid induced respiratory depression and sedation. Naloxone is non-selective opiod antagonist and can precipitate sudden severe pain. It has a very fast onset of action with peak effect in 1-2 minutes and effect of total dose of 0.4 to 0.8 mg lasting for 1 to 4 hours. Incremental dose of 20 to 40 μg may be given every few minutes till the ventilation of the patient improves. Infusion rate between 3-10 μg/hr may be started if prolonged ventilatory depression is anticipated.

Flumazenil: It is a pure benzodiazepine antagonist which promptly reverses the hypnotic effect of benzodiazepine. This drug has chemical structure which is similar to benzodiazepine, except that it has carbonyl group in place of phenyl. It's onset of action is less than one minute, and undergoes rapid hepatic metabolism with a half life of 1 hour. When it's used to antagonize the action of benzodiazepine with long duration of action, there are chances of recurrence of the symptoms. The usual total dose is 0.6 to 1.0 mg given as a gradual titrated dose of 0.2 mg / minute until the desired level of reversal is achieved. It is given as IV infusion if over dosage with a long-acting benzodiazepine is suspected. This review will not be complete without adding a note of caution that use of flumazenil may precipitate seizure activity that are being chronically treated with benzodiazepine or in those group of patients who are being treated with drugs that reduces seizure threshold like tricyclic antidepressants.

9. References

[1] Consensus conference. Anesthesia and sedation in the dental office. JAMA 1985;254(8):1073-1076.

[2] Green SM, Krauss B. Procedural sedation terminology: moving beyond "conscious sedation". Ann Emerg Med 2002;39(4):433-435.

[3] Godwin SA, Caro DA, Wolf SJ, et al. Clinical policy: procedural sedation and analgesia in the emergency department. Ann Emerg Med 2005;45(2):177-196.

[4] O'Connor RE, Sama A, Burton JH, et al. Procedural sedation and analgesia in the emergency department: recommendations for physician credentialing, privileging, and practice. Ann Emerg Med 2011;58(4):365-370.

[5] Thorpe RJ, Benger J. Pre-procedural fasting in emergency sedation. Emerg Med J;27(4):254-261.

[6] Zed PJ, Abu-Laban RB, Chan WW, et al. Efficacy, safety and patient satisfaction of propofol for procedural sedation and analgesia in the emergency department: a prospective study. CJEM 2007;9(6):421-427.

[7] Burton JH, Miner JR, Shipley ER, et al. Propofol for emergency department procedural sedation and analgesia: a tale of three centers. Acad Emerg Med 2006;13(1):24-30.

[8] Philip BK. The use of remifentanil in clinical anesthesia. Acta Anaesthesiol Scand Suppl 1996;109:170-173.

[9] Sacchetti A, Jachowski J, Heisler J, et al. Remifentanil use in emergency department patients: initial experience. Emerg Med J 2011.

[10] Dunn MJ, Mitchell R, Souza CD, et al. Evaluation of propofol and remifentanil for intravenous sedation for reducing shoulder dislocations in the emergency department. Emerg Med J 2006;23(1):57-58.

[11] Holas A, Krafft P, Marcovic M, et al. Remifentanil, propofol or both for conscious sedation during eye surgery under regional anaesthesia. Eur J Anaesthesiol 1999;16(11):741-748.

[12] Litman RS. Conscious sedation with remifentanil and midazolam during brief painful procedures in children. Arch Pediatr Adolesc Med 1999;153(10):1085-1088.

[13] TVSP Murthy, Singh R. Alpha 2 adrenoceptor agonist - Dexmedetomidine role in anaesthesia and intensive care: A clinical review. J Anaesth Clin Pharmacol 2009;25(3):267-272.

[14] Candiotti KA, Bergese SD, Bokesch PM, et al. Monitored anesthesia care with dexmedetomidine: a prospective, randomized, double-blind, multicenter trial. Anesth Analg 2010;110(1):47-56.

Permissions

The contributors of this book come from diverse backgrounds, making this book a truly international effort. This book will bring forth new frontiers with its revolutionizing research information and detailed analysis of the nascent developments around the world.

We would like to thank Dr. Michael Blaivas, for lending his expertise to make the book truly unique. He has played a crucial role in the development of this book. Without his invaluable contribution this book wouldn't have been possible. He has made vital efforts to compile up to date information on the varied aspects of this subject to make this book a valuable addition to the collection of many professionals and students.

This book was conceptualized with the vision of imparting up-to-date information and advanced data in this field. To ensure the same, a matchless editorial board was set up. Every individual on the board went through rigorous rounds of assessment to prove their worth. After which they invested a large part of their time researching and compiling the most relevant data for our readers. Conferences and sessions were held from time to time between the editorial board and the contributing authors to present the data in the most comprehensible form. The editorial team has worked tirelessly to provide valuable and valid information to help people across the globe.

Every chapter published in this book has been scrutinized by our experts. Their significance has been extensively debated. The topics covered herein carry significant findings which will fuel the growth of the discipline. They may even be implemented as practical applications or may be referred to as a beginning point for another development. Chapters in this book were first published by InTech; hereby published with permission under the Creative Commons Attribution License or equivalent.

The editorial board has been involved in producing this book since its inception. They have spent rigorous hours researching and exploring the diverse topics which have resulted in the successful publishing of this book. They have passed on their knowledge of decades through this book. To expedite this challenging task, the publisher supported the team at every step. A small team of assistant editors was also appointed to further simplify the editing procedure and attain best results for the readers.

Our editorial team has been hand-picked from every corner of the world. Their multi-ethnicity adds dynamic inputs to the discussions which result in innovative outcomes. These outcomes are then further discussed with the researchers and contributors who give their valuable feedback and opinion regarding the same. The feedback is then collaborated with the researches and they are edited in a comprehensive manner to aid the understanding of the subject.

Apart from the editorial board, the designing team has also invested a significant amount of their time in understanding the subject and creating the most relevant covers. They scrutinized every image to scout for the most suitable representation of the subject and create an appropriate cover for the book.

The publishing team has been involved in this book since its early stages. They were actively engaged in every process, be it collecting the data, connecting with the contributors or procuring relevant information. The team has been an ardent support to the editorial, designing and production team. Their endless efforts to recruit the best for this project, has resulted in the accomplishment of this book. They are a veteran in the field of academics and their pool of knowledge is as vast as their experience in printing. Their expertise and guidance has proved useful at every step. Their uncompromising quality standards have made this book an exceptional effort. Their encouragement from time to time has been an inspiration for everyone.

The publisher and the editorial board hope that this book will prove to be a valuable piece of knowledge for researchers, students, practitioners and scholars across the globe.

List of Contributors

Xiang-Yu Hou
School of Public Health, Queensland University of Technology, Brisbane, Australia
Department of Emergency Medicine, Royal Brisbane and Women's Hospital, Brisbane, Australia
School of Medicine, The University of Queensland, Brisbane, Australia

Akarsu Ayazoglu Tülin
Chief Asistant Kartal Kosuyolu Highly Specialized Education and Training Hospital İstanbul, Istanbul, Turkey

Özden Nihan
Göztepe Education and Training Hospital Istanbul, Turkey

Ali Moghtaderi
Neurology Department, Zahedan University of Medical Sciences, Iran

Roya Alavi-Naini and Saleheh Sanatinia
Research Center for Infectious Diseases and Tropical Medicine, University of Medical Sciences, Zahedan, Iran

Ernest E. Wang
North Shore University Health System, University of Chicago Pritzker School of Medicine, USA

Savas Ozsu
Karadeniz Technical University, Department of Chest Diseases School of Medicine, Trabzon, Turkey

Jiri Pokorny
POMAMED, Prague, Czech Republic

Silvia Marinozzi, Giuliano Bertazzoni and Valentina Gazzaniga
"Sapienza" University of Rome, Italy

Peter Aitken
Anton Breinl Centre for Public Health and Tropical Medicine, James Cook University, Townsville, Queensland, Australia

Peter Leggat
Anton Breinl Centre for Public Health and Tropical Medicine, James Cook University, Townsville, Queensland, Australia
School of Public Health, University of the Witwatersrand, Johannesburg, South Africa

Zahra Gardezi
University of Toledo, Toledo, Ohio, USA

Balwinder Singh
Division of Pulmonary & Critical Care Medicine, Mayo Clinic, Rochester, Minnesota, USA

Sanjay Kumar Verma
Department of Anesthesia, All India Instituteof Medical Sciences (A.I.I.M.S.), New Delhi, India

Akhilesh Kumar Tiwari
Department of Anesthesia, St. Stephen's Hospital New Delhi, India

Pedro Whatts
Department of Anesthesia, Saint Luke's Episcopal Hospital, Ponce, Puerto Rico

Dipti Agarwal
Department of Emergency Medicine, Mayo Clinic, Rochester, MN, USA

Subhash Chandra
Department of Medicine, Greater Baltimore Medical Center, Towson, MD, USA

Printed in the USA
CPSIA information can be obtained
at www.ICGtesting.com
JSHW011419221024
72173JS00004B/595

9 781632 421975